MANAGIN
INFECTIONS

•

decision-making

options

in clinical practice

•

MANAGING INFECTIONS

•

---

decision-making

---

options

---

in clinical practice

•

Editors

C.A. Bartzokas MD
Consultant in Medical Microbiology and Infection Prevention

G.W. Smith MRCP MRCPath
Consultant Senior Lecturer in Medical Microbiology

Consultant Editors

A.T. Leanord BSc MB ChB MD DTM&H MRCPath
Consultant in Medical Microbiology

N. Kennedy MB ChB MD MRCP DTM&H
Consultant in Infectious Diseases

C.W.R. Onion MB ChB MSc MD MRCGP MFPHM
Medical Director, Wirral Health Authority

*β*IOS
SCIENTIFIC
PUBLISHERS

Oxford • Washington DC

© BIOS Scientific Publishers Limited, 1998

First published 1998

A CIP catalogue record for this book is available from the British Library.

ISBN 1 85996 171 1

BIOS Scientific Publishers Ltd
9 Newtec Place, Magdalen Road, Oxford OX4 1RE, UK
Tel. +44 (0)1865 726286. Fax +44 (0)1865 246823
World Wide Web home page: http://www.bios.co.uk/

Important Note from the Publisher
The information contained within this book was obtained by BIOS Scientific Publishers Ltd from sources believed by us to be reliable. However, while every effort has been made to ensure its accuracy, no responsibility for loss or injury whatsoever occasioned to any person acting or refraining from action as a result of information contained herein can be accepted by the authors or publishers.

The reader should remember that medicine is a constantly evolving science and while the authors and publishers have ensured that all dosages, applications and practices are based on current indications, there may be specific practices which differ between communities. You should always follow the guidelines laid down by the manufacturers of specific products and the relevant authorities in the country in which you are practising.

Typeset by Saxon Graphics Ltd, Derby, UK
Printed by Biddles Ltd, Guildford, UK

CONTENTS

ADDRESS LIST

Editors

Dr C.A. Bartzokas MD
Consultant in Medical Microbiology and Infection Prevention, Tŷ Ucha, Hafod Road, Gwernymynydd CH7 5JS.

Dr G.W. Smith MRCP MRCPath
Consultant Senior Lecturer in Medical Microbiology, University of Liverpool, 8th Floor, Duncan Building, Daulby Street, Liverpool L69 3GA.

Consultant Editors

Dr A.T. Leanord BSc MB ChB MD DTM&H MRCPath
Consultant in Medical Microbiology, Law Hospital, Carluke ML8 5ER.

Dr N. Kennedy MB ChB MD MRCP DTM&H
Consultant in Infectious Diseases, Monklands Hospital, Monkscourt Avenue, Airdrie ML6 0JS.

Dr C.W.R. Onion MB ChB MSc MD MRCGP MFPHM
Medical Director, Wirral Health Authority, St Catherine's Hospital, Church Road, Birkenhead L42 0LQ.

Contributors

Dr B.L. Atkins MSc MRCP MRCPath
Senior Registrar in Microbiology, Oxford Public Health Laboratory, The John Radcliffe Hospital, Oxford OX3 9DU.

Dr R.G. Charles BSc FRCP FACC FESC
Consultant in Cardiology, The Cardio-Thoracic Centre, Thomas Drive, Liverpool L14 3PE.

Dr J.E. Coia BSc (Hon) MB ChB MD MRCPath
Consultant in Clinical Microbiology, Western General Hospital, Crewe Road, Edinburgh EH4 2XU.

Dr E.S.R. Darley MB ChB MRCP
Specialist Registrar in Medical Microbiology, Southmead Hospital, Westbury-on-Trym, Bristol BS10 5NB.

Dr N.G. Hunt MSc FRCGP
General Medical Practitioner, Rivermead Gate Medical Centre, 123 Rectory Lane, Chelmsford CM1 1TR.

Dr A.T. Leanord BSc MB ChB MD DTM&H MRCPath
Consultant in Medical Microbiology, Law Hospital, Carluke ML8 5ER.

Dr M.J. Ledson MB MRCP
Specialist Registrar in Respiratory Medicine, The Cardio-Thoracic Centre, Thomas Drive, Liverpool L14 3PE.

Dr M.V. Martin BDS BA PhD FRCPath
Senior Lecturer and Consultant in Oral Microbiology, Department of Clinical Dental Sciences, The University of Liverpool, Liverpool L69 3BX.

Dr P.J. Martin MA BM BCh MD MRCP
Senior Registrar in Neurology, Walton Centre for Neurology and Neurosurgery NHS Trust, Rice Lane, Liverpool L9 1AE.

Dr F.J. Nye MD FRCP
Consultant Physician, University Hospital Aintree, Lower Lane, Liverpool L9 7AL.

Dr C. O'Mahony MD FRCPI BSc DipVen
Consultant Physician in Genito-Urinary Medicine, Countess of Chester Hospital, The Countess of Chester Health Park, Liverpool Road, Chester CH2 1UL.

Dr W.S. Robles MD PhD
Consultant in Dermatology, Southend Hospital, Prittlewell Chase, Westcliff-on-Sea SS0 0RY.

Dr G.W. Smith MRCP MRCPath
Consultant Senior Lecturer in Medical Microbiology, University of Liverpool, 8th Floor, Duncan Building, Daulby Street, Liverpool L69 3GA.

Mr A.C. Swift ChM FRCS FRCSEd
Consultant Otorhinolaryngologist, University Hospital Aintree, Lower Lane, Liverpool L9 7AL.

Dr M.J. Walshaw MD FRCP
Consultant Chest Physician, The Cardio-Thoracic Centre, Thomas Drive, Liverpool L14 3PE.

Mr M.T. Watts FRCS FRCOphth
Consultant Ophthalmic Surgeon, Arrowe Park Hospital, Wirral Hospitals Trust, Arrowe Park Road, Upton, Wirral L49 5BE.

Dr C.L.C. Williams MB ChB MRCP MRCPath
Consultant in Medical Microbiology, Royal Alexandra Hospital, Corsebar Road, Paisley PA2 9PN.

Dr M.P. Wilson MB BS
Specialist Registrar in Medical Microbiology, Public Health Laboratory, Level 8, Bristol Royal Infirmary, Marlborough Street, Bristol BS2 8HW.

PREFACE

A paradox of our times is that as knowledge about medicine increases, less practical guidance is available to its practitioners. This is true in all fields of modern medicine but more so in the management of infections, where a great number of variable determinants must be weighed before an informed decision on an individual patient can be reached. There is no shortage of scientific knowledge on investigations and treatment. What is lacking is a framework within which clinical decisions can be informed by such knowledge.

Evidence-based medicine is "the conscientious, explicit and judicious use of current best evidence in making decisions about the care of individual patients" in the words of the gurus.[1] We believe that this book is the first attempt to address directly the issue of *judicious decision making* against a burgeoning background of systematic reviews and guidelines.

Micro-organisms do not respect administrative boundaries, and infections do pervade every single clinical activity. Therefore, we offer this book to all doctors – whether in primary, secondary, or tertiary health care. We have not made arbitrary distinctions between community and hospital practice: general practitioners may be interested to see how their patients are dealt with following referral to a hospital specialist, while consultants are given a broader perspective on the approaches adopted by those outside the ivory towers. We hope that medical students may also benefit from our analysis, and that their critical faculties will be enhanced by reflecting upon the art of, and the issues involved in, decision making.

Our overriding aim is to highlight *decision-making options* in clinical practice. We asked our authors, who are distinguished by their reputation for original thinking as well as their clinical expertise, to weigh arguments for and against a number of different courses of action for a range of common infections. The constituent actions of these *management options* are investigations, treatments, and referrals. We have refrained from compiling decision-making trees and algorithms. Such pathways have generally been eschewed to allow readers to make their own decisions, which only they can tailor to their patients, in the light of a host of arguments rarely discussed in conventional texts. In exploring the overall value of various options, our authors have taken into account the need to:

- Reconcile personal experience with published evidence.
- Impartially debate arguments for and against.
- Highlight impractical standards.
- Expose ineffective measures that have become rituals.
- Identify poor practices that (should) have earned a place in mythology.

All management options have been weighed impartially. However, the order in which they appear may hint at some sort of hierarchical ranking. Because it is not for us to decide what might constitute best practice for any individual patient, we have resisted the temptation to indicate a preference.

There are three distinct reasons for our approach to decision-making options in clinical practice:

1. Most of us are not inclined to follow somebody else's guidance, irrespective of their pedigree, or their scientific rationale. Guidance should not tell us what to do; rather, it should get us thinking about what we could do and point to the consequences of our actions.
2. In any case, the field of infections is so protean and complex, that there are few opportunities to provide robust and precise advice without ending up with a cumbersome tome that no-one in their right mind is likely to consult anyway.
3. The new millennium beckons us with educational clichés that problem-based learning and reflective practice change behaviour, whereas didactic teaching and rote-learning are anachronistic and of little practical value. We believe that both are of value if one can appreciate the relative effectiveness and psychological underpinnings of these polarized approaches.[2]

Other novel features of this book are:

- *History and examination checklists*, to provide pointers to specific clinical features which have a direct influence on decision making.
- *Rituals and myths*, to expose procedures that lack supporting evidence and measures that are contradicted by experiential or scientific evidence.
- *Pitfalls*, to forewarn of rare but significant mistakes, together with the explanations which tend to be used to justify their rationale.
- *Hints for investigators and prescribers*, to share the clinical experience of our authors. Once readers have decided why, when, and how to proceed further, detailed advice on which specimens they should collect, and which antibiotic they may prescribe is readily available from many reliable sources of reference, for example local microbiologists and laboratory handbooks, advisory committees on drugs and therapeutics, and national guidance such as the British National Formulary.

To avoid confusion we have purposely left the genus and species of bacterial pathogens in roman. The selection and titles of various settings of infection, as well as the general chapter layout, mirrors authors' preference. Searching through the contents should draw readers in to an informative and enjoyable scenic route. For rapid access, however, an alphabetical index of chapters, contents, key settings, specific infections and synonymous terms is provided at the end. Since infecting agents, investigations and prescriptions are peripheral to the Management options, the heart of the book, such references are not included in the index.

This work is the culmination of many years of discussion, debates, and our struggles with learning and practising medicine. We are grateful to Dr John C. Starakis, Lecturer in Infectious Diseases at the University of Patras Medical School, Greece, who has developed an invaluable starting framework for the book, by formulating systematic guidelines on infection management during a sabbatical year with CAB. We are also grateful to Mr John E. Corkill, Principal Scientist in Microbiology at the Royal Liverpool University Hospital, for his opinions and advice at critical stages of the preparation of the book. The secretarial contributions of Miss Joan Broster were borne with her customary grace and charm. We are all indebted to Dr Alistair T. Leanord, both for leading the consultant editorial team, and for providing the text on antimicrobial prophylaxis in selected chapters. If the creative thinking and synergy of all the authors prompt our readers to review their own decision making in the practical management of individual patients, our aim will have been fulfilled.

We warmly welcome comments on our philosophy and strategy to enhance clinical practice.

C.A. Bartzokas
G.W. Smith

---

[1] Sackett, D.L., Richardson, W.S., Rosenberg, W. and Haynes, R.B. (1997) *Evidence-based Medicine. How to Practice and Teach EBM*. Churchill Livingstone, Edinburgh.

[2] Petty, R.E. and Cacioppo, J.T. (1986) The elaboration likelihood model of persuasion. *Adv. Exp. Soc. Psychol.* **19**: 123–205.

Chapter 1
CARDIOVASCULAR INFECTIONS

R.G. Charles

Chapter contents

1 Infective endocarditis

Infective endocarditis (IE) is still a major worldwide problem. Valvular heart disease remains the most frequent underlying heart disease, and the majority (up to 80%) of patients with native valve endocarditis who do not use parenteral drugs have an identifiable predisposing cardiac lesion. As rheumatic fever has virtually disappeared in Western countries the spectrum of underlying cardiac lesions has changed. The most frequent, in descending order, are: mitral valve prolapse, no underlying disease, degenerative diseases of the aortic and mitral valves, congenital heart disease and rheumatic heart disease. Of increasing importance are special high risk populations – subjects with prosthetic valves, parenteral drug users, HIV-infected patients and the elderly.

- IE is infection of the endocardial surface of the heart, referring usually to bacterial or fungal infection, although chlamydial or rickettsial infections may occur.
- Infective endarteritis is infection of extracardiac endothelium – coarctation of the aorta, persistent ductus arteriosus, arterio-venous or arterio-arterial shunts – producing a clinical syndrome identical to IE.

Traditionally, IE has been classified according to its clinical course:

- *Acute IE* is a fulminating infection by a virulent organism (e.g. Staphylococcus aureus, Streptococcus pneumoniae, Streptococcus pyogenes, Haemophilus influenzae, Neisseria gonorrhoeae) with rapid valvular destruction, frequent metastatic foci, and death within weeks if untreated.
- *Subacute IE* is a more chronic course over months or years, with infrequent metastatic foci.

Today, a more practically useful classification refers to the underlying predisposition – native valve, prosthetic valve, parenteral drug user – and the specific organism isolated.

Management options
IE must be suspected in any patient with a persistent (>1 week) unexplained fever and a cardiac murmur, or in a parenteral drug user without a murmur. Persistent fever associated with suggestive extracardiac symptoms and signs, or in patients belonging to special risk groups must also arouse suspicion of IE.

Blood cultures and echocardiography are essential elements of management. The earlier the diagnosis is established and treatment started, the better the prognosis.

Management options in primary care
1. Investigate with blood cultures and open-access echocardiography, then start antibiotics.
2. Admit directly to hospital on grounds of clinical suspicion of IE.

Option 1. Investigate with blood cultures and open-access echocardiography, then start antibiotics.

✓ Hospital admission avoided if there is a simple intercurrent illness.

✗ Diagnosis of true IE likely to be delayed, with prognostic detriment.
✗ Antimicrobial therapy started before arranging for meticulously taken blood cultures will temporarily suppress bacteraemia and sometimes symptoms, causing major delay in subsequent definitive diagnosis.
✗ In-hospital observation required to document evolution of signs and development of complications.

Option 2. Admit directly to hospital on grounds of clinical suspicion of IE.

✓ Early definitive diagnosis and correct antimicrobial treatment of IE essential to optimize prognosis.

✓ Early decision can be made to refer for cardiac surgery if infection is not suppressed or complications develop.

✗ Unnecessary hospital admission, but this is a small price to pay for the early definitive exclusion of a life-threatening disease.

Management options in secondary care

Hospital management is well established. Every effort must be made to isolate the infecting organism by blood cultures. Echocardiography is extremely valuable in confirming the diagnosis by imaging vegetations, for identifying and detecting serial changes in the underlying cardiac lesion and assessing myocardial function.

1. Establish diagnosis of IE by properly taken blood cultures.
2. Initiate therapy before isolation of an organism.
3. Obtain echocardiography.
4. Consider differential diagnosis. If there is a strong initial clinical suspicion of IE, blood cultures and initiation of antimicrobial therapy must precede further specific investigations.

Option 1. Establish diagnosis of IE by properly taken blood cultures.

✓ In patients not exposed to previous antimicrobial therapy, cultures are positive in more than 95% of patients. Obtain three cultures, 1 hour apart, from separate venous sites.

✓ In patients exposed to previous antimicrobial therapy, and depending on clinical status, treatment may be delayed for up to 3 days or longer while obtaining two blood cultures each day.

✓ In acute IE, antimicrobial treatment should be delayed for no more than 3 hours while obtaining three blood cultures, since deterioration may be fulminant.

Option 2. Initiate therapy before isolation of an organism.

✓ Antimicrobial therapy should be commenced as soon as possible, usually within 3 hours, allowing for blood cultures.

✓ The choice of antimicrobial agents before isolation of an organism depends on the clinical circumstances which may predict the most likely organism.

✓ Involve clinical microbiologist at all stages of therapy.

Option 3. Obtain echocardiography.

✓ Demonstrates vegetations (60–80% cases).

✓ Documents current status of valvular lesions, and serial changes.

✓ Demonstrates structural complications such as aortic root abscess, sinus of Valsalva aneurysm.

✓ Assists in timing of surgery.

✓ Assists in differential diagnosis, e.g. exclusion of atrial myxoma.

Option 4. Consider differential diagnosis. If there is a strong initial clinical suspicion of IE, blood cultures and initiation of antimicrobial therapy must precede further specific investigations.

✓ Conditions which may exactly simulate IE include atrial myxoma, connective tissue diseases, acute rheumatic fever, thrombotic thrombocytopenic purpura, sickle cell disease, primary antiphospholipid syndrome and thrombotic lesions associated with extracardiac malignancies.

History checklist

General

- Onset of symptoms? Days, weeks or months ago? Symptoms usually start within 2 weeks of the index bacteraemia.
- Presenting symptoms? Malaise, fatigue, night sweats, weight loss, appetite loss, myalgia, headache, back pain.
- Recent invasive procedures? Dental extractions, periodontal surgery, upper airway instrumentation, upper and lower gastrointestinal, urological, and gynaecological procedures may all cause transient bacteraemia, and may give a clue to the organism responsible.
- Underlying general conditions? Diabetes mellitus, immunosuppression, HIV infection, i.v. drug abuse.
- Age of patient. Prevalence of IE in patients over the age of 60 is steadily increasing owing to the decline in rheumatic fever and increase in degenerative conditions as the predisposing lesion.

Specific

- Known cardiac lesion? Congenital, murmur discovered on previous routine medical examination (e.g. school, armed services, insurance), rheumatic valvular disease.
- Previous cardiac surgery? Prosthetic heart valve, palliative or corrective surgery for congenital heart disease.
- Symptoms of secondary clinical events? Emboli (stroke may be a presenting feature), congestive heart failure symptoms.

Examination checklist

General

- Fever? Almost invariable with IE, but may be absent in those previously treated with antibiotics, the elderly, the very ill or in congestive heart failure.
- Extracardiac signs? Splenomegaly (30%), finger clubbing (15%, chronic cases), systemic emboli (30%), especially cerebral emboli causing stroke, pulmonary emboli causing pneumonia or septic infarction common in intravenous drug users (>70%), metastatic abscess formation.
- Skin, mucous membrane, eye signs?
     Splinter haemorrhages in nail beds.
     Petechiae in conjuctivae and mouth.
     Osler's nodes: small painful nodules in pulp of fingers or toes.
     Roth spots: oval retinal haemorrhages with pale centre (canoe-shaped).
     Janeway lesions: flat, red, painless lesions on the palms or soles.

Specific

- Cardiac murmurs? Invariable, except in early acute infection. New regurgitant or changing murmurs may be noted.
- Congestive heart failure? The most common complication of IE. Mandatory to consider early or emergency cardiac surgery.

Rituals and myths

- There is no advantage in taking blood cultures at any particular time or body temperature (e.g. when rising, at peak) since the bacteraemia in IE is continuous.
- Arterial blood cultures have no advantage over venous blood cultures.
- Taking blood cultures more than 60 minutes apart causes unnecessary delay in the initiation of treatment in patients who have not received out-patient antimicrobials within the previous 2 weeks.

- Fastidious organisms are commonly suspected as a cause of negative cultures. In fact, prior exposure to antimicrobials is a much more common cause.

Pitfalls
- Cardiac surgery is an early, not a late resort in IE management. Major indications are congestive heart failure secondary to valve dysfunction, myocardial or valve ring abscess, uncontrolled infection despite antibiotics and prosthetic valve dysfunction.

Hints for investigators and prescribers
- If out-patient antibiotics were given for only a few days, cultures may become positive again within 24 hours. After longer periods of treatment, cultures will generally be positive when the fever recurs.
- Negative blood cultures may uncommonly be due to fastidious organisms.
- Fungi should be considered in patients with prosthetic valves, immunosuppression, and those with very large vegetations on echocardiography, or large peripheral emboli (from which the responsible fungus may be isolated from a surgical specimen).
- Arrange serology for Q-fever and psittacosis in 'culture negative' IE.
- Although oral antimicrobial therapy has been described, the failure rate is higher. Do not use oral therapy in IE unless it is unavoidable (i.v. drug users with isolated right-sided staphylococcal IE **may** be an exception).
- Subacute presentation/non-parenteral drug user: high dose penicillin G or ampicillin with gentamicin.
- Acute onset/non-parenteral drug user: antistaphylococcal penicillin or cephalosporin.
- If intracardiac prosthesis present, or parenteral drug user: include vancomycin since S. aureus strains isolated are usually resistant to all β-lactam antibiotics.
- Endocarditis in patients who have damaged or prosthetic heart valves, or have anatomical heart defects, and who are undergoing procedures that are prone to cause bacteraemia can be prevented with antibiotics. The protective efficacy of prophylaxis against first episodes of endocarditis was 49% in one study, while another showed a protective efficacy of 91% in native heart valves. Only 15% of endocarditis cases follow dental therapy and, therefore, only a small proportion of procedures capable of producing a clinical endocarditis are at present being covered by prophylaxis. Spontaneous bacteraemias occur on a regular basis with such activities as teeth brushing causing a transient bacteraemia in 30% of cases. It is therefore impossible to predict with any accuracy which procedures will lead to a significant bacteraemia posing a significant risk, and when to protect against such a risk. It is also not known whether the transient appearance of bacteria more associated with endocarditis, e.g. streptococci, has a higher significance than one that is less commonly associated with IE. The risk of developing IE after a dental procedure has been estimated to be between 1:500 to over 1:100 000. Prophylaxis must be balanced against the loss of patient days due to the side-effects (mainly anaphylaxis) of any antibiotics given.

1.1 Infective endocarditis in special risk groups

Prosthetic valves
The prognosis of IE associated with prosthetic valves (PV) is worse than in native valve endocarditis. The risk of endocarditis is the same for both mechanical and bioprosthetic valves.

Intravenous drug abusers
- IE is common (5% per year).
- Right-sided IE is classical, but there is probably also a high incidence of left-sided IE.
- Microbiology is different from native valve IE: higher prevalence of staphylococci, Gram-negative organisms and fungi.

- Recent studies indicate that isolated right-sided endocarditis due to staphylococci could be cured by a 28-day course of oral ciprofloxin and rifampicin at a rate equivalent to a standard parenteral regime.

The elderly
- Prevalence of IE in patients over the age of 60 has increased steadily.
- IE in the elderly is frequently associated with few clinical symptoms and signs, leading to delayed diagnosis.
- Transoesophageal echocardiography has improved diagnostic sensitivity and specificity in the elderly.

History checklist
The key historical feature is the time relationship to prior cardiac surgery, either *early* (<60 days post-operatively) or *late* (>60 days post-operatively).

- Early PV endocarditis is usually acquired in hospital, and is associated with staphylococci, diphtheroids, fungi or Gram-negative organisms. It has the worst prognosis (30–80% mortality).
- Late PV endocarditis is associated with the same organisms as native valve endocarditis and has a mortality of 20–40%.

Examination checklist
- Early PV endocarditis rarely shows the classic peripheral signs of IE.
- Persisting post-operative fever should be assumed to be early PV endocarditis until proved otherwise.
- Signs of new or changing murmurs, new or worsening heart failure, persisting fever, new conduction abnormalities and neurological signs carry an adverse prognosis.

Hints for investigators and prescribers
- Begin antimicrobial therapy before definitive culture results are available.
- Involve the clinical microbiologist from the outset.

Further reading
Fowler, N.O. (1991) Infective endocarditis. In: *Diagnosis of Heart Disease*. Springer-Verlag, New York, NY, pp. 410–416.

Erbel, R., Liu, F., Ge, J., Rohmann, S. and Kupferwasser, L. (1995) Identification of high risk subgroups in infective endocarditis and the role of echocardiography. *Eur. Heart J.* **16**: 588–602.

Korzeniowski, O.M. and Kay, D. (1992) Infective endocarditis. In: *Heart Disease. A Textbook of Cardiovascular Medicine* (ed. E. Braunwald). WB Saunders, Philadelphia, PA, pp. 1078–1105.

Vongpatanasin, W., Hillis, L. and Lange, R. (1996) Prosthetic heart valves. *N. Engl. J. Med.* **335**: 407–416.

2 Implantable device-associated infections

Cardiac pacemakers are implanted for the treatment of symptomatic or prognostically important bradyarrhythmias. Implantable cardioverter defibrillators (ICD) are utilized for the treatment of life-threatening malignant ventricular tachyarrhythmias, sometimes associated with bradycardia. Virtually all cardiac pacemakers and ICDs are now implanted in the pectoral region, usually in a subcutaneous, but occasionally a submuscular, pocket. The leads connecting them to the heart are inserted transvenously by percutaneous puncture of the subclavian vein or by cut-down on the cephalic vein in the deltopectoral groove.

The procedures are undertaken with antistaphylococcal antibiotic prophylaxis and a subsequent infection rate of around 1% is expected. Device-related infections may occur early or late following implantation, and may be superficial, deep within the pocket with the risk of septicaemia or associated with skin erosion by the device. Pacemaker or ICD system infection is potentially fatal so it is essential that it be managed promptly and correctly.

- A superficial wound infection is an infection contained within the surgical wound itself, with no systemic features of infection.
- Pocket infection is infection within the generator implant pocket. Direct communication, via the lead(s) to the heart, into the central circulation promotes the development of septicaemia.
- Erosion is exteriorization of the device due to loss of integrity of the overlying skin. Management is primarily surgical.
- Pre-erosion occurs when skin over the generator pocket becomes fixed and tethered, dusky red, and sometimes shiny and thin before it is breached. At this stage bacteria can cross the compromised skin and contaminate the pocket. Management is primarily surgical.

Management options for superficial wound infections

1. Manage in primary care setting. Assume staphylococcal infection and treat with penicillinase-resistant antibiotic.
2. Start antistaphylococcal antibiotic in primary care, but refer promptly back to the implant centre.

Option 1. Manage in primary care setting. Assume staphylococcal infection and treat with penicillinase-resistant antibiotic.

✓ Conservative therapy with antibiotics in truly superficial wound infection is often successful.
✓ Avoids unnecessary return to hospital.

✗ Time consuming, since frequent repeat observation is required, with referral to implant centre if prompt improvement over a few days is not seen.
✗ Unfamiliarity with device-related infections may permit misdiagnosis and thus delayed treatment of pocket infection.

Option 2. Start antistaphylococcal antibiotic in primary care, but refer promptly back to the implant centre.

✓ Conservative therapy with antibiotics is often successful.
✓ Shared care early in the infection enlists the greater experience of the implant centre in the management of device-related infection.
✓ Many implant centres advise the patient to return to the hospital as soon as infection is suspected.

✗ Infection may have been successfully treated without inconvenience and expense of further hospital visits.

History checklist

- When was the implant performed? Superficial wound infection invariably occurs within days to a couple of weeks of the primary implant, or generator change.
- Any symptoms of systemic infection? If yes, associated deep pocket infection must be suspected and managed accordingly.

Examination checklist

General

Signs of systemic infection require management as deep pocket infection, even if specific examination at the implant site reveals only minor signs of infection.

Specific

- Superficial reddening directly associated with the incision line, partial failure of union of the wound edges, mild purulent discharge.
- Exclude presence of infected skin stitch, or parts of subcutaneous suture knots poking through the wound site.

Management option for pocket infections

Remove the entire system and abandon the pocket.

✓ There is only one management option and it is urgent. The patient must be referred to the implant centre for urgent removal of the generator and all leads present, drainage of the site and systemic antibiotic therapy. Temporary pacing is required for patients who have no underlying intrinsic cardiac rhythm.

History checklist

- When was the implant performed? Acute infection of an otherwise healthy new implant site is usually due to a failure of sterile procedure or antibiotic prophylaxis. S. aureus is frequently involved. Infection in a chronic implant site – months to years after implant – is more common. Staphylococcus epidermidis is more often responsible.
- Any symptoms of systemic infection? In addition to tenderness and pain at the implant site, fever, rigor, malaise, anorexia and debility may be described.

Examination checklist

- Signs of systemic infection? Fever and general signs of infection are common. Pocket infections which discharge episodically into the central venous system may cause pulmonary infection.
- Signs of local infection?
    Reddening and tension of skin overlying the pocket.
    Tenderness, sometimes exquisite.
    Swelling, sometimes tense.

Rituals and myths

- Inappropriate conservatism in primary care. The author has seen many cases of device-related infection treated with multiple courses of antibiotics, and local toilet with dressings by the district nurse in cases which are irretrievable by conservative measures. The threshold for referral of a superficial device-related wound infection must be low.
- Inappropriate conservatism at implant centres. Attempts at conserving an infected pocket by drainage, antibiotics and surgical revision at the same site have a low success rate and should now be an anachronism. The system must be explanted and infection eradicated with appropriate antibiotics before re-implantation at a different site.

Hints for investigators and prescribers

- Occasionally, a grossly infected pacemaker pocket causing systemic infection may show no local symptoms or signs. An implanted foreign body must always be viewed with suspicion as a source of infection despite beguiling appearances of innocence.
- Surgical explantation of an infected device system must include **all** leads, even those abandoned at previous procedures. Leads may be coated in a biofilm of infection and act as a persisting source.

Further reading

Byrd, C.L. (1995) Management of implant complications. In: *Clinical Cardiac Pacing* (eds K.A. Ellenbogen, G.N. Kay and B. Wilkoff). WB Saunders, Philadelphia, PA, pp. 491–522.

3 Pericarditis

Acute pericarditis is a constellation of symptoms and signs due to inflammation of the pericardium, characterized by chest pain, a pericardial friction rub and abnormalities of the ECG. It may be due to infectious or non-infectious causes. In the out-patient setting, the most common causes are idiopathic (non-specific) or viral infection. Other infectious causes include bacteria (pneumococci, staphylococci, streptococci, Gram-negative organisms, Neisseria spp. and Legionella spp.), tuberculosis, and fungal and protozoal infections. Many of the clinical features of acute pericarditis are common to many causes.

Management options

1. Establish clinical diagnosis and ECG confirmation. Manage conservatively with rest and non-steroidal anti-inflammatory drugs (NSAID) in primary care.
2. Admit directly to hospital. Establish diagnosis, exclude underlying disease requiring specific therapy. Institute symptomatic or specific therapy according to aetiology.

Option 1. Establish clinical diagnosis and ECG confirmation. Manage conservatively with rest and non-steroidal anti-inflammatory drugs (NSAID) in primary care.

✓ Viral and idiopathic pericarditis are usually self-limited, aided by rest and pain relief, over 2–6 weeks. These are the commonest causes of acute pericarditis.
✓ Unnecessary hospital admission can be avoided.
✓ Patients with recurrent episodes of pericardial inflammation known not to be related to any other underlying abnormality can be treated symptomatically.

✗ Hospital observation is desirable initially to exclude acute myocardial infarct, pyogenic pericarditis, and the development of pericardial tamponade (15% of cases).
✗ Typical ECG confirmation (widespread upwardly concave S-T segment elevation) and even pericardial friction may be absent in acutely ill patients.

Option 2. Admit directly to hospital. Establish diagnosis, exclude underlying disease requiring specific therapy. Institute symptomatic or specific therapy according to aetiology.

✓ Symptomatic treatment, as above, may require the addition or substitution of corticosteroids if pain is severe and does not respond to NSAIDs.
✓ Urgent pericardiocentesis can be performed promptly for symptomatic relief, and for cardiac tamponade. In such cases, the diagnostic yield from laboratory examination of the fluid is high.

History checklist

- Flu-like prodrome. Common in viral and idiopathic pericarditis.
- Chest pain. The main complaint. Typically precordial radiating to the left trapezius ridge or neck. Sharp, pleuritic or dull quality. Increased by movements of the chest wall, and lying flat. Relieved by sitting forward.
- Breathlessness. Mainly due to rapid, shallow breathing due to pleuritic pain. May be worsened by a large pericardial effusion, sometimes causing life-threatening cardiac tamponade.

Examination checklist

General
In bacterial pericarditis the patient is often acutely ill and toxic; the course of tuberculous pericarditis is insidious with less florid signs.

Specific

A pericardial friction rub, described by Collin as 'the squeak of leather of a new saddle under the rider' is pathognomonic.

Rituals and myths

- The chest X-ray is of little diagnostic value. If the heart is enlarged suspect pericardial effusion and arrange echocardiography.
- Pericardiocentesis for purely diagnostic purposes gives a yield of only 5%, and is not justified. The sole exception is where a high suspicion of purulent pericarditis exists.

Hints for investigators and prescribers

- Ask about recent travel. Some patients require more extensive investigation to rule out a specific underlying cause.
- Characteristic ECG changes occur in 90% of cases of acute pericarditis, even when other clinical features are atypical.
- Oral anticoagulants must not be given during acute pericarditis. If anticoagulation must be continued, e.g. presence of a mechanical heart valve prosthesis, use heparin. Watch for evidence of cardiac tamponade and reverse heparin with protamine if required.
- Antibiotics must be used only for documented pyogenic pericarditis.

Further reading

Gizton, L.E. and Laks, M.M. (1982) The differential diagnosis of acute pericarditis. *Circulation* **65**: 1004.

Lorrell, B.H. and Braunwald, E. (1992) Pericardial disease. In: *Heart Disease. A Textbook of Cardiovascular Medicine* (ed. E. Braunwald). WB Saunders, Philadelphia, PA, pp. 1465–1516.

Chapter 2

CENTRAL NERVOUS SYSTEM INFECTIONS

P.J. Martin

Infections of the CNS must be managed as neurological emergencies. The greater the delay in instituting appropriate treatment, the worse the outcome.

In general, the site of the infection within the nervous system will dictate the symptoms and signs. Appreciating where the infection is will guide appropriate investigation and thus result in microbiological confirmation and optimum treatment.

Abnormalities of the host's immune response may impede the expression of the characteristic clinical features of that infection. In addition a number of alternative CNS pathologies may mimic acute CNS infections. It is important not to overlook these, as some are completely reversible with appropriate treatment.

Besides therapies targeted towards the CNS infection itself, adequate care must be provided for the secondary effects of the infection, e.g. control of seizures, management of the obtunded patient.

Chapter contents

1 Meningitis

Bacterial meningitis

Symptoms and signs develop over a few hours with potential deterioration to death. Thus the onset is more rapid than other infections of the nervous system. In the elderly or immunosuppressed, symptoms and signs are less florid and the onset more insidious. Meningitis must be suspected in a newborn or infant with non-specific signs of systemic illness: fever, drowsiness, irritability, vomiting, seizures and a tense or bulging anterior fontanelle.

In adults or children, fever, severe headache, drowsiness and neck stiffness are characteristic. Stupor, coma, seizures and circulatory shock may develop. Neck stiffness on passive flexion of the neck is the best sign of a meningitic process. The presence of a petechial or purpuric rash in combination with the above features is the hallmark of meningococcal septicaemia, although the rash may be absent or atypical.

Viral meningitis

The dominant features are headache, fever and meningism arising within 24 hours. Meningism is often milder than in purulent meningitis although this is not a reliable clinical indicator. Lethargy, drowsiness and irritability are common, but confusion, impairment of consciousness (stupor or coma) and focal signs are extremely rare and should alert the clinician to the fact that the patient almost certainly does not have a viral meningitis. Accompanying symptoms include sore throat, nausea, aches in the back and muscles, vague malaise and weakness.

Tuberculous meningitis

Symptoms usually arise over 7–14 days, sometimes even longer. Thus the onset is usually more insidious than bacterial meningitis, although tuberculous meningitis can sometimes be equally acute. Low grade fever, headache, neck stiffness, general malaise and confusion are the earliest features. As the illness progresses, impairment of consciousness, from somnolence through to coma, develop. Seizures, papilloedema and cranial nerve palsies (of the ocular nerves, facial or acoustic nerves) frequently develop. Cranial nerve lesions indicate a severe basal meningitis, but sixth nerve palsies (particularly in the presence of papilloedema) may also be due to raised intracranial pressure. Tuberculomas are rare in developed countries but are one of the commonest space occupying lesions in developing nations. They present with seizures or progressive neurological deficit. They may be multiple.

Management options

1. Prescribe i.v./i.m. antibiotics to all cases but do no tests.
2. Prescribe all suspected cases i.v./i.m. antibiotics, then investigate.
3. Prescribe selected (rapidly deteriorating) cases i.v./i.m. antibiotics, otherwise investigate first.
4. Investigate first, then prescribe i.v./i.m. antibiotics.

Option 1. Prescribe i.v./i.m. antibiotics to all cases but do no tests.

Tell the patient that treatment is being commenced on the suspicion of meningitis but the true diagnosis is unclear.

✓ Bacterial meningitides sensitive to the chosen antibiotics will be treated.

✗ Viral meningitis will be inappropriately treated with antibiotics.
✗ Tuberculous and fungal meningitis will not respond.
✗ Bacterial meningitis of unusual aetiology will be partially or incompletely treated.

✗ No formal diagnosis will ever be reached and mimicking conditions such as subarachnoid haemorrhage will be missed.

Option 2. Prescribe all suspected cases i.v/i.m antibiotics, then investigate.

Tell the patient that appropriate treatment is being commenced and that confirmatory investigations will be commenced as soon as possible afterwards.

✓ The common pathogens will be covered by an empirical choice.
✓ Treatment is instituted as early as possible, providing the best chance of a favourable outcome.
✓ Even if cerebrospinal fluid (CSF) culture is ultimately negative, if CSF analysis is performed within 24 hours of antibiotic therapy, the CSF cell count, protein, glucose and Gram stain may not be affected. Up to 38% of specimens may remain positive on culture.
✓ Lumbar puncture (LP) should always be possible within 6 hours of initiating treatment in most areas.
✓ Assay for pneumo- and meningococcal antigen can still confirm the diagnosis in some cases.

✗ With a delay of 12 or more hours between antibiotics and LP, the greater is the likelihood of the CSF findings being obscured.
✗ If the CSF findings are not characteristic, culture is negative and the patient fails to improve, then directing future treatment is speculative rather than evidence-based.

Option 3. Prescribe selected (rapidly deteriorating) case i.v/i.m antibiotics, otherwise investigate first.

Tell the patient that there is time to safely obtain a diagnostic CSF specimen before treatment is started, which may be useful in case of future clinical uncertainty. Deteriorating patients will be told they need treatment immediately, before any tests.

✓ Patients who need early (life-saving) treatment will receive it.
✓ Utilize the window of opportunity for diagnostic CSF specimen.
✓ Obtain a reliable CSF for future reference in case of future management dilemma (patient fails to improve as expected).

✗ Patients may deteriorate whilst awaiting investigation, hence 'emergency' approach to LP is vital.

Option 4. Investigate first, then prescribe i.v/i.m antibiotics.

Tell the patient that a CSF sample is needed before treatment is started.

✓ Diagnostic specimens of CSF in all cases.

✗ Some patients may deteriorate or die because of unacceptable delay in commencing treatment.

History checklist

General
- Establish how old the patient is (different pathogens occurring in different age groups, see below) and, if appropriate, whether they have chronically abused alcohol.
- Usual general health (any suggestion of immunosuppression).

Specific
- Enquire about headache, fever, neck stiffness, photophobia, drowsiness, vomiting and seizures.

- Has a rash been seen?
- Has there been any double vision (to implicate nerves III, IV or VI in a basal meningitis process, or VI as a false localizing feature of raised intracranial pressure).
- Ask about recent contacts, recent travel and recent middle ear and mastoid infections.
- Has there been recent head trauma, CSF rhinorrhoea, or does the patient have an *in situ* ventriculoperitoneal shunt?
- Has the patient had previous courses of oral antibiotics?

Examination checklist

- The level of consciousness should be ascertained and recorded either as descriptive terms or as a formal coma score. The time of the observations should be clearly stated to allow subsequent comparative assessments.
- Every inch of the skin should be searched for early signs of a macular or petechial rash.
- Neck stiffness and Kernig's sign.
- Presence of papilloedema, which should preclude LP.
- A systematic and comprehensive neurological examination should be undertaken so that early warning signs of an abscess are not missed. Focal signs indicate sinister complications.
- Examine the auditory canal and tympanic membranes.
- Classical features of meningism may be absent in the elderly in whom confusion and fluctuating conscious level may be the prominent features.

Referrals

- All patients with suspected meningitis must be admitted to hospital as an emergency.
- Specialist opinions (infectious diseases/neurology) should be sought in atypical cases (immunosuppressed patient, CSF picture inconclusive, difficulty managing complications, e.g. seizures, doubt about diagnosis etc.).

Rituals and myths

- Antibiotic treatment for meningococcal meningitis is often continued beyond a week. In cases without complications, 5–7 days is all that is needed.
- A fall in serum sodium is often attributed to inappropriate antidiuretic hormone (ADH) secretion secondary to the meningitis and is treated by fluid restriction. More frequently, this electrolyte imbalance reflects total salt and therefore water depletion and the ADH levels are an appropriate response to hypovolaemia. Adequate fluid balance must be maintained.

Pitfalls

- Not all patients with meningitis have typical clinical features of meningism. This is particularly so in patients at the extremes of age and the immunocompromised. Bacterial meningitis in adolescents and young adults can present as an acute confusional state in which meningism may not yet have developed or may be difficult to elicit.
- Tuberculous meningitis may present as an acute, subacute, or more protracted illness, characterized predominantly by headache, meningism or by progressive encephalopathy, respectively. In 20% of cases, the CSF glucose is normal (potentially mimicking viral meningitis). Ziehl-Nielsen stain is frequently negative.
- In the presence of papilloedema, focal neurological signs, progressive reduction in conscious level or coma, or prolonged seizures in adults, a CT scan of the brain must be performed before LP. In this situation, if bacterial meningitis is suspected, empirical antibiotics must be commenced before CT scanning, otherwise unacceptable delay will ensue.
- Failure to measure CSF pressure is a common oversight. Alternative diagnoses (e.g. venous sinus thromboses) may be missed.

- HIV seroconversion can be accompanied by aseptic lymphocytic meningitis, which is clinically indistinguishable from other viral meningitis. Resolution of symptoms is usually complete in 10 days. Most HIV patients have a chronic, asymptomatic meningeal reaction with mild elevations of protein and lymphocytes and evidence of intrathecal Ig synthesis (oligoclonal bands). Syphilitic meningitis has been increasingly prevalent in AIDS patients in the USA in whom it runs an extremely aggressive course.
- Misinterpreting a lymphocytic CSF with markedly elevated protein as being due to viral meningitis. Also think about partially treated bacterial meningitis, chronic meningitis with atypical organisms (tuberculosis, fungi, Borrelia spp.) or non-infective CSF inflammatory processes (e.g. sarcoid, lupus).

Hints for investigators and prescribers

- The dominant cell type in malignant meningitis can be lymphocytes, and cytological examination is often necessary on three or four large volume CSF samples taken on separate occasions before malignant cells are demonstrated.
- Patients with tuberculous meningitis who initially improve may suddenly deteriorate. This may be due to the development of hydrocephalus secondary to basal meningitis, or the development of a tuberculoma. Such patients must undergo repeat imaging with CT or MRI.
- Adjunctive corticosteroid therapy: certain controlled trials of adjunctive dexamethasone in children with bacterial meningitis have shown a reduction in neurological complications, predominantly sensorineural deafness. The effect seems to be greatest in patients with Haemophilus influenzae infections, and in patients presenting late with the most severe disease. There is a possible lesser effect in pneumococcal meningitis but not in meningococcal disease.
- A close contact of an index case has a 500–1000 times greater chance of developing meningitis. The risk of developing meningitis is greatest immediately after contact with the index case, with the majority of cases arising in the first week of contact, although subsequent secondary cases have been reported after 2 months. The prevalence of nasopharyngeal carriage is 5–10% in non-epidemic situations, and up to 90% in closed communities, e.g. army barracks, monasteries. All close contacts of the index case, defined as all people sleeping in the same household, close contacts in a closed community (e.g. boarding school), and kissing and saliva exchanging contacts, should be offered prophylaxis. During an epidemic, chemoprophylaxis does not modify the course of the outbreak. The index case should also get a course of chemoprophylaxis. Prophylaxis should not be given to casual contacts or to health care workers tending the affected patient unless mouth-to-mouth resuscitation has been performed. Rifampicin has a 95% efficacy in eradicating meningococci from carriers. Up to 25% of patients become recolonized with rifampicin-resistant meningococci which may subsequently cause invasive disease. Rifampicin is contraindicated in pregnancy, liver disease and people with alcoholism. Patients should be warned that the efficacy of the oral contraceptive may be compromised and barrier methods of contraception should be used, that staining of contact lenses is possible and that the urine may change colour to reddy-orange. Ciprofloxacin has up to a 97% eradication rate. Its use is contra indicated in pregnancy and in children. It has, however, become more readily used in children, especially to treat patients with cystic fibrosis, with no ill effects, and it is unlikely that a single dose would produce significant damage to developing cartilage. Meningitis prophylaxis is not a licensed indication for ciprofloxacin use.
- Vaccination. In an outbreak where meningococci of serogroups A or C are implicated, quadravalent vaccine can be used in conjunction with chemoprophylaxis in close contacts.

Further reading

Bonadio, W.A. (1996) Adjunctive dexamethasone therapy for pediatric bacterial meningitis. *J. Emergency Med.* **14**: 165–172.

Harvey, D.R. and Stevens, J.P. (1995) What is the role of corticosteroids in meningitis? *Drugs* **50**: 945–950.

Humphries, M. (1992) The management of tuberculous meningitis. *Thorax* **47**: 577–581.

Lambert, H.P. (1994) Meningitis. *J. Neurol. Neurosurg. Psychiatry* **57**: 405–415.

Odio, C.M., Faingezicht, I., Paris, M., Nassar, M., Baltodano, A., Rogers, J., Xavier-Llorens, S., Olsen, K.D. and McCracken, G.H. (1991) The beneficial effects of early dexamethasone administration in infants and children with bacterial meningitis. *N. Engl. J. Med.* **324**: 1525–1531.

Phuapradit, P. and Vejjajiva, A. (1987) Treatment of tuberculous meningitis: role of short-course chemotherapy. *Q. J. Med.* **239**: 249–258.

Prasad, K. and Haines, T. (1995) Dexamethasone treatment for acute bacterial meningitis: how strong is the evidence for routine use? *J. Neurol. Neurosurg. Psychiatry* **59**: 31–37.

Quagliarell, V.J. and Scheld, W.M. (1997) Treatment of bacterial meningitis. *N. Engl. J. Med.* **336**: 716.

Rockowitz, J. and Tunkel, A.R. (1995) Bacterial meningitis: practical guidelines for management. *Drugs* **50**: 838–853.

2 Brain abscess

The development of cerebral abscess may follow an exacerbation of a primary infection (e.g. suppurative otitis media). Otherwise, it may develop on a background of general malaise over the preceding few weeks. Symptoms referable to the abscess itself may develop rapidly over 3–4 days with new features arising daily, or the onset may be more gradual, over a few weeks. Headache, drowsiness, confusion and seizures are the most common manifestations. Fever is common early, but may remit as the abscess becomes encapsulated. The development of progressive focal signs is governed by the site of the intracranial infection:

- temporal lobe: upper homonymous quadrantanopia, dysphasia if dominant temporal lobe.
- frontal lobe: altered personality, hemiparesis.
- parietal lobe: inattention, higher sensory loss.
- occipital lobe: homonymous hemianopia.

In cerebellar abscesses the features of raised intracranial pressure are usually dominant due to the development of obstructive hydrocephalus (headache, vomiting, drowsiness, papilloedema) and these may obscure the focal signs (nystagmus, dysathria, limb and gait ataxia).

Management options
1. Refer all suspected cases to a neurologist/neurosurgeon before investigation or treatment.
2. Investigate and refer radiologically all suspected cases to a neurologist/neurosurgeon.
3. Investigate, treat with i.v. antibiotics and refer if patient fails to improve.

Option 1. Refer all suspected cases to a neurologist/neurosurgeon before investigation or treatment.

Tell the patient that they are being referred to a specialist for appropriate investigation and treatment.

✓ A specialist opinion would be gained on all potential cases.

✗ Relative paucity of neuroscience units in the UK means that existing services would be swamped.

✗ Appropriate patients would have an unacceptable delay in transfer due to the workload generated by inappropriate referrals. These patients would deteriorate pending treatment.

Option 2. Investigate and refer radiologically all suspected cases to a neurologist/neurosurgeon.

Tell the patient that if preliminary investigations suggest a neurosurgical condition then appropriate and prompt referral will be undertaken.

✓ CT scanning is now available in the majority of general hospitals.
✓ The CT appearance of cerebral abscess is easily recognized.
✓ The differential diagnosis (cystic glioma/metastasis) also requires neurosurgical referral.
✓ Best management of cerebral abscess requires close neurosurgical supervision, with stereotactic drainage/aspiration necessary for diagnostic and therapeutic purposes.
✓ Repeat imaging studies best undertaken and interpreted by neuroradiologists in conjunction with neurosurgeons.
✓ Neurological complications (e.g. seizures) suitably managed by liaising neurologist.
✓ Readily available neuro-intensive care unit (ITU) if needed.

✗ Can be a delay in arranging CT scan on overworked hospital scanners.

✗ Can be a delay in transfer due to bed shortages in neuroscience units.

Option 3. Investigate, treat with i.v. antibiotics and refer if patient fails to improve.

Tell the patient that treatment will be initiated and that if their condition fails to respond they will subsequently be referred.

✓ Some patients will respond to i.v. antibiotics alone without neurosurgical intervention (small or multiple abscesses, <2.5 cm diameter, without significant mass effect).

✓ Will not overload scarce neuroscience facilities.

✗ If medical management is insufficient and the patient deteriorates, neurosurgical intervention carries a greater risk.

✗ Window of therapeutic opportunity may well be lost.

✗ Does not allow an early microbiological diagnosis since stereotactic aspiration cannot be performed.

History checklist

General
- General health of the patient (weight loss, fever, malaise).
- Fever is present in only 50% of patients, more commonly in acute cases, and probably results from the primary source of infection rather than from the abscess itself.

Specific
- Ask about headache (up to 75%) associated with nausea or vomiting, seizures (up to 50%, focal or secondary generalized) and focal neurological symptoms, for example weakness (motor cortex), balance (posterior fossa), memory and speech (temporal lobe) or personality change (frontal lobe).
- In determining the site of the primary infection, enquire specifically about chronic middle ear infection, sinusitis, dental abscess, chronic lung disease, cardiac disease (native or prosthetic valve disease, ventricular septal defect, etc.) and recent penetrating cranial trauma.

Examination checklist
- General signs (e.g. fever, level of consciousness).
- Examine the ears, mouth, heart and chest and look for stigmata of infective endocarditis (IE) or hereditary haemorrhagic telangiectasia (pulmonary arterio-venous shunts associated with cerebral abscess).
- Neurological signs depend on the location of the abscess.
- Look carefully for papilloedema, nystagmus, hemiparesis (often mild), dysphasia, hemi- or quadrantanopia, and ataxia.

Referrals
Patients with suspected intracranial abscess can suddenly deteriorate due to brain stem herniation or acute ventriculitis, hence they must be referred to a neurosurgeon at once.

Rituals and myths
- Prophylactic treatment with anticonvulsants is often used to inhibit the risk of epilepsy in patients undergoing craniotomy. At least 80% of patients who undergo surgery for supratentorial abscess will subsequently develop seizures (often delayed in onset for years). Studies showing a lower risk of seizures have not followed the patients for long enough. Yet there is no evidence that phenytoin or carabamazepine prevent either the occurrence of seizures or the persistence of epilepsy if given routinely to all high-risk patients who undergo craniotomy. Prophylactic anticonvulsant prescribing merely brings adverse drug effects.

- Steroids (dexamethasone) are frequently used to reduce intracranial pressure in the presence of intracranial mass lesions. In animal studies of intracranial abscess, steroids are of no definite benefit. They may inhibit the penetration of some antibiotics into the CNS and can inhibit the encapsulation of the abscess due to inhibition of the inflammatory response. Nevertheless, they are used in the presence of surrounding oedema pending more definitive measures (abscess aspiration) to reduce intracranial pressure.

Pitfalls
- Focal neurological symptoms and signs may be absent.
- Papilloedema may be absent.
- Pyrexia may not be apparent.

Hints for investigators and prescribers
- LP in patients with large abscesses if there is significant oedema and mass effect is dangerous. It rarely provides any useful information, and given improvements in stereotactic or image directed neurosurgery, CSF analysis should not be performed, thus reducing the high risks of iatrogenic tentorial herniation.
- At the time the intracranial abscess is identified, a search must commence for its source. Failure to aggressively treat the primary site of infection leads to further local and remote sequelae.
- In AIDS patients with suspected cerebral toxoplasma, failure to respond to appropriate treatment within 7 days necessitates repeat imaging and biopsy to exclude lymphoma. In addition, multiple intracranial pathologies can exist in patients with AIDS. Hence, toxoplasmosis may coexist with cerebral lymphoma. The clinician should have a low threshold for repeating investigations.
- The risk of recurrence of cerebral toxoplasma in AIDS patients is 30%. Hence, acute therapy should be succeeded by secondary prophylactic treatment.

Further reading

Foy, P.M., Chadwick, D.W., Rajgopolan, N., Johnson, A.L. and Shaw, M.D.M. (1992) Do prophylactic anticonvulsant drugs alter the pattern of seizures following craniotomy? *J. Neurol. Neurosurg. Psychiatry* 55: 753–757.

Legg, N.J., Gupta, P.C. and Scott, D.F. (1973) Epilepsy following cerebral abscess: a clinical and EEG study of 70 patients. *Brain* 96: 259–268.

Mamelak, A.N., Mampalam, T.J., Obana, W.G. and Rosenblum M.L. (1995) Improved management of multiple brain abscesses: a combined surgical and medical approach. *Neurosurgery* 36: 76–86.

Mampalam, T.J. and Rosenblum, M.L. (1991) Trends in the management of bacterial brain abscesses; a review of 102 cases over 17 years. *Neurosurgery* 23: 451–458.

Nielsen, H., Glydensted, C. and Harmsen, A. (1982) Cerebral abscess: etiology and pathogenesis, symptoms, diagnosis and treatment. *Acta Neurol. Scanda.* 65: 609–622.

Rosenblum, M.L., Mampalam, T.J. and Pons, V.G. (1986) Controversies in the management of brain abscesses. *Clin. Neurosurg.* 33: 603–632.

3 Encephalitis

An acute, febrile illness evolving over several days. The dominant features are headache, vomiting, lethargy, personality and mental changes and confusion. The patient seems uncooperative and irritable. As the illness develops, the patient becomes more somnolent, stuporose or eventually comatose. Seizures are common. These may be generalized, but initially can be brief partial seizures and reflect the part of the brain afflicted. Thus patients with herpes simplex encephalitis often have simple (consciousness preserved) or complex (consciousness impaired) partial seizures characterized by olfactory of gustatory phenomena, automatisms and confusion. Personality change, psychosis, dysphasia and the development of focal motor signs (e.g. hemiparesis) must alert the physician to the possibility of encephalitis.

Management options
1. Admit all suspected cases and start aciclovir.
2. Admit and investigate all suspected cases and start potential/proven cases on aciclovir.

Option 1. Admit all suspected cases and start aciclovir.

Tell the patient that optimal treatment is being provided pending confirmation of the suspected diagnosis by specialist investigations.

✓ The long-term consequences (cognitive impairment, refractory seizures) of untreated herpes simplex encephalitis can be devastating, hence all possible cases should be treated.
✓ Fatality of herpes simplex encephalitis without treatment is 60–70%. With treatment, the mortality is under 30%.
✓ Aciclovir is relatively safe, thus a protocol of treating suspected cases should not bring excessive adverse events.
✓ If appropriate investigation reveals alternative pathology, then aciclovir can be discontinued and other therapy commenced as appropriate.

✗ Acute focal encephalitis is usually, though not invariably, due to herpes simplex virus (HSV). A minority of patients will be unnecessarily treated.
✗ Aciclovir can cause renal impairment particularly in the dehydrated patient, thus renal function must be monitored in all cases.

Option 2. Admit and investigate all suspected cases and start potential/proven cases on aciclovir.

Tell the patient that only if they are shown to have a brain infection will treatment be prescribed.

✓ Only appropriate cases will be treated.

✗ Definite proof of herpes simplex encephalitis requires specialist investigations, which are not always available without unacceptable time delay.
✗ While awaiting diagnostic confirmation, potentially reversible cases may irreversibly deteriorate.

History checklist

General
The earliest feature of most patients with viral encephalitis is headache. It is important to ascertain whether the presenting headache is usual for that patient – or if it is out of character and has features to suggest a sinister nature.

Specific
- Ask about features associated with the headache, particularly vomiting.
- Is the headache becoming progressively worse?
- Has there been any personality change, irritability, brief lapses in consciousness or concentration (to suggest partial seizures), or speech disturbance (dysphasia)?
- Has there been lethargy, confusion, memory disturbance, prolonged or fluctuating drowsiness or impaired level of consciousness or fever?

Examination checklist
- Is there fever and what is the conscious level?
- Assess whether the patient is fully alert and orientated, or drowsy and confused.
- Is there evidence of a visual field deficit (upper quadrantanopia to suggest temporal lobe involvement) or dysphasia?
- Long tract signs are usually absent.
- Generalized seizures are obvious, but brief partial (simple or complex) seizures may be subtle.
- Is there any meningism to suggest a meningoencephalitis?

Referrals
- All patients with suspected viral encephalitis must be admitted to hospital.
- Specialist referral to a neurologist is advisable since MRI, EEG and careful CSF analysis are required.
- Assessment of the potential longer-term sequelae (cognitive impairment, partial seizures) is probably better undertaken in specialist units.

Rituals and myths
Although recent cold sores have been suggested to be associated with herpes simplex encephalitis, they are usually irrelevant.

Pitfalls
- Herpes simplex encephalitis may present as a subacute or even chronic neuropsychiatric state (confusion, psychosis, cognitive deterioration). It must be considered in the patient who acutely or subacutely acquires refractory seizures without other cause.
- Renal function must be monitored in patients given aciclovir; adequate i.v. hydration is necessary in the confused or drowsy patient.
- Cerebral venous thrombosis can exactly mimic herpes simplex encephalitis.

Hints for investigators and prescribers
- The CSF is abnormal in the majority of patients with herpes simplex encephalitis. Depending on the severity of the condition and the degree of brain swelling, the CSF pressure may be mildly to markedly elevated. About 90% of patients have a lymphocytic pleocytosis with cell counts of 10–1000 per mm³. There may also be a slight excess of red cells due to haemorrhagic inflammation on the surfaces of the temporal lobes. The protein is typically mildly elevated ($0.5–1.5$ g l⁻¹). The CSF glucose is usually normal. In a proportion of cases, only some of the above parameters are abnormal, and in a minority of cases (5%) the CSF may be entirely normal.
- Management of the patient with viral encephalitis relies on supportive and specific measures. Agitation may necessitate sedation, particularly for investigation, impaired conscious level may necessitate ventilation, and seizures require adequate emergency management. Repeated doses of benzodiazepines are hazardous and the patient should be loaded with 15–18 mg kg⁻¹ of phenytoin with subsequent maintenance doses according to regular blood levels. There is no trial data to support the use of dexamethasone or mannitol in the management of raised intracranial pressure in encephalitis. The

likelihood of this occurring is, however, reduced by the rapid institution of antiviral therapy.

- Aciclovir is only of proven benefit in patients with herpes simplex encephalitis. It reduces the mortality from 60–70% to less than 30% and it increases the number of patients surviving with no or minor sequelae from 15% to over 40%. Renal function must be monitored; profound but usually reversible renal impairment is a complication of therapy particularly in the dehydrated patient (which is usually the case in the confused, agitated or obtunded).

Further reading

Cinque, P., Cleator, G.M., Weber, T., Monteyne, P., Sindic, C.J, van Loon, A.M. for the EU Concerted Action on Virus Meningitis and Encephalitis. (1996) The role of laboratory investigation in the diagnosis and management of patients with suspected herpes simplex encephalitis: a consensus report. *J. Neurol. Neurosurg. Psychiatry* **61**: 339–345.

Lipkin, W.I. (1997) European consensus on viral encephalitis. *Lancet* **349**: 299–300.

Skoldenberg, B., Forsgren, M., Alestig, K., Bergstrom, T., Burnan, L., Dahlqvist, E. *et al.* (1984) Acyclovir versus vidarabine therapy in herpes simplex encephalitis: a randomised multicentre study in consecutive Swedish patients. *Lancet* **ii**: 707–711.

Whitley R.J. (1990) Viral encephalitis. *N. Engl. J. Med.* **323**: 242–250.

Whitley, R.J., Alford, C.A., Hirsch, M.S., Scooley, R.T., Luby, J.P., Aoki, F.Y., *et al.* and the NIAID Collaborative Antiviral Study Group. (1986) Vidarabine versus aciclovir therapy in herpes simplex encephalitis. *N. Engl. J. Med.* **314**: 144–149.

Whitley, R.J., Cobbs, C.G., Alford, C.A. Jr, Soong, S-J., Hirsch, M.S., Connor, J.D. *et al.* for the NIAID Collaborative Antiviral Study Group. (1989) Diseases that mimic herpes simplex encephalitis: diagnosis, presentation, and outcome. *JAMA* **262**: 234–239.

4 Transmissible neurodegenerative diseases

Creutzfeld-Jakob disease (CJD)
Initial symptoms lasting a few weeks are often vague and include changes in mood (often mild depression), personality and sleep disturbance. These progress to a rapidly evolving dementia (over the course of several weeks to a few months) with disturbance of balance (ataxia), visual distortions, visual hallucinations, dysarthria and the development of stimulus sensitive myoclonus. Patients become mute, axially rigid and comatose but the myoclonus often persists until death. The rapid progression helps distinguish CJD from other neurodegenerative conditions.

Whereas CJD is typically a disease of middle age onwards, the new variant (nv) CJD is seen in a younger age group (teens onwards). Mental changes (mimicking depression) dominate, and paraesthesia in hands and feet are common. Dementia and rigidity develop more slowly than in classical CJD and myoclonus is often absent.

Subacute sclerosing panencephalitis (SSPE)
Occurs primarily in children and adolescents up to the age of 20 years. Rarely it occurs in young adults. Patients have usually suffered measles at a young age (under 2 years). Initial symptoms are of progressive cognitive decline with impaired school performance, followed by personality changes, seizures, ataxia, myoclonus. Progression to rigidity with decorticate posturing and extensor plantars occurs over 1–3 years. In 10% of cases, the disease may be more fulminant, and in a further 10% more protracted with apparent 'remissions'.

Progressive multifocal leucoencephalopathy (PML)
The vast majority of cases now occur in AIDS patients in whom the incidence of PML approaches 5%. Rarely it occurs in patients with chronic neoplastic conditions such as chronic lymphocytic leukaemia (CLL), Hodgkin's lymphoma and the myeloproliferative disorders. The illness is subacute with initial personality and cognitive changes progressing over several weeks. Focal neurological signs, e.g. dysarthria, hemi- or tetraparesis, visual field defects, or cortical blindness then develop. Progression to coma and death usually occurs over 3–6 months from symptom onset.

Management options
1. All neurodegenerative diseases are untreatable, therefore do nothing.
2. Neurodegenerative disorders are uncommon, therefore suspected cases should be referred to a neurologist.

Option 1. All neurodegenerative diseases are untreatable, therefore do nothing.

Tell the patient that you think their condition is untreatable and, therefore, you are powerless to help.

✓ Limited resources will not be wasted on patients with untreatable conditions.
✓ No risk of contamination via infected instruments or CNS biopsy material.

✗ Cases are sufficiently rare that the extra caseload will have virtually no overall impact on resources.
✗ Patients and relatives will not accept this approach.
✗ No diagnosis ever reached until post-mortem.
✗ Other potentially treatable conditions may be missed.

Option 2. Neurodegenerative disorders are uncommon, therefore suspected cases should be referred to a neurologist.

Tell the patient that you have little or no experience of their suspected condition, hence specialist assessment is necessary.

✓ General physicians or GPs may never see a case of CJD, PML or SSPE in their practising careers; the only way to develop expertise in diagnosis is therefore by specialist referral to maintain caseload throughput to neurologists.

✓ Specialist and carefully interpreted investigation is needed for all cases (MRI, EEG, and possibly CSF analysis and brain biopsy) which can only be undertaken in neurological units.

✓ Other conditions mimicking CJD, SSPE or PML will not be missed.

History checklist

General
- Is the patient immunocompromised (PML) or have they previously had measles (SSPE)?
- How old is the patient (SSPE usually develops between the ages of 5 and 15 years)?

Specific
- Features common to SSPE, PML and CJD are insidious mental changes (memory, confusion, behavioural and personality changes, progressing to a dementing state).
- Enquire about involuntary movements, particularly myoclonic jerks (SSPE and CJD). Visual disturbances (hemianopia, visuospatial disorientation, ocular apraxia, and cortical blindness) may be seen in PML and to a lesser extent in CJD. Poor balance and clumsiness are features of all three disorders.

Examination checklist
- The cardinal clinical features of CJD are dementia, myoclonus and ataxia.
- In PML, dementia, visual deficits, motor weakness, ataxia and dysarthria or dysphasia are the prominent signs.
- SSPE is characterized by dementia, involuntary movements (myoclonus, chorea, tremor, dyskinesia), then progression to decerebrate rigidity and finally loss of cortical functions.

Referrals
All suspected cases of SSPE, PML or CJD should be referred to a neurologist.

Rituals and myths
- Measles vaccine can provoke subsequent development of SSPE. However, the risk of SSPE after measles itself is 8.5 cases per 1 million measles cases versus 0.7 SSPE cases per 1 million measles vaccinations. Since routine measles vaccination was undertaken in the USA, the incidence of SSPE has fallen tenfold to 0.06 cases per million population.
- Prion diseases cannot cross species barriers. Unfortunately, this is not true and there is concern that nv CJD may be related to exposure to beef infected with bovine spongiform encephalopathy (BSE).

Pitfalls
- Lithium toxicity can mimic CJD.
- Signs of lithium toxicity can occur with apparently normal serum lithium concentrations.

Hints for investigators and prescribers
- In SSPE the serum measles antibody titres are usually significantly elevated. CSF protein becomes elevated as the illness develops, with the presence of oligoclonal bands indicating local immunoglobulin synthesis within the CNS. Fifty to eighty per cent of the CSF IgG is

measles-specific and as the disease progresses the ratio of CSF measles antibody to serum measles-antibody rises. The EEG in SSPE shows high amplitude slow waves with a periodicity of 5–15 seconds and becomes diffusely slow as the disease develops. MRI shows initially discrete and then confluent white matter lesions according to the stage of the disease.

- The demonstration of antibodies to the JC virus in suspected PML is only helpful if titres rise rapidly, as many of the normal population show positive titres. MRI shows numerous non-enhancing white matter lesions in the cerebral hemispheres, cerebellum and brainstem. It may be necessary to confirm the diagnosis by brain biopsy.
- CJD remains a post-mortem diagnosis unless brain biopsy is performed. Ante-mortem suspicion rests on the clinical features, the EEG (characteristically showing repetitive triphasic periodic complexes) and evidence of cerebral atrophy on MRI. It may soon be possible to reliably diagnose CJD by CSF examination with analysis for the 14–0–3 brain protein or even by tonsillar biopsy.
- No proven treatment exists for PML, CJD or SSPE, although interferons have been tried in the latter condition but without definitive success. Symptomatic treatment can be offered for myoclonus (with clonazepam) or generalized seizures.

Further reading

Collinge, J., Sidles, K.C.L., Meads, J., Ironside, J. and Hill, A.F. (1996) Molecular analysis of prion strain variation and the aetiology of 'new variant' CJD. *Nature* 383: 685–690.

Hill, A.F., Zeidler, M.Z., Ironside, J. and Collinge, J. (1997) Diagnosis of new variant Creutzfeldt-Jakob disease by tonsil biopsy. *Lancet* 349: 99–100.

Hsich, G., Kenney, K., Gibbs, C.J., Lee, K.H. and Harrington, M.G. (1996) The 14–03–3 brain protein in cerebrospinal fluid as a marker for transmissible spongiform encephalopathies. *N. Engl. J. Med.* 335: 924–930.

Palmer, M.S., Dryden, A.J., Hughes, J.T. and Collinge, J. (1991) Homozygous prion protein genotype predisposes to sporadic Creutzfeldt-Jakob disease. *Nature* 352: 340–341.

Will, R.G., Ironside, J.W., Zeidler Cousens, S.N., Estibeiro, K., Alperovitch, A., Poser, S., Pocchiari, M. and Hofman, A. (1996) A new variant of Creutzfeld-Jakob disease in the UK. *Lancet* 347: 921–925.

Chapter 3
CHRONIC FATIGUE SYNDROME

N.G. Hunt

This chapter principally concerns chronic fatigue syndrome (CFS). Over the years this condition has aroused much debate and controversy. Many questions still remain with regard to making the diagnosis, the aetiology and management of the condition. What follows is an attempt to encapsulate current thinking regarding this illness complex. Inevitably it will raise many more questions than it answers.

Definitions

Chronic fatigue syndrome
This new term for what is a heterogeneous condition was proposed in 1988 by a consensus group in the USA. It was formerly known as chronic Epstein–Barr virus (EBV) syndrome. The change in name was because of doubts over the causal role of EBV in patients who had been diagnosed as suffering from chronic EBV syndrome.

Variations to this original criterion-based definition have been developed for research purposes in Australia, the UK and the USA. Differences between these proposed definitions relate principally to the inclusion criteria used for pre-existing psychiatric problems. It follows that given the heterogenous nature of CFS, coupled with the fact that different research groups use different CFS definitions, interpretation and comparison of research results needs particular caution – something which continues to hamper epidemiological research in this field.

Despite this problem, all the definitions are characterized by a minimum of 6 months of medically unexplained severe, disabling physical and mental fatigue and fatigability – fatigue after exertion. Symptoms such as muscle pain, mood disturbance and sleep disorder are also usually present. Other common causes of chronic fatigue should be excluded before labelling a patient with this diagnosis.

Encephalomyelitis
Acute inflammation of the brain and spinal cord.

Fatigability
The onset of symptoms in the continuum of tiredness or weariness through to exhaustion occurring after exertion.

Fatigue
The subjective feeling of physical and/or mental weariness resulting from exertion and which settles with rest. It can be a normal everyday experience but is also a symptom present in a large number of illnesses. There is no objective measurement for the degree of fatigue, which is perhaps best viewed as a continuum from tiredness or weariness to profound exhaustion.

The threshold at which fatigue becomes abnormal is dependent upon the clinician's interpretation of the patient's reported complaint. It is likely that under such circumstances of excessive fatigue, patients would describe significant impairments in their physical and mental functioning.

Myalgic encephalomyelitis (ME)

An expression used to describe an outbreak of uncertain aetiology involving staff at the Royal Free Hospital in 1955. Subsequently, it was used to describe other outbreaks in the world in which paralysis was a significant feature, but no cause was found.

Over time, the use of the term has diversified to describe cases apparently triggered by known virus infection; although the term post-viral fatigue syndrome is best used to describe this group. It has also been used to describe cases where there is no paralysis.

There is little evidence to support the specific pathological entity encephalomyelitis occurring in these cases, and myalgia is by no means universally found. Thus, although the term ME is popular with the lay press and widely known by the public, its continued use is being discouraged by the medical profession.

The patient populations suffering from CFS and ME by their various definitions are not the same, although there is undoubtedly a degree of overlap. Some authors have referred to this subset as CFS(ME). In the USA some specialists have referred to this subset as CFS with encephalopathy or chronic fatigue immune dysfunction.

Neurasthenia

An old-fashioned medical expression first described in 1869 but listed in the 10th edition of the *International Classification of Diseases*; covering a number of conditions, some with features common to CFS.

Post-viral fatigue syndrome

An expression reserved to describe cases of CFS where there is clear evidence that the condition has been triggered by a viral infection.

Somatization

Often seen in association with depression and/or anxiety. The patient attributes physical symptoms to a physical cause. However, in reality there is an underlying mental health problem.

As CFS is a heterogenous condition, it is likely that at the present time more than one condition is being identified. There is also a degree of overlap between the symptomatology of CFS and that of psychological conditions. For example, depression and anxiety are associated with many cases of CFS. Having said this, between 20 and 40% of CFS patients do not have depression or any other psychiatric condition. The relationship between psychiatric illness and CFS is not yet fully understood. Depression and CFS are clinical entities in their own right.

The current situation for both professionals and patients is therefore rather confusing – researchers have used at least four different criterion-based definitions, there are difficulties in teasing out co-morbid psychiatric complaints, and questions concerning aetiology still divide the profession, often resulting in different management pathways. Attempts at estimating the prevalence of CFS vary greatly from 0.05% to 1.8% for the population. There is a female preponderance, with the main peak presenting between the ages of 30 and 40 for both sexes and an earlier smaller peak in women aged 15–25. Cases in children under 12 appear to be much less common.

The majority of cases of CFS can be managed in the primary care setting. The natural course of CFS is not yet fully understood. What can be said is that children have better and quicker recovery rates than adults. In teenagers the average illness lasts approximately 4.5 years, while in adults this can be much longer. Overall about 20% make a complete recovery within 2 years. Another 60% go through a fluctuating illness but will stabilize at lower energy levels. The other 20% have a more severe and debilitating illness. The risk of relapses appears to be lifelong.

Orientation

While it is important to be aware of the various definitions, at a pragmatic level in primary care we need to be able to tease out the important points which could lead us to consider CFS when confronted with a patient complaining of tiredness or fatigue.

Fatigue, or one of its synonyms, is a very common presentation in primary care. It can be the prodromal symptom of numerous illnesses: a presenting symptom in those suffering from anxiety and depression, insomniacs, those with chronic pain, and can also occur as the result of treatment.

Currently there are no clinically recommended diagnostic criteria for CFS, although several research diagnostic criteria are available. Pending the development of 'gold standard recommendations', the clinician confronted with a patient who complains of fatigue may like to consider the approach given on p. 35.

Chapter contents

1 Chronic fatigue syndrome in adults

Management options

1. Do nothing, no investigations and no treatment.
2. Do not bother to investigate, referring all patients regardless of severity to a local secondary care centre.
3. Investigate all patients with baseline tests, offer symptomatic treatment and refer selected cases to a local specialist.
4. Investigate all patients with baseline tests, offer symptomatic treatment and refer selected cases to a tertiary chronic fatigue/ME centre.

Option 1. Do nothing, no investigations and no treatment.

Tell the patient that the clinical examination was entirely normal, that the symptoms are all in the mind and there is nothing you can do about it.

✗ Such a dismissive statement is totally unacceptable and does nothing to help the chronically fatigued patient. You need to keep an open mind. Accept and acknowledge that the patient is unwell. A supportive and positive attitude is essential.

✗ The absence of baseline investigations does not exclude other treatable causes of chronic fatigue, does nothing to lessen the diagnostic uncertainty and possibly compromises the doctor–patient relationship.

✗ The implication that the condition is entirely psychological, again may adversely affect the doctor–patient relationship. Any perceived mismatch in patient ideas and expectations at this stage may be storing up further problems for the GP and his future interaction with the patient and carers.

✗ In terms of health economics, such a strategy is unlikely to be cost-effective in terms of maximizing patient functioning in as shorter a time as possible.

Option 2. Do not bother to investigate, referring all patients regardless of severity to a local secondary care centre.

✗ Unlikely to be very cost-efficient as there is a general consensus on the baseline investigations which can be arranged in the primary care setting.

✗ Investigations will filter out a number of treatable causes of chronic fatigue. These individuals can then be offered specific treatment and appropriate referral if warranted.

✗ Referring all patients regardless of severity of chronic fatigue, if repeated all over the district, is likely to produce a log jam in the out-patients department of the local hospital. There is a lot the general practitioner and his/her primary care team can do to support these patients, rather than consigning them to the therapeutic vacuum of the NHS waiting list.

✗ GPs should remember that not all consultants to whom these patients might be referred necessarily have the expertise or interest in dealing with patients with CFS. Moreover, this may result in inappropriate forms of treatment being offered.

Option 3. Investigate all patients with baseline tests, offer symptomatic treatment and refer selected cases to a local specialist.

✓ A second opinion may be helpful to the doctor in confirming a suspicion, and reassuring to the patient who may feel more comfortable in having a specialist confirm the diagnosis. On occasions, it can ease pressure on the doctor incurred from carers.

✓ If the clinician is doubtful about the diagnosis or there are aspects of the presentation which are atypical, then referral is entirely appropriate.

✗ Patients are often referred to a number of specialities depending upon presentation, consultant availability and interest. Frequently these referrals are to physicians or neurologists. It is important to refer to a specialist who has an interest in this area. The ME associations keep lists of specialists with expertise in this field.

Option 4. Investigate all patients with baseline tests, offer symptomatic treatment and refer selected cases to a tertiary chronic fatigue/ME centre.

✓ Management in the primary care setting is appropriate for many sufferers. Appropriate management depends on proper assessment of the patients level of disability, psychological state and illness beliefs.

✓ Refer in cases where there are atypical features, particularly those with neurological signs, difficulty in walking, weight loss, older patients and those with any abnormal investigations.

✗ In the current internal market of the NHS, some patients have found difficulty in obtaining extra contractual referral funding from their health authority or in some cases from GP fundholders for tertiary referrals. With the change in government in the UK and the subsequent publication and forthcoming implementation of 'The New NHS' white paper, this problem is likely to recede.

History checklist

General

- A biopsychosocial approach should be adopted, looking not just from the medical perspective but also taking into account how psychological and social factors have affected an individual's illness.
- Enquire about the patient's past medical history, paying particular attention to any history of severe depression, recent life events and any stressors.
- Ask about any recent illnesses, alcohol or substance abuse, foreign travel and whether any medications including vitamins and supplements are being taken.

Specific

- Taking time to take a careful history and elucidating exactly what a patient's problems are will help enormously in narrowing down the differential diagnoses. During history-taking, time should be taken to explore the patient's problems and their own health beliefs. Patients suffering from CFS often emphasize their physical problems and make light of their psychological problems in order to add credence to their story or to avoid the stigma of being labelled as having a psychological problem.
- Is the patient feeling weary? If yes, remember that different patients will use different synonyms to describe how they feel. Since there is no objective measure of the feeling of fatigue you need to assess the severity of their complaint. Asking a question such as whether they would be able to dig the garden and if so, how long it would take for them to recover from this exertion, can be used to gauge their level of fatigue. An understanding of the patients level of functionality is essential. Patients may describe a physical fatigue complaining of a lack of stamina, lack of energy and muscle weakness, while mental fatigue may variously be described as complaining of poor memory, impaired concentration, depressed mood, disinterest or abnormal sleepiness.
- What makes this tiredness abnormal and debilitating for the patient? Ask how it impairs their day-to-day activities. CFS patients will often describe a worsening of fatigue if exposed to any physical or mental exertion. Patients may describe periods of improvement followed by relapses in their symptoms.
- What was the patient's level of physical activity prior to the onset of fatigue and what is their attitude to physical activity now? This is an important area to explore and can give a useful insight into what a patient's (possibly unrealistic) expectations may be, and to the

activities which they might like to do but are avoiding because of their current level of physical dysfunction.

- How long has the fatigue been apparent? The general consensus is that for adults the fatigue should have lasted 6 months or more before a diagnosis of CFS can be entertained. Fatigue of shorter duration is common after many illnesses.
- Can they recall any precipitating infection which triggered the fatigue? If yes, look for evidence suggestive of a particular infection. For example, one of glandular fever if confirmed by serological tests could lead to a diagnosis of post-viral fatigue syndrome being made. CFS suffers will often describe an acute onset of the illness.
- Any there any associated symptoms? There are various different criterion-based definitions of CFS, so the patient populations will be different depending on the particular set of criteria being followed. Common symptoms are recurrent sore throat, headache, nausea, muscle and joint pain, flu-like symptoms and tender cervical and axillary lymph nodes. Intolerance to alcohol may be described. Postural hypotension may be noted on examination.
- Could the patient be suffering from anxiety or depression? Psychological symptoms are very common in CFS, depression being found in half of all CFS patients. At the present time the exact explanation for this association is not known, but it is not simply that the depression is secondary to the disability. Other psychosocial stressors should be identified.
- It has been recognized that in the primary care setting GPs often miss cases of depression particularly with somatizing patients. In order to increase the uptake of recognized psychological distress, screening questionnaires such as the General Health Questionnaire and the Hospital Anxiety and Depression Scale have been used.
- Explore the patient's health beliefs. This is important as negative health beliefs about their symptoms can affect mood, behaviour and level of disability. Illness attribution and the strength of such feeling can give some indication of the possible long-term outcome. For example, in patients followed up in the tertiary care sector poorer outcome has been associated with those patients who believe that their symptoms are due solely to a physical cause. Fortunately, in the primary care setting such strong physical attributional health beliefs are unusual, patients being much more likely to cite psychosocial factors.
- What are their coping mechanisms? The key here is to attempt to tease out any dysfunctional aspects in the history. A common finding is failure to rest adequately at the start of the illness. Sometimes there are descriptions of protracted periods of rest and/or inconsistent activity oscillating between prolonged rest and excessive activity, which is too much too soon. Dysfunctional strategies such as these can result in a perpetuation of the problem.

Examination checklist
- Physical and psychological assessment is mandatory. Remember that the diagnosis of CFS is one of exclusion.

Rituals and myths
- The stereotype of 'yuppie flu' is an artefact of referral bias. According to one study, CFS sufferers in the primary care setting show no social class bias.

Pitfalls
- Mismatch in doctor–patient perception of the problem.
- Rest, which is crucial in the acute phase, if too prolonged can become counterproductive.
- Over zealous physiotherapy can be counterproductive.
- Failure to tackle psychosocial stressors or treat any co-morbid depression will delay recovery.
- Confounding problems with conditions other than CFS, but which have some overlapping symptoms. For example, patients with somatization disorder being misdiagnosed as CFS (ME).
- Negative health beliefs can help to perpetuate CFS.

Hints for investigators and prescribers

Aetiology
- The aetiology of CFS remains unknown.

Diagnostic criteria
- Several case definitions for CFS have been published in the USA, Australia and the UK. All have their limitations and also lack specificity, identifying a number of disorders rather than just one. A suggested clinical approach for chronic fatigue presentation is shown in *Figure 1*. Included within the flow diagram is also a summary of the latest USA diagnostic criteria for CFS from the Centers for Disease Control and Prevention (CDC) (after Fukuda *et al.*, 1994). Having excluded other causes of fatigue (ADOPTS screen), a

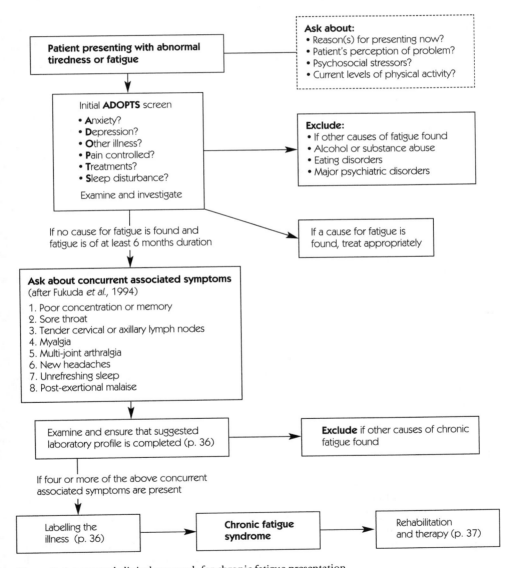

Figure 1. A suggested clinical approach for chronic fatigue presentation.

history of relapsing or persistent fatigue lasting more than 6 consecutive months can be termed chronic fatigue. A diagnosis of CFS also requires at least four of the eight concurrent associated symptoms suggested by Fukuda *et al.* (1994), listed in *Figure 1*.

- In the UK, the Oxford criteria have been used extensively. Like the CDC criteria, they are intended for use as a research tool and are not currently recommended for clinical use. The Oxford criteria are as follows:
  (i)   fatigue as the principle symptom;
  (ii)   definite onset, not life long;
  (iii) substantial physical and mental functional impairment;
  (iv)   a history of at least 6 months of fatigue, which has been present for over 50% of the time;
  (v)   may be associated with myalgia, mood and sleep problems.
  (vi)   exclusion criteria: identified medical causes of fatigue, patients currently suffering from schizophrenia, bipolar disorder, substance abuse, eating disorder.

- The Oxford criteria go on to identify a subgroup of CFS which has followed or is associated with an infection. This is termed post-infectious fatigue syndrome (PIFS). Criteria additional to those up for CFS reported for inclusion in the PIFS group are:
  (i)   definite evidence of infection at onset or at presentation;
  (ii)   syndrome are present for at least 6 months from the start of the infection;
  (iii) infection confirmed by laboratory evidence.

- Both groups should also be assessed for concurrent psychiatric disorder. It should be noted that depressive and anxiety states are not necessarily grounds for exclusion.

- The Oxford criteria have some drawbacks: lack of specificity, poor predictive validity, certain patients are excluded because there is no definite onset in their history and the inherent difficulties of knowing whether fatigue has been present for more than 50% of the time.

Initial investigations

A suggested laboratory profile:

- FBC;
- acute phase proteins (erythrocyte sedimentation rate or C-reactive protein);
- urea and electrolytes;
- creatine kinase;
- liver function tests;
- calcium and phosphate;
- thyroid-stimulating hormone and free thyroxine;
- urine dipstick test for protein and sugar.

Other tests which may be considered depending on history:

- serological tests (i.e. Epstein–Barr virus/cytomegalovirus, respiratory viruses and enteroviral IgM), if requested within 3 months of onset;
- autoantibody screen;
- chest X-ray;
- HIV screen.

Labelling the illness

- Should one 'label' the illness? Assuming that a patient fulfils the diagnostic criteria for CFS and other treatable causes of chronic fatigue have been excluded, there seems little point in not sharing this diagnosis with the patient. By using the descriptive term CFS, you are acknowledging that there is a problem but without endorsing any particular illness causation. It is best to avoid using the term ME which incorrectly suggests an inflammatory disorder in the brain and spinal column. Shared understanding of the patient's illness beliefs can then be explored and appropriate management of the condition discussed.

Rehabilitation and therapy

Given the heterogenous nature of CFS, rehabilitation programmes should be patient-specific, focusing on individual needs.

Initial assessment should include:

- Establishing what the current level of activity is.
- Stabilizing activity to a level which conserves some energy reserves. For some individuals who were previously operating at the upper threshold of their activity this will involve a reduction in activity, they need to slow down their pace of life, while others will have the capacity for modest gradual increases in activity.
- Rest is very important in the acute phase of the illness.
- Stress should be minimized.

Following this initial stabilization, a flexible programme is then developed with the patient, involving paced graded activity within a routine which has balanced periods for rest and such activity.

- Exercise goals or targets should be chosen to reflect current fitness and level of activity and not based on past pre-illness performance.
- Sleep problems and depression should be treated according to standard clinical proto-cols, and this may involve both psychological therapies and drug treatments. Many CFS sufferers are particularly sensitive to antidepressants. In addition to helping with depression, some antidepressants act by improving sleep and/or decreasing pain. Tricyclic anti-depressants should be commenced at a low dose which is then gradually increased to therapeutic levels.
- Alternatively, recent reports suggest that the new selective serotonin re-uptake inhibitors (SSRIs) have been of benefit to certain patients. As with tricyclic antidepressants, any SSRI should be commenced starting at one-tenth to one-quarter of the usual clinical dose. They should not be abruptly withdrawn.
- Non-steroidal anti-inflammatory drugs can be used to deal with myalgia and arthralgic pains.
- Relaxation techniques are very helpful, but not tense and releasing muscle exercises, as in the initial phase these can be particularly energy draining and painful.
- Patients should be warned to expect temporary exacerbations of physical symptoms as the programme progresses. A resurgence of neurological symptoms, however, might indicate the beginning of a CFS relapse. In this situation, rest, as in the acute phase, is advised.
- Some patients will benefit from CFS self-help groups.
- For those patients who have dysfunctional coping behaviours or inappropriate illness perceptions which are inhibiting recovery, then referral for cognitive behavioural therapy may be helpful.
- Expect improvement over months rather than weeks.

Further reading

Chalder, T. (1995) *Coping with Chronic Fatigue*. Sheldon Press, London.

Chalder, T., Berelowitz, G., Pawlikowska, T., Watts, L., Wessely, S., Wright, D. and Wallace, E.P. (1993) Development of a fatigue scale. *J. Psychosom. Res.* **37**: 147–153.

Colby, J. (1996) *ME. The New Plague*. First and Best in Education Ltd., Peterborough.

David, A.S., Wessely, S. and Pelosi, A.J. (1991) Chronic fatigue syndrome: signs of a new approach. *Br. J. Hosp. Med.* **45**: 158–163.

Dowsett, E.G. (1997) *What is ME/CFS?* South Essex Health Trust, Brentwood.

Euba, R., Chalder, T., Deale, A. and Wessely, S. (1996) A comparison of the characteristics of chronic fatigue syndrome in primary and tertiary care. *Br. J. Psychiat.* **168**: 121–126.

Fukuda, K., Straus, S., Hickie, I. *et al.* (1994) The chronic fatigue syndrome: a comprehensive approach to its definition and study. *Ann. Int. Med.* **121**: 953–959.

Goldberg, D. and Williams, P. (1988) *A User's Guide to the General Health Questionnaire*. NFER-Nelson, Windsor.

Holmes, G., Kaplan, J., Gantz, N. *et al.* (1988) Chronic fatigue syndrome: a working case definition. *Ann. Int. Med.* **108**: 387–389.

Ho-Yen, D. (1993) *Better Recovery from Viral Illness*, 3rd Edn. Dodona Books, Inverness.

Jason, L.A., Richman, J.A., Friedberg, F, Wagner, L., Taylor, R. and Jordan, K.M. (1997) Politics, science and the emergence of a new disease. The case of chronic fatigue syndrome. *Am. Psychol.* **52**: 973–983.

Lewis, G. and Wessely, S. (1992) The epidemiology of fatigue: more questions than answers. *J. Epid. Comm. Health* **46**: 92–97.

Lloyd, A.R., Hickie, I., Boughton, C.R. *et al.* (1990) Prevalence of chronic fatigue syndrome in an Australian population. *Med. J. Aust.* **153**: 524–528.

Medical staff of the Royal Free Hospital. (1957) An outbreak of encephalomyelitis in the Royal Free Hospital Group, London, in 1955. *Br. Med. J.* **2**: 895–904.

National Institute of Allergy and Infectious Diseases. (1996) *Chronic Fatigue Syndrome – Information for Physicians.* Public Health Service, US Department of Health and Human Services.

National Task Force on Chronic Fatigue Syndrome (CFS), Post Viral Fatigue Syndrome (PVFS), Myalgic Encephalomyelitis (ME). (1994) Report. Westcare, Bristol.

Pawlikowska, T., Chalder, T., Hirsch, S.R., Wallace, P., Wright, D.J.M. and Wessely, S.C. (1994) Population-based study of fatigue and psychological distress. *Br. Med. J.* **308**: 763–766.

Ridsdale, L. (1995) A critical appraisal of the literature on tiredness. In: *Evidence-Based General Practice*, W.B. Saunders Company Ltd, London, pp.148–159.

Royal Colleges of Physicians, Psychiatrists and General Practitioners. (1996) *Chronic Fatigue Syndrome. Report of a Joint Working Group.* Royal College of Physicians Publication Unit, London.

Sharpe, M., Archard, L., Banatvala, J. *et al.* (1991) Chronic fatigue syndrome: guidelines for research. *J. R. Soc. Med.* **84**: 118–121.

Sharpe, M., Hawton K., Simkin S. *et al.* (1996) Cognitive behaviour therapy for chronic fatigue syndrome: a randomised controlled trial. *Br. Med. J.* **312**: 22–26.

Shepherd, C. (1995) *Myalgic Encephalomyelitis: Post-Viral Fatigue Syndrome. Guidelines for the care of patients*, 2nd Edn. M.E. Association, Stanford le Hope.

Wessely, S. (1995) The epidemiology of chronic fatigue syndrome. *Epidemiol. Rev.* **17**: 139–151.

Wessely, S., Hotopf, M. and Sharpe, M. (1998) Chronic fatigue and its syndromes. Oxford University Press, Oxford.

Wilson, A., Hickie, I., Lloyd, A., Hadzi-Pavlovic, D., Boughton, C., Dwyer, J. and Wakefield, D. (1994) Longitudinal study of outcome of chronic fatigue syndrome. *Br. Med. J.* **308**: 756–759.

World Health Organisation. (1993) *The ICD-10 Classification of Mental and Behavioural Disorders: Diagnostic Criteria for Research.* World Health Organisation, Geneva, Switzerland.

Zigmond, A.S. and Snaith, R.P. (1983) The hospital anxiety and depression scale. *Acta Psychiatr. Scand.* **67**: 361–370.

Useful addresses (UK)

Action for ME
PO Box 1302
Wells
Somerset BA5 2WE
Tel: 01749 670799

ME Association
Stanhope House
High Street
Stanford le Hope
Essex SS17 0HA
Tel: 01375 642466

National ME Support Centre
Disablement Services Centre
Harold Wood Hospital
Romford
Essex RM3 9AR
Tel: 01708 378050

Persistent Virus Disease Research
Foundation
4 One Tree Lane
Beaconsfield
Bucks HP9 2BU
Tel: 01494 674769

Westcare
155 Whiteladies Road
Clifton
Bristol BS8 2RF
Tel: 0117 923 9341

2 Chronic fatigue syndrome in children

The general approach is similar to that of adults. Fortunately recovery is often much quicker than in adults. Again it is a diagnosis by exclusion of other causes of fatigue. In this age group, school phobia should be considered in the differential diagnosis. The criterion-based definitions of CFS can be applied, but there is concern that the 6-month duration criterion is too long and that 3 months may be more appropriate. This clearly gives the opportunity for earlier intervention but needs to be balanced against the possible risks of misdiagnosis with all the problems this can cause.

Management overview
- As with adults limited blood tests are justified, along with EBV serology. A negative screen coupled with a normal physical examination can be very reassuring for family and child alike.
- Management of children suffering from CFS is possible in the primary care setting for all but the most severely affected.
- The mainstays of the management approach in children are reassurance, explanation emotional support and regular frequent monitoring, which may initially be on a weekly basis.
- Management revolves around resting in the acute phase, and thereafter paced graded exercise with rest periods. Coupling this with realistic goal setting is encouraged, depending on the health of the child.
- The key is for the child to live within his energy limits imposed by CFS by conserving energy and resting when needed. Activities should be prioritized avoiding any mental or physical activities which are particularly energy draining, for example, sport and excessive homework.
- Education provision should be flexible according to the child's stage of recovery. For example, schooling may be on a part-time basis targeting selected lessons, while in the case of some relapses and in severe cases, home-based tuition during the child's most productive part of the day will be needed. Consideration should be given to assessing the child's special educational needs. The overall aim is to resume normal schooling gradually where possible.
- Communication and cooperation between members of the primary care team, local child psychiatric services, child psychology workers, teachers and education authority representatives, parents and the sufferer is vital to ensure the best possible management.
- GPs should be aware of the need to detect family adaptation to the illness which can lead to secondary gain on the part of the child. This secondary gain should be actively discouraged.
- Referral to a specialist team should be made if there is severe and protracted disability, specific psychiatric disorders and family factors which have resulted in secondary gain. These latter cases should be admitted for rehabilitation.
- Parental stress in dealing with a chronically ill child needs to be recognized and appropriate counselling arranged.
- Occupational health aids such as wheelchairs, transport and Benefits Agency allowances should not be overlooked.

History checklist

General
- As with adults, a holistic approach should be adopted. Such a 'whole person' approach to clinical decision making is vital if we are to unravel the full potential of the consultation process.

- Exploration of family dynamics and psychosocial aspects requires particular care and sensitivity. It is important to explore the family's and child's health beliefs, especially as many families see the problem as a purely physical one.

Specific
- As with the adult approach. Specific enquiry should be made about schooling and the child's degree of attendance at school. This aspect needs thorough evaluation as school phobia can be a complication of CFS in children.
- Depression and anxiety are common symptoms which should be explored along with any other psychological stressors.

Examination checklist
- Physical and psychological assessment is mandatory. See also 'Hints for investigators and prescribers', p. 35.

Further reading
Franklin, A. (1995) *Children with ME. Guidelines for School Doctors and General Practitioners.* M.E. Association, Stanford le Hope.

Chapter 4
EAR, NOSE AND THROAT INFECTIONS

A.C. Swift

The upper respiratory tract is constantly exposed to potential airborne pathogens, which include bacteria, viruses and fungi. However, infection is prevented in most instances by the natural defence provided by the nasal mucosa, saliva and the commensal population of resident bacterial flora. Infection will ensue however if the natural defence is breached or impaired and if the bacterial inoculum is large or virulent.

Orientation
This chapter sets out to provide a basic but up to date outline of the most important details in common infections of the head and neck. The specific infections are presented by region.

For each condition in this chapter the management options have been arranged in the following sequence:

Option 1. Do nothing.
Option 2. Advise.
Option 3. Investigate.
Option 4. Prescribe antibiotics.
Option 5. Refer.
Option 6. Operate.

Clearly, options 5 and 6 do not apply to every condition and are therefore, not always included. In an attempt to make the major decisions that have to be made easy-to-identify, no attempt has been made to weigh different combinations of these options.

Chapter contents

1 Common cold

The common cold is a viral infection of the upper respiratory tract. Rhinoviruses account for 30% of common colds, but only 60% of people infected with the virus will be affected.

Typical symptoms include a blocked runny nose, sore throat and hoarse voice. There may also be an associated general illness. The severity and pattern of symptoms varies according to the particular infecting virus. Bacterial sinusitis may ensue, but the incidence of this is unknown.

Management options

Option 1. Do nothing.

✓ Most people will recover within 1–2 weeks.

✗ Bacterial superinfection may supersede the viral infection.

Option 2. Advise.

✓ Recovery will be encouraged by rest. Physical exertion should be avoided since this may impair the immune response.

✓ Continuing with a normal working lifestyle may disseminate the viral infection to other colleagues.

✗ Most people will recover without any specific problems.

Option 3. Investigate.

✗ There is no need to investigate unless bacterial superinfection or an unusual viral infection is suspected. A throat swab or viral titres may then be appropriate.

Option 4. Prescribe antibiotics.

✓ The only justification for antibiotic treatment is where bacterial superinfection is thought to have occurred with subsequent sinusitis, pharyngotonsillitis, persistent laryngitis or a chest infection.

✗ Prescribing antibiotics in the absence of bacterial infection will lead to overtreatment, encourage bacterial resistance and cause unnecessary side-effects or possible anaphylaxis in some patients.

History checklist
- How long have the symptoms been present?
- Prolonged cold-like symptoms may be caused by bacterial superinfection. This may result in either bronchitis, pharyngotonsillitis or sinusitis.

Examination checklist
The following are indicative of bacterial superinfection or suggest an alternative diagnosis such as infectious mononucleosis or cytomegalovirus (CMV) infection:
- Purulent secretions in the nasal cavities and inflammation of the pharynx and tonsils.
- Associated cervical lymphadenopathy.

Rituals and myths
Antibiotics should not be prescribed unless there is good evidence for bacterial superinfection.

Pitfalls
- Other underlying upper respiratory tract pathology may be assumed to be due to the cold and delay the recognition of the correct diagnosis. Examples include an early laryngeal tumour, nasal polyps or low grade chronic sinusitis.

Referrals
Only necessary if secondary purulent sinusitis or laryngitis fails to resolve.

Hints for investigators and prescribers
- Anti-inflammatory agents or paracetamol will give symptomatic relief.

Further reading
Lindberg, S. (1994) Morphology and functional studies of the mucociliary system during infections in the upper airways. *Acta Oto-Laryngol.* (suppl. 515): 22–25.

Naclerio, R.M., Proud, D., Lichenstein, L.M., Kagey-Sobotka, A., Hendley, J.O., Sorrentino, J. and Gwaltney, J.M. (1987) Kinins are generated during experimental rhinovirus colds. *J. Infect. Dis.* **157**: 133–140.

2 Laryngitis

Laryngitis can be acute, recurrent or chronic. Acute laryngitis is most commonly caused by a respiratory tract viral infection associated with a common cold. Laryngitis can also occur after exposure to irritants or vocal abuse. However, the latter is more commonly associated with recurrent or chronic laryngitis, which is not normally infective in origin, unless there is an unusual chronic infection such as tuberculosis (TB).

Most patients will present with hoarseness or voice loss. The voice quality may be deeper, have a variable strength and pitch, and tire easily with use. In some patients, the voice may be reduced to a whisper. Soreness and pain on swallowing often accompany acute laryngitis.

Management options

Option 1. Do nothing.

✓ Acute laryngitis will resolve spontaneously in most patients within a couple of weeks.

✗ Effect of delayed treatment: an acute laryngeal disorder may become chronic or leave residual problems, such as functional dysphonia.

✗ Chronic laryngitis may result in some patients.

✗ The diagnosis of a laryngeal tumour may be delayed or missed.

Option 2. Advise.

✓ Vocal rest and avoiding irritants such as cigarette smoke will speed recovery and prevent chronic laryngitis from developing.

✗ Most patients will recover spontaneously.

Option 3. Investigate.

✓ Laryngoscope with a flexible endoscope under local anaesthesia will exclude other laryngeal pathology or nasal/sinus disease early in the course of the illness.

✓ X-rays of the chest or sinuses may identify a compounding source of infection.

✗ Laryngitis will resolve quickly in most patients and investigation would have been unnecessary.

✗ X-rays expose patients to irradiation and have cost implications. They are therefore best reserved for patients in whom laryngitis does not resolve.

Option 4. Prescribe antibiotics.

✓ Antibiotics are indicated if there is bacterial superinfection. This is likely if there is a history of purulent sputum production or increasing pain and soreness.

✓ Antibiotics are indicated if there is a coexisting sinusitis or chest infection.

✗ Most cases are viral and prescribing antibiotics would lead to overtreatment.
Patients would be exposed to unnecessary side-effects and possible anaphylaxis.
Effects of treating without investigation: there is a risk of delaying the diagnosis of a laryngeal tumour.

Option 5. Refer.

✓ Microlaryngoscopy and biopsy is indicated if a specific laryngeal lesion is seen on outpatient laryngoscopy.

✗ Laryngeal inflammation will be exacerbated by intubation and surgical manipulation or biopsy if the larynx is acutely inflamed. This may precipitate stridor and airway distress.

History checklist

- Is there a history of a respiratory tract infection, or an episode of vocal abuse or irritant exposure?
- Is there a history of smoking or alcohol excess? What is the duration of hoarseness? If the hoarseness does not show signs of resolution after 3 weeks, then consider urgent referral for laryngoscopy so that a tumour or other chronic inflammatory disorder can be excluded.

Examination checklist

- Assess the degree of hoarseness and the voice strength and quality.
- Examine the vocal cords either with a mirror or preferably with a flexible laryngoscope.
- Check the nose and throat for evidence of infection.
- Exclude cervical lymphadenopathy in case there is an underlying laryngeal malignancy.
- If there is suggestion of a chest infection, listen to the chest.

Rituals and myths

- Patients often request antibiotic treatment, but this is not necessary in most cases.

Pitfalls

- Keep a high index of suspicion regarding the possibility of other laryngeal pathology.
- Although the main concern is to exclude a malignant laryngeal tumour, other chronic inflammatory disorders can also affect the larynx, and may mimic malignancy. These non-malignant conditions include TB, syphilis, non-infective granulomatous diseases such as Wegener's granulomatosis, sarcoidosis and fungal infection.
- Do not overlook a coexisting chest infection or purulent sinusitis.

Referrals

- Referral is usually not necessary unless there is a failure to improve after about 3 weeks. If resolution does not occur, the patient should be referred for a specialist opinion to exclude a laryngeal malignancy or chronic inflammatory disorder.
- If the patient has stridor then refer immediately since another pathology is likely.

Hints for investigators and prescribers

Sputum should be cultured if there is a productive cough and bacterial infection is thought likely.

Further reading

Van den Broek, P. (1998) Acute and chronic laryngitis. In: *Scott-Brown's Otolaryngology, 1998, Laryngology and Head and Neck Surgery*, 6th Edn (ed. J. Hibbert). Butterworths, London, pp. 99–118.

3 Croup

Laryngotracheobronchitis, or croup, is a viral infection which affects young children, particularly between the ages of 6 months and 3 years. The infection occurs in epidemics and the incidence peaks in the autumn and winter months. Most children recover within a few days. The key features of croup in a child are barking cough, hoarseness, stridor, pyrexia and restlessness. The onset tends to be less acute, developing over a couple of days, and less severe, when compared to acute epiglottitis.

Management options

Option 1. Do nothing.

✓ Providing the child does not have airway distress, recovery should be uneventful.

✗ The parents will not thank you.
✗ Failure to recognize airway obstruction or progression of airway distress could lead to disaster.

Option 2. Advise.

✓ If the child is managed at home, keeping the bedroom warm and humid with steam will help clearance of mucus secretions.
✓ If there is concern regarding the airway, the child should be taken immediately to hospital. This is particularly appropriate for very young children.
✓ The child should be kept well hydrated.

Option 3. Investigate.

✓ Oxygen saturation can be monitored non-invasively by oximetry. Subglottic narrowing may be demonstrated by plain X-ray.

✗ Effects of delayed treatment: this could have serious consequences if the airway becomes compromised. Investigations before treatment could waste precious time.
✗ The diagnosis is clinical and inappropriate investigation will increase the child's distress.
✗ Blood cultures are usually sterile.

Option 4. Prescribe antibiotics.

✓ Not indicated unless there is bacterial superinfection.

✗ Effects of treating before investigating: the diagnosis is based on the clinical features and it would be advantageous to treat before investigating.
✗ Antibiotics are generally not required because the disease is viral.
✗ Recovery will occur without steroids.

Option 5. Operate.

✓ Tracheotomy will relieve severe airway obstruction.

✗ Tracheotomy is invasive and has associated complications and morbidity.
✗ Endotracheal intubation has generally superseded tracheotomy.

Examination checklist
- Is the child pyrexial? Is the child restless? Is there concomitant toxaemia?

- Is the child stridulous? There may be biphasic stridor due to mucosal oedema in the sub-glottis.

Pitfalls
- Infections are not always viral. Bacterial superinfection can occur.
- Do not confuse with acute epiglottitis.
- Do not underestimate airway obstruction: if in doubt refer immediately to hospital.

Referrals
- Children should be referred immediately to hospital if there is the slightest doubt about the safety of the airway. This is particularly important in very young children.

Hints for investigators and prescribers
- The white cell count is usually normal.
- A throat swab is unhelpful.
- Steroids used to be controversial but are now accepted as being beneficial at relieving moderate to severe airway obstruction (Schroeder and Knapp, 1995). A single dose of dexamethasone sodium phosphate (0.6 mg kg^{-1}) has been shown to be effective.

Further reading
Cressman, W.R.Y and Myer, C.M. (1994) Diagnosis and management of croup and epiglottitis. *Respir. Med.* **41**: 265–276.

Schroeder, L.L. and Knapp, J.F. (1995) Recognition and emergency management of infectious causes of upper airway obstruction in children. *Semin. Respir. Infect.* **10**: 21–30.

4 Epiglottitis

This is an acute infective condition of the supraglottis, which primarily affects the epiglottis but may include the lingual tonsil, aryepiglottic folds and false cords.

It usually affects young children but can occur at any age. The incidence of epiglottitis has fallen dramatically since the introduction of Hib vaccination programmes for meningitis.

Epiglottitis is an acute illness with the following key features: altered voice, pain on swallowing, distressed child, stridor and pyrexia. In young children the illness develops and progresses rapidly, causing respiratory distress, drooling, and toxicity and pyrexia. The onset is less acute in adults, but features include painful swallowing, pyrexia, cervical lymphadenopathy and oedema of the soft palate and palatine arches.

Management options

Option 1. Advise.

✓ Urgent transfer and admission to hospital where the airway can be safely managed; 100% humidified oxygen will give considerable relief.

Option 2. Investigate.

✓ Oximetry will be of value in assessment and monitoring progress.
✓ Blood cultures are often positive.
✓ A lateral X-ray of the neck may show a swollen epiglottis.

✗ In young children, X-rays are unnecessary and can lose vital time in which the airway obstruction may progress.

Option 3. Prescribe antibiotics.

✓ Since the condition results from a bacterial infection (most commonly Haemophilus influenzae) antibiotics are required and should be given intravenously.
✓ Often infection will progress and prove fatal if unabated.

Option 4. Operate.

✓ Tracheotomy will relieve airway obstruction but most children are now managed by intubation.

✗ In children with potentially dangerous airway obstruction, the airway is maintained and controlled over the acute period by intubation. The latter is now considered the ideal method of management rather than tracheotomy.
✗ A more conservative approach is justifiable in adults since they will often respond to medication before the airway is impaired sufficiently to require intubation.

History checklist
• Fluid intake and swallowing?

Examination checklist
• Assess the upper airway and look for airway obstruction. Children will often sit upright to try to ease their breathing difficulty. However, do not distress children by trying to examine the throat since this may induce severe airway obstruction.
• Is the child dehydrated?
• Fibreoptic laryngoscopy is useful in adults and older children but should be avoided in young children.

Rituals and myths
- It is a myth that a calm pale child is improving. The opposite is true, and a calm pale child is indicative of imminent disaster.

Pitfalls
- Do not underestimate upper airway obstruction, particularly in children. Cyanosis in the latter is a late and inconsistent sign.
- Effects of delayed treatment: very dangerous in children and may result in death.

Referrals
- Urgent hospital admission is essential.

Hints for investigators and prescribers.
- Trying to swab the throat in children may induce airway obstruction but may be suitable to collect in adults.
- Blood gases in airway obstruction. Blood cultures are often positive.
- Third generation cephalosporins have become the drugs of choice.
- There is no evidence that steroids are beneficial.

Further reading
Cressman, W.R.Y. and Myer, C.M. (1994) Diagnosis and management of croup and epiglottitis. *Respir. Med.* **41**: 265–276.

Torkkeli, T., Ruoppi, P., Nutinen, J. and Kari, A. (1994) Changed clinical course and current treatment of acute epiglottitis in adults: a 12 year experience. *Laryngoscope* **104**: 1503–1506.

5 Sore throat

Acute sore throats are one of the commonest medical complaints. A diagnosis of tonsillitis, pharyngitis or tonsillopharyngitis is made according to where the site of inflammation/infection is most intense.

Most sore throats are caused by viral infections but bacteria are responsible for a lesser number or cause superinfection after a viral infection.

Group A β-haemolytic streptococcal infection is the most common bacterial cause of acute tonsillitis/pharyngitis, but it has been estimated that fewer than 10% of adults and 30% of children with sore throats actually have a streptococcal infection. Thus the condition is over-diagnosed and antibiotics are prescribed more than actually necessary (Pichichero, 1995).

Less common causes of throat infections include Neisseria gonorrhoeae, Mycoplasma pneumoniae, Chlamydia pneumoniae, Archanobacterium haemolyticum and infection from non-group A streptococci C and G.

Acute pharyngotonsillitis due to group A β-haemolytic streptococci occurs primarily in children between the ages of 5 and 15 years and is most common during the late winter and spring. A carrier rate of 22% has been reported by the age of 5 years (Denny, 1994).

Acute tonsillitis is characterized by severe acute sore throat, swollen inflamed tonsils which may be covered by patchy exudate, tender large jugulodigastric lymph nodes and pyrexia.

Management options

Option 1. Do nothing.

✓ Many acute sore throats are viral and will resolve spontaneously within a few days.

✗ Bacterial infections may persist.

✗ There is a small risk of complications.

Option 2. Advise.

✓ Reassurance may be the ideal management policy. Two or three sore throats per year are quite normal. Recurrent infrequent tonsillitis may well resolve or be accepted without further active treatment.

✗ To give no advice is likely to increase demands on health care.

Option 3. Investigate.

✓ Blood tests may confirm a diagnosis of infectious mononucleosis.

✓ A throat swab may identify an acute streptococcal sore throat but results will not be immediately available. Antistreptolysin antigen may be detected when the infection is caused by Lancefield group A β-haemolytic streptococci.

✗ The results from a throat swab do not correlate well with pathogens within the tonsils.

✗ Most patients will recover completely without the need for investigation.

Option 4. Prescribe antibiotics.

✓ If the tonsils are obviously infected with a mucopurulent exudate then antibiotics should be prescribed.

✗ If there is a pharyngitis, but the tonsils are not obviously infected then the infection is likely to be viral and antibiotics are not required. A recent controlled study into the effect of antibiotics for 'sore throats' in general practice has shown that complications are rare even when antibiotics are delayed or not used. It also showed that prescribing antibiotics increases the likelihood of the patient re-attending with a similar problem in the future (Little *et al.*, 1997).

✗ Prescribing antibiotics for all patients presenting with sore throats will lead to increased bacterial resistance and expose patients unnecessarily to the risk of side-effects and anaphylaxis.

Option 5. Refer.

Advise tonsillectomy, combined in some cases with adenoidectomy. If there is an associated sinusitis, antral washout should also be considered.

✓ Tonsillectomy is indicated if there is a history of four to five severe episodes of tonsillitis for 1 year. Each patient should be assessed individually according to the severity and frequency of their throat problems.

✓ Tonsillectomy may also be recommended because of tonsillar size and airway obstruction. This is more likely to occur in children.

✓ Tonsillectomy should also be recommended in patients with rheumatic heart disease and where tonsillitis has been complicated by glomerulonephritis.

✗ Caution should be observed in advising tonsillectomy/adenoidectomy in very young children (<3 years old) in case surgery is complicated by haemorrhage.

✗ Advising tonsillectomy for infrequent tonsillitis will lead to unnecessary surgery in many patients. Spontaneous resolution may occur with age.

History checklist
- Details of the severity and frequency of attacks should be obtained.
- Is there any suggestion of chronic airway obstruction? This is more likely to occur in children, and will present with a history of loud snoring with possible apnoeic episodes. Large adenoids should be considered. Airway obstruction may become apparent only during episodes of acute tonsillitis.
- Is there a history of rhinosinusitis? Rhinitis and sinusitis are likely to predispose to recurrent throat infection and must be considered when assessing the patient.
- Is there a history of failure to thrive or difficulty eating during acute episodes?

Examination checklist
- The classic triad of features are a pyrexia, tonsillar exudate and tender cervical lymphadenopathy.
- What do the tonsils look like? During an episode of infection the tonsils may be smooth, inflamed and swollen or they may be covered by exudate and have pus exuding from the crypts. Between attacks the tonsils usually appear normal.
- Are the tonsils enlarged? Large tonsils may cause substantial airway obstruction in young children. They may sometimes meet in the midline, particularly during acute tonsillitis.
- Are the adenoids large? Chronic airway obstruction due to large adenoids often accompanies tonsillar enlargement. The adenoids can be examined indirectly with a mirror or directly with an endoscope. The post nasal airway can also be assessed from a lateral plain X-ray.
- Are there other features which may suggest infectious mononucleosis? Characteristic features include marked cervical lymphadenopathy, malaise and pyrexia. Palatal petechiae, oral ulcers and hepatosplenomegaly may occur.

Rituals and myths
- It is a myth that most cases of bacterial sore throat can be reliably distinguished clinically from viral infection.

- The ritual combination of adenoidectomy with tonsillectomy in children is no longer valid, because there is an added risk of bleeding with adenoidectomy. The decision to remove the adenoids should be assessed on an individual basis.

Pitfalls
- A severe episode of tonsillitis associated with marked lymphadenopathy may be due to infectious mononucleosis.
- If infectious mononucleosis is a possibility, ampicillin, amoxycillin and amoxycillin/clavulanate should be avoided since they may induce the development of a rash, and this is now regarded medicolegally as indefensible.

Referrals
- Specialist referral is only indicated for frequent recurrent tonsillitis, which is likely to require treatment by tonsillectomy.
- Severe tonsillitis, which is not responding to oral antibiotics, may need hospital admission for intravenous therapy.

Hints for investigators and prescribers
The antibiotic of choice for acute tonsillitis due to β-haemolytic streptococci is penicillin (erythromycin in patients with penicillin allergy). However, after several courses of penicillin, the bacterial flora of the tonsil changes and resistant organisms emerge. In patients undergoing elective tonsillectomy, β-lactamase producing bacteria were recovered in 82% of tonsil cultures, and anaerobes were isolated in 98% of cases (Mitchelmore *et al.*, 1994). Therefore, in patients with recurrent infections and a history of multiple courses of antibiotics, a better choice would be a β-lactamase-resistant antibiotic such as amoxycillin/clavulanate. (If patients are penicillin allergic, alternative antibiotics that would be effective include clindamycin or cefuroxime.)

Further reading
Denny, F.W. Jr. (1994) Tonsillopharyngitis. *Pediatr. Rev.* **15**: 185–191.

Little, P., Gold, C., Williamson, I., Warner, G., Gantlet, M. and Kinmonth, A.L. (1997) Re-attendance and complications in a randomized trial of prescribing strategies for sore throat: the medicalising effect of prescribing antibiotics. *Br. Med. J.* **315**: 350–352.

Mitchelmore, I.J., Reilly, P.G., Hay, A.J. and Tabaqchali, S. (1994) Tonsil surface and core cultures in recurrent tonsillitis: prevalence of anaerobes and beta-lactamase producing organisms. *Eur. J. Clin. Microbiol. Infect. Dis.* **13**: 542–548.

Pichichero, M.E.. (1995) Group A Streptococcal tonsillopharyngitis: cost-effective diagnosis and treatment. *Ann. Emergency Med.* **25**: 390–403.

6 Quinsy

Quinsy is a peritonsillar abscess. It is usually unilateral and affects young adults either *de novo* or as a complication of acute tonsillitis. Before the formation of an abscess there is peritonsillar cellulitis. It has been proposed that the infection arises in mucous salivary tissue in the supratonsillar space.

Common features of quinsy are severe unilateral sore throat, rapid onset, pyrexia, ipsilateral cervical lymphadenopathy, trismus and salivation.

Management options

Option 1. Do nothing.

✓ The patient will eventually develop an abscess cavity, which will discharge and then resolve.

✗ The duration of illness will be prolonged.

✗ Morbidity will be worse and complications may ensue.

Option 2. Advise.

✗ Serious complications may develop if a quinsy is left untreated.

Option 3. Investigate.

✓ Culture of the pus will often reveal pathogenic bacteria and antibiotic sensitivities can be assessed.

✗ Culturing pus from the abscess cavity sometimes fails to grow any pathogens.

✗ Culturing pus does not affect the outcome.

Option 4. Prescribe antibiotics.

✓ High doses of a broad-spectrum antibiotic are necessary. Failure to do this may lead to progression of the infection and the subsequent development of complications such as a parapharyngeal abscess, airway obstruction or the consequences of severe septicaemia.

✗ Resolution will eventually occur without antibiotics once an abscess forms, points and discharges, but recovery will be delayed and complications may ensue.

Option 5. Refer.

✓ It is not always easy to differentiate between cellulitis and abscess formation. However, if an abscess cavity has formed then drainage is preferable. Once pus is released, the patient will experience immediate relief.

✗ If an abscess is not drained it will eventually point superior to the tonsil and drain spontaneously. However, this could take several days and trismus will persist during this time.

Option 6. Operate.

Drain abscess cavity

✓ The abscess cavity can be drained after topical anaesthesia by either an intraoral incision with a guarded scalpel blade or needle aspiration. The site of incision is above the affected tonsil at the level of the soft palate.

✓ Needle aspiration is a good alternative to incision and has been shown to be effective in 94–96% of patients (Herzon, 1995).

Tonsillectomy à chaud

✓ Tonsillectomy is sometimes performed at the time of the acute illness. The justification for this is that the patient has just one period of illness, recovery is not prolonged and the risk of recurrence is removed. Care must be taken at the time of anaesthesia since the airway may be difficult and the abscess could rupture at an inappropriate time. It is probably sensible to remove the tonsil from the non-affected side at the same time, particularly if there is a history of recurrent tonsillitis.

✗ If tonsillectomy à chaud is applied routinely, many patients will undergo it unnecessarily. Patients should therefore be carefully selected according to their previous history.

Elective tonsillectomy (6–8 weeks after the acute illness)

✓ Tonsillectomy should prevent recurrent quinsy.

✗ With the advent of effective antibiotics, the development of serious complications can be prevented without recourse to surgery.

History checklist
- Sore throat and tonsillitis are very common in general practice. Symptoms that should alert one to the possibility of quinsy are:
  (i) rapid onset of general malaise;
  (ii) severe sore throat which is usually worse on one side;
  (iii) increased salivation and difficulty swallowing.
- Is there a history of recurrent tonsillitis? This will help determine the subsequent management. In particular, have antibiotics been prescribed regularly for recurrent tonsillitis? These could have induced bacterial resistance.
- Have antibiotics been taken over the preceding few days? Oral antibiotics may not achieve effective blood levels for adequate tissue penetration if an abscess has formed.

Examination checklist
- Tender enlarged unilateral jugulodigastric lymph nodes.
- Trismus.
- Medially displaced tonsil.
- Soft palate swelling.
- Altered phonation.
- Speech may sound as if there is a 'ball in the throat'.
- Airway impairment.
- Stridor will occur if there is coexisting laryngeal oedema.
- Look for signs of septicaemia.

Rituals and myths
- Routine culturing of pus from the abscess does not affect the outcome (Herzon, 1995).
- It is a myth that tonsillectomy is always necessary. Only 13% of patients develop a further quinsy and indiscriminate tonsillectomy results in many patients undergoing the procedure unnecessarily.
- If tonsillectomy is undertaken, both tonsils should be removed: neither morbidity, nor recovery will be affected by this.

Pitfalls
- Quinsy may be considered similar to severe tonsillitis and is not a serious illness. However, a quinsy is a specific disorder and carries a risk of serious complications. Such complications are now unusual with the advent of antibiotic therapy, but a high index of suspicion must nevertheless be maintained.

Referrals
- Refer all patients urgently, particularly if there are signs of airway impairment.

Hints for investigators and prescribers
- Routine cultures are of dubious value, but may be useful if the patient fails to respond.
- The standard treatment is a course of high dose penicillin. Metronidazole is often combined with this but the latter does not increase the speed of resolution (MacDougall and Denholm, 1995). Amoxycillin/clavulanate is also effective. Various broad-spectrum antibiotics have been used but there is no data available that compares the efficacy of different regimes.

Further reading

Herzon, F. (1995) Peritonsillar abscess: incidence, current management practices an a proposal for treatment guidelines. *Laryngoscope* **105** (suppl. 74): 1–17.

McDougall, G. and Denholm, S.W. (1995) Audit of the treatment of tonsillar and peritonsillar sepsis in an ear, nose and throat unit. *J. Laryngol. Otol.* **109**: 531–533.

Passy, V. (1994) Pathogenesis of peritonsillar abscess. *Laryngoscope* **104**: 185–190.

Savolainen, S., Jousiies-Somer, H.R, Makitie, A.A. and Ylikoski, J.S. (1993) Peritonsillar abscess. Clinical and microbiological aspects and treatment regimens. *Arch. Otolaryngol. Head Neck Surg.* **119**: 521–524.

7 Acute sinusitis

Acute sinusitis most commonly follows an upper respiratory tract viral infection and may become clinically significant if bacterial superinfection occurs. The most common bacteria are Streptococcus pneumoniae and H. influenzae. Dental infection is a less common cause and anaerobes are then likely to be involved.

Adults are primarily affected and the maxillary sinus is most commonly involved. Symptoms include facial pain and a purulent nasal discharge, and although most cases resolve within a couple of weeks, occasionally the infection may be fulminant and complications such as orbital or intracranial infection may ensue.

Management options

Option 1. Do nothing.

✓ Resolution will occur spontaneously in most patients and there is recent evidence that antibiotics do not speed recovery (Philpot, 1997).

✗ Morbidity may be increased and complications may ensue.

Option 2. Advise.

✓ Reassurance that recovery will occur without antibiotics will avoid such treatment in many patients.

✗ The outcome is unlikely to be affected in most cases.

Option 3. Investigate.

✓ Endoscopy will confirm the diagnosis and confirm the presence of a purulent infection.
✓ A plain sinus X-ray will confirm evidence of sinusitis.

✗ Most patients will recover without the need for investigation.
✗ A plain sinus X-ray will expose the patient to irradiation. Endoscopy will usually confirm the pathology and may avert the need for radiology.
✗ A culture of pus from the nasal cavity may not truly reflect the pathogens within the maxillary sinus.

Option 4. Prescribe antibiotics.

✓ Antibiotics are generally prescribed in patients seeking medical advice for acute sinusitis. Although short courses have been shown to be effective, it is generally recommended that antibiotics are prescribed for 10–14 days to adequately treat the infection (Haye et al., 1996; Kennedy, 1995). They should also be of suitable activity to cover the likely pathogens, particularly since treatment will normally be empirical. It is important to remember that β-lactamase-resistant bacteria are becoming more common, particularly in the USA (Kennedy, 1995).

✗ Frequent use of antibiotics in the community will increase the resistant rate of many commonly found bacteria. There is also a small risk of anaphylaxis and other side-effects.

Option 5. Operate.

✓ A simple antral lavage will give rapid relief in patients with a severe maxillary sinus. Drainage can be maintained by an irrigating tube or an inferior meatal antrostomy.
✓ It is sometimes necessary to drain pus from the frontal sinus by trephination.

✗ Most patients will recover without the need for surgical drainage.

✗ Any surgical procedure in the presence of acute infection will be associated with a risk of bleeding.

✗ More extensive surgical procedures, such as external frontoethmoidectomy, are usually not necessary.

History checklist

- Is there a history of recurrent acute sinusitis? If infections keep recurring frequently, this may be due to narrow sinus ostia and obstruction within the ostiomeatal complex.
- Is there associated facial pain or headache? Pain over the cheek, nasal bridge or forehead is likely with acute infection.
- Is there a history of dental pain?

Examination checklist

- Check for facial swelling and localized tenderness.
- Check that the eye is not swollen, since periorbital cellulitis is a complication of sinusitis.
- Look for a dental abscess if there is not a clear history of a recent head cold.
- Is the nasal septum deviated? A septal spur impacted in the middle meatus may well predispose to recurrent purulent sinusitis.

Rituals and myths

- Antibiotics are not always required and spontaneous resolution is reported to occur in 30–40% of patients (Haye *et al.*, 1996).

Pitfalls

- Other causes of facial pain may lead to diagnostic confusion.
- Do not overlook pre-existing but undiagnosed nasal pathology such as nasal polyposis or a low grade chronic sinusitis.
- Failure to respond to initial antibiotic therapy is likely to be due to bacterial resistance. The bacterial flora changes after the acute infective stage and becomes polymicrobial with emergence of resistant aerobic and anaerobic bacteria (Brook *et al.*, 1996). β-lactamase resistant antibiotics should be prescribed.
- Effects of delayed treatment: may prolong morbidity.
- Effects of treating before investigation: unlikely to affect outcome.

Referrals

- Only necessary when the infection is fulminant, fails to resolve or recurs frequently.

Hints for investigators and prescribers

- Nasal swabs do not accurately reflect the bacteria within the sinuses and are probably not worthwhile. A nasal swab may be helpful if it can be taken directly from the middle meatus lateral to the middle turbinate under endoscopic control. However, this will only be possible in a specialized clinic.
- If patients undergo antral lavage, the aspirate should be sent for culture. Ideally, a β-lactamase resistant antibiotic such as amoxycillin/clavulanate should be prescribed. However, amoxycillin and ampicillin are commonly used. For patients who are penicillin-allergic, clarithromycin is recommended.
- The duration of treatment should ideally be 10–14 days. Shorter courses are often prescribed, although these could lead to inadequate treatment of the infection.
- Topical decongestant medication (0.05% ephedrine or oxymetazoline) may help relieve mucosal congestion if used during the acute episode for a few days, but rebound congestion is likely to occur if used for longer than a week.
- Topical steroids will counteract the effect of local inflammation and should reduce

mucosal swelling. Steroid drops are likely to be more effective than sprays in the ethmoidal region. However, there is no proof that topical steroids are effective in acute sinusitis.

Further reading

Brook, I., Frazier, E.H. and Foote, P.A. (1996) Microbiology of the transition from acute to chronic maxillary sinusitis. *Clin. Microbiol.* **45**: 372–375.

Daley, C.L. and Sand, M. (1988) The runny nose: infection of the paranasal sinuses. *Inf. Dis. Clin. N. Am.* **2**: 131–136.

Haye, R., Lingaas, E., Hoivik, H.O. and Odegard, T. (1996) Efficacy and safety of azithromycin versus phenoxymethylpenicillin in the treatment of acute maxillary sinusitis. *Eur. J. Clin. Microbiol. Infect. Dis.* **15**: 849–853.

Kennedy, D.W., Gwaltney, J.M. and Jones, J.G. (1995) Medical management of sinusitis: educational goals and management guidelines. *Ann. Otol. Rhinol. Laryngol.* **167** (suppl.): 22–30.

Philpot, C.R. (1997) Antibiotic treatment in acute bacterial sinusitis. *Lancet* **349**: 1476–1477.

Wald, E.R., Milmoe, G.J., Bowen, A.D., Ledesma-Medina, J., Salamon, N. and Bluestone, C.D. (1981). Acute maxillary sinusitis in children. *N. Engl. J. Med.* **304**: 749–754.

8 Chronic sinusitis

Chronic sinusitis normally presents with various combinations of symptoms which include nasal obstruction, or a sensation of nasal congestion, nasal mucus, facial discomfort, frontal headaches and impairment of smell. However, symptoms can often be mild or non-specific, leading to chronic sinusitis not being recognized as the true cause of the patients problems.

There may be co-existing nasal allergy which is suggested by excessive sneezing, nasal and ocular itching and watery rhinorrhoea. However, it has been suggested that allergy is not of major importance in the pathogenesis of chronic sinusitis (Kennedy *et al.*, 1995).

Management options

Option 1. Do nothing.

✓ Many patients will tolerate their symptoms for many years.

✗ Symptoms are likely to persist and there may be associated acute exacerbations.

✗ Orbital or intracranial complications will occasionally occur.

Option 2. Advise.

✓ Patients should be advised that they have a chronic condition of the nasal mucosa and that significant improvement is possible with therapy, but recurrent problems may occur.

✗ If the above advice is not explained, the patient may be over-optimistic about what can be realistically achieved.

Option 3. Investigate.

✓ Nasal endoscopy is essential for a complete assessment of the nose.

✓ The extent of disease is best shown by a CT scan. This also gives anatomical detail. However, a scan should be restricted to those patients who do not respond sufficiently to medical treatment and in whom surgery is contemplated.

✗ Nasal culture is unlikely to be truly representative of the pathogens.

✗ Plain sinus X-rays grossly underestimate sinus disease and can generally be avoided. Endoscopy usually provides sufficient information for diagnostic purposes.

Option 4. Prescribe antibiotics.

✓ Antibiotics will often give considerable symptomatic relief. Prolonged and repeated courses are usually necessary. It has recently been suggested that the ideal duration of treatment should be 3–6 weeks. Treating first, before investigation, may give temporary relief. However, without correct assessment the condition will not be fully appreciated and treatment is likely to be inadequate.

✗ Treatment with other forms of medication without antibiotics are likely to be ineffective.

✗ Prolonged courses of broad-spectrum antibiotics are more likely to cause side-effects such as gastrointestinal upset and candidosis in addition to the risk of anaphylaxis and inducing bacterial resistance.

Option 5. Operate.

✓ With careful patient assessment, sinus surgery is very effective and symptoms are usually relieved.

✓ If there is a significant deviation of the nasal septum this should be corrected both for surgical access and symptomatic relief.

✗ Maxillary sinus washout is unlikely to give long-term relief in chronic sinusitis.

✗ Sinus surgery is associated with risks and complications. These include bleeding, skull base penetration and orbital complications. Fortunately, these problems are uncommon.

✗ Although functional endoscopic sinus surgery is effective in obtaining relief and control in most cases, it is time-consuming and expensive.

Surgery should be offered to patients who still have significant symptoms following prolonged medication. Ideally, they should have persevered with medical treatment for at least 3 months.

There have been significant advances in sinus surgery over recent years with the development of functional endoscopic sinus surgery. This technique facilitates very precise surgery in the ethmoid sinus so that natural drainage pathways to the large paranasal sinuses can be opened, ethmoid cells can be drained and ventilated and polyps and disease tissue removed as required without stripping the entire lining of the sinus.

The latter technique has resulted in a great reduction in the indications for external sinus surgery such as external ethmoidectomy and the Caldwell-Luc operation on the maxillary sinus.

History checklist
- Enquiry should be made about whether the nasal mucus is purulent. In addition, a history of recurrent acute sinusitis should be sought.
- A history of loss of smell should also be looked for.

Examination checklist
- Is there evidence of rhinitis with mucosal swelling and inflammation?
- Is the nasal septum deviated?
- Are nasal polyps present?
- What is the nature of any nasal discharge?
- Ideally, the nasal cavities should be examined after vasoconstriction and with an endoscope.
- Plain sinus X-rays have a limited role, but much more detail is provided by a CT scan set specifically for sinuses to show both the fine bony architecture and the soft tissues. A combination of both coronal and axial views is ideal.

Rituals and myths
- It is often assumed that patients with sinusitis need to undergo antral washout. Although this may be helpful diagnostically, it is unlikely to give more than temporary relief in chronic sinusitis, and the benefits are therefore limited.

Pitfalls
- Chronic sinusitis does not always cause facial discomfort or pain. There are many causes of headache and facial pain and these patients can be diagnostically challenging.
- Inflammatory sinus disease within the ethmoid sinus may not be visible on anterior rhinoscopy and may require careful endoscopy to see subtle signs such as localized mucosal oedema, polyp formation or mucus tracks. However, the true extent of the disease is sometimes only revealed by a CT scan.
- If sinusitis does not respond to antibiotics exclude a fungal infection.

Referrals
- All patients who do not respond to a prolonged course of medical treatment with topical steroids and antibiotics.

Hints for investigators and prescribers

- Nasal cultures are not generally necessary and may not truly reflect the pathogens within the sinuses.
- If a nasal swab is done, the specimen can be taken specifically from the middle meatus under endoscopic control. Bacterial isolates may be commensals and should be interpreted in the light of the overall clinical picture. Cultures may also be negative or not truly reflective of the bacteria within the actual sinuses.
- If a fungal infection is suspected, send whole crusts and concretions for culture. Tissue samples may also show fungal hyphae in invasive disease.
- If allergy is suspected, a total IgE and radioallergoadsorbent test to inhaled allergens may be helpful.
- Amoxycillin/clavulanate for at least 14 days is recommended. For patients who are allergic to penicillin, clarithromycin may be used.
- Amoxycillin, ampicillin, erythromycin, tetracycline and second-generation cephalosporins may not give adequate cover (Kennedy *et al.*, 1995).

Steroids

Topical betamethasone nasal drops are an effective means of reducing inflammation in the middle meatus and ethmoid and are associated with a reduction in symptoms in practise although controlled trials are lacking. They should be inserted in a head down/forward position in order to reach the ethmoid sinus, and should be continued for 2–3 months.

- Steroid sprays are easier to use but do not appear to be as effective as drops and their cost is considerably more.
- Occasionally, a short course of systemic steroids is indicated if sinusitis is associated with severe polyposis.
- Overuse of steroids can lead to interference with natural steroid control by affecting the hypothalamic-adrenal axis. Patients should therefore be advised not to exceed the recommended dose of topical steroids.
- Long-term use of steroid nasal sprays occasionally induces a candida infection.

Antihistamines

- Topical or oral antihistamines are helpful if there is an associated allergic problem.
- Antihistamines can increase the viscosity of mucus and make it harder to clear.
- Oral antihistamines can induce drowsiness, but this is less likely with more recent preparations.

Decongestants

- Oral or topical decongestants can give effective relief of nasal obstruction if this is caused primarily by rhinitis.
- Topical decongestants will cause rebound congestion if used for longer than 1 week. Long-term use will induce rhinitis medicamentosa.

Further reading

Erkan, M., Aslan, T., Ozcan, M. and Koc, N. (1994) Bacteriology of antrum in adults with chronic maxillary sinusitis. *Laryngoscope* **104**: 321–324.

Hartog, B., Degener, J.E., van Benthem, P.P.G. and Hordijk, G.J. (1995) Microbiology of chronic maxillary sinusitis in adults: isolated aerobic and anaerobic bacteria and their susceptibility to twenty antibiotics. *Acta Otolaryngol.* (Stockh) **115**: 672–677.

Kennedy, D.W., Gwaltney, J.M. and Jones, J.G. (1995) Medical management of sinusitis: educational goals and management guidelines. *Ann. Otol. Rhinol. Laryngol.* **167** (suppl.): 22–30.

Swift, A.C. and Denning, D. (1998) Osteitis of the skull base following fungal sinusitis. *J. Laryngol. Otol.* **112**: 92–97.

9 Vestibulitis and furunculosis

Vestibulitis is a chronic infection of the skin of the nasal vestibule. Itching, crusting and excoriation of both nasal vestibules are the key symptoms. A nasal furuncle is an acute infection of a hair follicle within the anterior nares, usually caused by Staphylococcus aureus and characterized by an acutely painful 'spot' in the lateral wall of the nasal vestibule.

Management options

Option 1. Do nothing.

✓ Not appropriate. Vestibulitis is likely to persist.

✗ Infection from a furuncle could possibly spread intracranially.

Option 2. Advise.

✓ Avoidance of nose picking and external irritants may result in spontaneous resolution of vestibulitis.

✓ Patients with a furuncle should be cautioned against squeezing it and should seek urgent advice if any untoward symptoms develop.

Option 3. Investigate.

✓ In patients with a severe furuncle or a history of recurrent furuncles, blood dyscrasias and diabetes should be excluded.

✓ A swab from the nasal vestibule will often yield the particular pathogen. This is usually S. aureus.

✗ The infection usually responds to local treatment whether a swab is cultured or not.

Option 4. Prescribe antibiotics.

✓ Topical treatment is effective for both conditions. If the infection from a furuncle is severe or persistent, or if there is local cellulitis, a systemic antistaphylococcal antibiotic may be required.

History checklist
- Is there a history of local trauma from nose picking?
- Is there a history of nasal discharge, which would predispose to infection?
- Is there a history of eczema?
- If the patient presents with a furuncle, exclude a history of diabetes or immunosuppression.

Examination checklist
- Look for nasal crusts attached to vibrisae in nasal vestibules.
- Is the columellar edge of the nasal septum projecting into the nares and being subjected to local trauma?
- A furuncle will be intensely painful and tender and the surrounding soft tissue will be swollen.

Pitfalls
- A nasal furuncle is potentially dangerous since infection can spread intracranially via the ophthalmic veins and cause cavernous sinus thrombosis.

Hints for investigators and prescribers

- Apply chlorhexidine/neomycin cream four times daily for at least 10 days.
- An alternative preparation is mupirocin ointment, but this should be reserved for resistant cases or when methicillin-resistant S. aureus is cultured.

Further reading

O'Donnell, B.F. and Black, A.K. (1998) Conditions of the external nose. In: *Scott-Brown's Otolaryngology, 1998, Rhinology*, 6th Edn (eds I.S. Mackay and T.R. Bull). Butterworths, London, pp. 6–7.

10 Recurrent salivary gland infections

Salivary gland tissue is widespread throughout the oral cavity, but infection affects primarily the two major salivary glands, namely the submandibular and parotid glands. These are the only glands with a substantial duct, which can become blocked and lead to infection.

Submandibular gland

Submandibular sialadenitis is usually secondary to a calculus blocking the duct. The patient will complain of recurrent episodes of swelling and pain localized to the gland, which becomes worse with eating. A stone may be palpable within the duct in the floor of the mouth and is typically radio-opaque on plain X-ray.

The key feature of submandibular sialadenitis is an acutely swollen, unilateral submandibular gland which swells after eating. A calculus may be palpable in the floor of the mouth.

Parotid gland

Similar infections may occur within the parotid gland due to duct obstruction from either a calculus or a stricture. Calculi within the parotid duct are usually radiologically non-opaque. Some patients will have recurrent parotitis without duct obstruction due to sialectasia. Many of these patients will have an autoimmune disorder and display features of Sjogren's syndrome such as dry eyes, dry mouth, arthralgia and bilateral parotid swelling.

Rarely, a single episode of acute suppurative parotitis may occur. This usually affects elderly, debilitated, diabetic or immunosuppressed patients, and classically used to occur after abdominal surgery.

The clinical feature of recurrent parotitis is subacute parotid swelling which is often bilateral. It often starts in childhood and in adults may be associated with dry eyes or a dry mouth.

Management options

Option 1. Do nothing.

✓ Many patients with recurrent parotitis without duct obstruction will eventually improve spontaneously.

✗ Recurrent parotitis due to duct obstruction will usually need surgical intervention to clear the obstruction or remove the gland. However, resolution may occur in patients with mild symptoms.

✗ Recurrent submandibular sialadenitis is unlikely to resolve without operative intervention.

Option 2. Advise.

✓ Regular parotid massage is often effective in controlling recurrent parotitis.
✓ Drinking plenty and using sialogogues such as lemon juice helps to promote salivary flow and prevent recurrent parotitis.

Option 3. Investigate.

✓ Plain X-rays will usually demonstrate submandibular duct stones, but parotid duct calculi are generally radiolucent and contrast studies are required.
✓ Sialectasia will be demonstrated by a sialogram.
✓ If Sjogren's disease is suspected, a blood test for nuclear autoantibodies (SS-A, SS-B) is

often positive. Dry eyes can be demonstrated by Schirmer's test. A labial biopsy will often show a lymphocytic infiltrate.

✓ CT/MRI will demonstrate calculi and dilated duct systems.

✗ Not to investigate will leave doubt about the correct diagnosis.

Option 4. Prescribe antibiotics.

✓ Antibiotics will relieve severe or prolonged infections.

✗ Many patients with recurrent sialadenitis of the submandibular or parotid glands will improve without resorting to antibiotics.

Option 5. Operate.

Excision of the parotid or submandibular gland

✓ Excision of a submandibular or parotid gland, which is causing severe problems, will control the problem locally. Patients with salivary gland duct obstruction will benefit most from this approach.

✗ Patients with non-obstructive sialadenitis will often improve spontaneously without resorting to surgery.

✗ Patients with mild symptoms from duct obstruction will usually improve without surgery.

Calculus removal without gland excision

✓ If a single calculus can be palpated within the duct it may be possible to remove it by incising the duct, thus avoiding gland excision. Until recently, this was really only feasible for calculi in the submandibular duct in the floor of the mouth. However, with recent advances, it is now possible to remove calculi from within the parotid duct endoscopically by shattering the calculus with a Holmium laser. Calculi have also been reduced to small fragments and extruded by lithotripsy using external ultrasound. These techniques require specialized equipment, which is not freely available.

✗ Removing calculi by local incision in the duct may leave remnants behind which will cause recurrent infection.

✗ During the process of incision into the submandibular duct, there is a risk of damaging the lingual nerve.

Other forms of management of non-obstructive recurrent parotitis include radiotherapy, duct ligation and tympanic neurectomy. The effectiveness of these techniques is questionable. Recently, the successful use of intraduct lavage with tetracycline has been reported.

History checklist

- Is the gland painful? Pain related to meals and periods of abatement are more suggestive of sialadenitis secondary to duct obstruction. Persistent discomfort with less marked exacerbation's occurs with sialectasis and chronic infection from salivary stasis. Severe pain of rapid onset in an ill patient suggests acute suppurative parotitis.
- Is the swelling recurrent or persistent? Recurrent swelling of the submandibular gland is likely to be caused by a calculus blocking the submandibular duct. Recurrent painful swelling of the parotid gland occurs in recurrent parotitis, which may be due to obstructive or non-obstructive causes. Patients in the latter category will often have an autoimmune disorder and go on to develop Sjogren's syndrome, the symptoms of which include keratoconjunctivitis sicca, symmetrical arthralgia and xerostomia. Persistent swelling of the parotid gland occurs with tumours, chronic sialadenitis, or granulomatous conditions such as sarcoidosis and TB.

Examination checklist

- Is the affected salivary gland enlarged or tender?
- Are the other salivary glands enlarged? This may imply an autoimmune disease.
- Examine the mouth and palpate the duct intraorally. A calculus may be palpable in the parotid or submandibular duct.
- Check for cervical lymphadenopathy (this may occur with either acute infection or malignancy).
- The external ear canal should be examined when assessing the parotid gland. A malignant tumour may invade the external ear canal.
- Assess facial nerve function. Facial nerve paralysis occurs with either malignant tumours or sarcoidosis.

Rituals and myths

- In patients with recurrent parotitis due to duct obstruction, it is often considered necessary to excise the entire gland. However, superficial parotidectomy has been found effective and the extent of surgery should be guided by the extent of the disease.

Pitfalls

- Always be aware that an enlarged salivary gland may be due to a tumour.
- Patients with autoimmune parotitis have an increased risk of developing a lymphoma in the affected gland.

Referrals

- Seek specialist advice if the symptoms become severe, frequent or fail to resolve.

Hints for investigators and prescribers

- If there is a discharge from the duct orifice then a sample should be cultured.
- Antibiotics will usually be prescribed without knowledge of the infecting agent. A broad-spectrum antibiotic that covers oral anaerobes is ideal.
- Mycobacterial infections should be considered in refractory cases.

Further reading

O'Brien, C.J. and Murrant, N.J. (1993) Surgical management of chronic parotitis. *Head Neck* **15**: 445–449.

Watkin, G.T. and Hobsley, M. (1986) Natural history of patients with recurrent parotitis and punctate sialectasis. *Br. J. Surg.* **73**: 745–748.

11 Acute parotitis

Acute bacterial parotitis used to be a recognized complication of gastrointestinal surgery and probably arose due to dehydration and poor oral hygiene. However, it is now much less common and less severe. Other predisposing factors include general debility, old age, oral neoplasms, calculi, immunosuppression, and drugs which reduce salivary secretion.

The key features are an ill pyrexial patient with an acutely swollen tender parotid gland (usually unilateral). Pus may be expressible from the parotid duct.

Management options

Option 1. Do nothing.

✗ This would be totally inappropriate and negligent practice.
✗ Acute suppurative parotitis can be fatal, even when treated well.

Option 2. Advise.

✓ Inform relatives of the seriousness of the condition and emphasize the need for the patient to drink a lot and pay attention to good oral hygiene.

Option 3. Investigate.

✓ Identifying the pathogens by culture of pus sampled from the parotid duct orifice or via a percutaneous needle aspirate is helpful in deciding which antibiotic to use.
✓ Imaging by CT or preferably MRI will help delineate the extent of the infection and identify any underlying abscess formation, particularly in the deep lobe.
✓ A blood culture may be positive if the patient has a bacteraemia.

✗ Sialography is contraindicated in the acute stage of infection and may well compound the situation.

Option 4. Prescribe antibiotics.

✓ High dose i.v. antibiotics are essential. Without such treatment, complications will ensue and the patient may die.

✗ The arguments against antibiotics in this situation are far outweighed by the benefits.
✗ Effect of delayed treatment: an abscess cavity may form. Complications may develop.
✗ Effect of treating with antibiotics before investigating: pathogens may not be identified. However, this is unlikely to have any significant effect on the clinical outcome.

Option 5. Operate.

✓ Abscess cavities should be drained.

✗ The facial nerve may be damaged.

History checklist
- Acute suppurative parotitis may be uni- or bilateral.
- Is the patient immunosuppressed?

Examination checklist
- Is the patient pyrexial? Is the patient dehydrated?
- Examine the oral cavity and try and express pus from within the gland by external pressure.

- Look for evidence of a coexisting infection. Acute parotitis can occur with a peritonsillar abscess, tonsillitis or a dental abscess. Suppuration may occur in the contralateral gland.
- Is there evidence of a complication such as thrombophlebitis, osteomyelitis, facial nerve paralysis, pneumonia, mediastinitis or airway obstruction?

Pitfalls
- Always look for a cause. There may be a calculus or infection elsewhere.
- Remember that a parotid swelling could be a tumour, and skin discolouration associated with an aggressive malignant tumour could mimic the appearance of an abscess. Mycobacterial infection is a rare possibility.

Hints for investigators and prescribers
- Blood should be collected for a white cell and differential count.
- Blood for culture should be considered.
- If pus can be expressed via the duct, a sample should be sent for culture.
- If there is a superficial abscess, pus can be aspirated and sent for culture.
- Pus should be cultured for aerobes, anaerobes, fungi and mycobacteria.
- If a local cause for infection cannot be found, consider an immune deficiency disorder.
- Samples should ideally be obtained before commencing antibiotics.
- Intraoral pus can be collected either in a syringe or by a swab, which is then placed in transport medium. The sample should reach the laboratory quickly and a Gram stain and anaerobic culture requested. β-lactamase-resistant bacteria have been reported in 75% of patients (Brook, 1992).
- Erythromycin, ampicillin or a cephalosporin have been recommended (Lamey *et al.*, 1987). However, anaerobic cover and β-lactamase-resistance should be considered; suitable choices include amoxycillin/clavulanate or cefuroxime combined with metronidazole until sensitivities are available.

Further reading
Brook, I. (1992) Diagnosis and management of parotitis. *Arch. Otolaryngol. Head Neck Surg.* **118**: 469–471.

Lamey, P.J., Boil, M.A., Macfarlane, T.W.O. and Samaranayake, L.P. (1987) Acute suppurative parotitis in outpatients: microbiology and post treatment sialographic findings. *Oral Surg. Oral Med. Oral Path.* **63**: 37–41.

Pou, A.M., Johnson, J.T. and Weissman, J. (1995) Management decisions in parotitis. *Compr. Ther.* **21**: 85–92.

12 Otitis externa

This is an inflammatory or infective condition of the skin of the external ear canal. It may be acute or chronic and range from mild to severe. With mild infection, the only complaint will be aural itching. Moderate infection is painful and the ear discharges. If the infection progresses to severe, the ear canal becomes very swollen and narrow and pain can be intense. Hearing may be impaired.

Management options

Option 1. Do nothing.

✓ Why waste time on a trivial irritation? Mild infection or inflammation may resolve spontaneously.

✗ Infection is likely to establish chronicity.

Option 2. Advise.

✓ Patients should be advised to avoid scratching the ear if itchy and to keep the ear dry. In mild cases, this may relieve the problem. In more severe cases, it will help prevent recurrence.

✗ Not to give the above advice will lead to recurrent infection.

Option 3. Investigate.

✓ Culture of infected debris will often provide information about the pathogens and their antibiotic sensitivity.

✓ If the condition fails to respond to local treatment, the possibility of a yeast or fungal infection should be considered and a culture may confirm that this is the case.

✓ If malignant otitis externa is suspected, cultures should be obtained as soon as possible, looking specifically for Pseudomonas spp. Detailed imaging by high resolution CT or isotope scans should be considered, particularly if there is cranial nerve involvement.

✓ Diabetes should be excluded in patients with malignant otitis externa.

✗ One can expect a wide range of bacteria to be reported by the microbiology laboratory.

✗ Otitis externa responds to local cleaning and topical treatment in most cases without knowledge of the pathogens, and a culture is therefore not necessary.

Option 4. Prescribe antibiotics.

✓ Topical preparations containing antibiotics are usually effective. Many of these preparations contain steroids, which help reduce local inflammation and swelling.

✓ Systemic antibiotics are indicated if the infection is severe or if it has spread to affect the pinna and surrounding skin.

✓ Systemic anti-pseudomonal antibiotics should be prescribed in high doses if malignant otitis externa is suspected.

✗ If topical antibiotic drops are used without first cleaning the ear, they are less likely to work and bacterial resistance or selection is likely. Pseudomonas often predominates when this has occurred. Fungal infection is also more likely.

✗ Prolonged use of neomycin-containing preparations can lead to a local allergic reaction.

✗ Mild infections may resolve without antibiotics once the ear is thoroughly cleaned.

✗ Astringents such as glycerine and icthammol or aluminium acetate may be as effective as antibiotics.

Option 5. Operate.

Microscopic suction clearance

✓ The most important factor in treating this condition successfully is to clean the ear canal thoroughly. This is best performed with a microscope in an out-patient department. Cleaning may need to be repeated regularly until the infection resolves.

✗ Microscopic clearance may be painful and may traumatize the ear canal if not done carefully.

Surgery of external auditory canal

✓ Surgery may be indicated on rare occasions in patients with stenozed ear canals and hyperplastic epithelium. If a severe bacterial infection fails to respond, there may be underlying cartilage necrosis and this may need to be excised.

✗ Surgery to a stenosed ear canal carries a risk to the facial nerve if the bone of the external canal needs to be drilled. However, this risk should be small.

History checklist
- Is there a history of infection after swimming?
- Has the patient been abroad? Hot humid atmospheres will predispose to infection, and otitis externa is particularly likely after swimming in polluted or unclean water.
- Is there a history of any other chronic skin disorder such as eczema or psoriasis? The protective cutaneous barrier is breached in these skin disorders and infection is likely, particularly with scratching due to itching.

Examination checklist
- Is the ear canal clean but inflamed, or full of moist, macerated squamous debris or exudate?
- Is the external canal narrow due to oedematous skin in the outer cartilaginous section of the canal?
- Is there stenosis of the ear canal due to chronic infection/inflammation? Such stenosis may affect either the external meatus or the inner section of the bony canal.
- Is there surrounding cellulitis of the concha or pinna?
- Is there an associated tympanic membrane perforation or associated otitis media?
- Is there associated lymphadenopathy or pyrexia?

Malignant otitis externa refers to deep-seated infection with Pseudomonas aeruginosa in which cranial nerve paralysis is likely. The facial nerve is affected most often but the trigeminal, vagus and hypoglossal may also be affected. The condition is more likely to occur in elderly diabetics.

Pitfalls
- The advice that nothing smaller than an elbow should go near the ear is correct. Infection is often introduced into the ear by fingers while scratching an itchy ear.
- Do not underestimate malignant otitis externa. The onset may be insidious but it can become rapidly progressive and is fatal in some cases.
- Infection is not always bacterial. Fungi are likely if local/systemic antibiotic treatment has been prolonged.
- Prescribing a systemic antibiotic without cleaning the ear regularly is likely to encourage the emergence of resistant bacteria.

Referrals
- Patients with malignant otitis media, chronic incalcitrant infections, or diabetic patients.

Hints for investigators and prescribers

- An ear culture is ideal but not always necessary since most infections will respond to local therapy. However, a culture is indicated for recalcitrant infections or severe infection where systemic antibiotics are required.
- Fungal cultures may need to be requested.
- Although the external ear canal is not sterile, the pathogens listed above are rarely isolated from healthy ears.
- A variety of topical ear preparations is available. These may be combined with a steroid, which is useful in chronic eczematous skin conditions.
- Otomize spray (neomycin/acetic acid/dexamethasone) is useful for restoring the natural acid environment of the external canal and thus inhibits bacterial growth.
- Genticin or Gentisone HC and polymyxin preparations such as Otosporin are useful for Pseudomonas infections. Canesten is used specifically for fungal infections.
- Patients with malignant otitis externa should be treated with an antipseudomonal antibiotic. Oral ciprofloxacin in high dosage is effective and penetrates bone well, but 6 weeks' treatment is still recommended (Sade *et al.*, 1989; Lang *et al.*, 1990).
- If otitis externa fails to respond to antibiotic therapy and a fungal infection is suspected, the ear canal should be thoroughly cleaned and a topical antimycotic agent such as clotrimazole prescribed. Systemic therapy is rarely indicated (Lucente, 1993).

Further reading

Lang, R., Goshen, S., Kitzes-Cohen, R. and Sade, J. (1990) Successful treatment of malignant external otitis with oral ciprofloxacin: report of experience with 23 patients. *J. Infect. Dis.* **161**: 537–540.

Lucente, F.E. (1993) Fungal infections of the external ear. *Otolaryngol. Clin. N. Am.* **26**: 995–1006.

Sade, J., Lang, R., Goshen, S. and Kitzes-Cohen, R. (1989) Ciprofloxacin treatment of malignant external otitis. *Am. J. Med.* **87** (suppl. 5a): 138–141.

13 Acute otitis media

Acute otitis media (AOM) is normally a disease of childhood, which presents with acute otalgia, pyrexia and malaise, with or without discharge. However, not all acutely-ill children present with specific ear-related symptoms, particularly if younger than 2 years old (Niemela *et al.*, 1994). An upper respiratory viral infection often predisposes to acute bacterial infection and viruses have been detected in approximately 16% of patients (Brook and van de Heyning, 1994).

The condition affects 62% of children within their first year and 80% by 3 years. Boys are affected more than girls, there is a genetic predisposition, and it is more common in children with a midline cleft palate (Cantor, 1995). Risk factors include child care outside of the home, parental smoking, and a sibling with a history of AOM and the use of dummies or pacifiers (Uhari, 1996). The risk is reduced in children breast-fed for longer than 3 months.

The eardrum often perforates during the course of the illness and the ear then discharges. The infection usually resolves within a few days, although a persistent effusion may remain in the middle ear for several months.

Management options

Option 1. Do nothing.

✓ Spontaneous resolution is likely in most cases.

✗ Intracranial complication may develop.
✗ The otalgia may cause undue distress.

Option 2. Advise.

✓ Parents should be reassured that the condition is self-limiting and will resolve within a few days.
✓ Factors, which should reduce the recurrence, should be encouraged. These include breast feeding, avoiding tobacco smoke and preventing viral transmission by hand washing and using virucidal agents to wash surfaces in day care centres.

Option 3. Investigate.

✓ If there is a purulent discharge, the pathogen may be identified. This is particularly important if the infection fails to resolve and otorrhoea persists.

✗ Most cases will resolve spontaneously and culture is unnecessary.
✗ Bacteria are not recovered from about 25% of cultures from children with acute otitis media.

Option 4. Prescribe antibiotics.

✓ Pain and discharge should resolve within a few days and complications or persistent discharge should be prevented.

✗ The infection is likely to resolve within a few days without antibiotics. There has recently been controversy about whether antibiotics are required in treating AOM. Some research studies have failed to show any beneficial effect from antibiotics and found 85% of children pain-free within 24 hours of the acute infection without antibiotics (Browning, 1990; Brook and van de Heyning, 1994; Froom *et al.*, 1997).
✗ There is inconclusive evidence that antibiotics improve outcome or that they prevent the unusual complications of meningitis or mastoiditis (Froom *et al.*, 1997).

✗ The optimum duration of antimicrobial treatment is unknown. It has been recommended that the course does not exceed 10 days (Froom *et al.*, 1997).

✗ Antibiotics are associated with side-effects and possible anaphylaxis.

✗ Antibiotic use for a common condition is more likely to induce bacterial resistance and the total cost of treating a community will be expensive.

History checklist
- Is there a history of previous earache or discharge?
- Are there any associated problems with the nose or throat?
- Is there a history of hearing loss? Has balance been affected?

Examination checklist
- Is the child ill?
- Is the eardrum red or bulging?
- Is the drum perforated?

Rituals and myths
- It is often thought that antibiotics are always needed. Recent evidence has shown however, that resolution occurs spontaneously in over 80% of children and that recovery occurs at the same rate whether or not antibiotics are used.

Pitfalls
- If the external ear canal is inflamed the eardrum may not be visible and an underlying AOM may not be recognized.
- If there is no clinical improvement with antibiotics or if pyrexia persists or the child has a chronic headache, an intracranial complication should be suspected. The incidence is, however, low (0.15%).
- Acute mastoiditis remains a possible but rare complication in children with acute otitis media (Nadal *et al.*, 1990).
- Effect of delayed treatment: unlikely to have any significant effect. Otalgia may be prolonged.
- Effect of treating before investigation: no significant effects.

Referrals
- Referral is appropriate when there is history of frequent recurrent infection or if an intracranial complication is suspected.

Hints for investigators and prescribers
- No bacterial growth can be expected in 25% of cultures from ear swabs. Any bacterial isolate from a discharging ear is likely to be a pathogen.
- The current recommendation in the UK is for a 10-day course of amoxycillin. This should be changed to amoxycillin/clavulanate if there is no response within 3 days. If there is a history of penicillin allergy, a macrolide or trimethoprin should be prescribed. Second generation cephalosporins are a suitable alternative to penicillin-based antibiotics.
- It has recently been suggested that doctors should perhaps consider antibiotics as optional and discuss their use with parents before they are prescribed (Del Mar *et al.*, 1997).
- Acute mastoiditis should be treated with i.v. amoxycillin/clavulanate. If an abscess has developed, this should be drained. Mastoid surgery should be considered if there is no improvement within a couple of days.

Further reading
Brook, I. and van de Heyning, P. (1994) Microbiology and management of otitis media. *Scand. J. Infect. Dis.* (suppl. 93): 20–32.

Browning, G. (1990) Childhood otalgia: acute otitis media. *Br. Med. J.* **300**: 1005–1006.

Cantor, R.M. (1995) Otitis externa and otitis media. A new look at old problems. *Pediatr. Emerg.* **13**: 445–455.

Del Mar, C., Glasziou, P. and Hayem, M. (1997) Are antibiotics indicated as initial treatment for children with acute otitis media? A meta-analysis. *Br. Med. J.* **314**: 1526–1529.

Froom, J., Culpepper, L., Jacobs, M., DeMelker, R.A., Green, L.A., van Buchem, L., Grob, P. and Heeren, T. (1997) Antimicrobials for acute otitis media? A review from the International Primary Care Network. *Br. Med. J.* **315**: 98–101.

Nadal, D., Herrmann, P., Baumann, A. and Fanconi, A. (1990) Acute mastoiditis: clinical, microbiological, and therapeutic aspects. *Eur. J. Pediatr.* **149**: 560–564.

Niemela, M., Uhari, M., Jounio-Ervasti, K., Luotenen, J., Alho, O. and Vierimaa, E. (1994) Lack of specific symptomatology in children with acute otitis media. *Pediatr. Infect. Dis. J.* **13**: 765–768.

Uhari M., Mantysaari K. and Niemela M. (1996) A meta-analytic review of the risk factors for acute otitis media. *Clin. Infect. Dis.* **22**: 1079–1083.

14 Chronic suppurative otitis media

Chronic suppurative otitis media (CSOM) without cholesteatoma is defined as chronic inflammation of the middle ear and mastoid, in which a discharge persists for over 6 weeks. Untreated, the condition leads to destructive changes and irreversible sequelae, which develop insidiously. Clinically it is separated into two distinct groups according to whether or not a cholesteatoma is present.

The key features are hearing loss, smelly discharge, intermittent vertigo, perforation of attic, or pars tensa, and cholesteatoma.

Management options

Option 1. Do nothing.

✓ The patient may go deaf, but you will be hearing the complaints.

✗ A discharge is likely to persist. If a cholesteatoma is present there will be slow insidious progression and local destruction.

✗ Intracranial complications may occur.

Option 2. Advise.

✓ Without an understanding of the outcome and possible complications the patient may become complacent about the ear and avoid treatment.

✗ The patient will suffer the consequences of ignoring the ear.

Option 3. Investigate.

Culture

✓ Culture may indicate the pathogens and their antibiotic sensitivity.

✗ Most cases of CSOM without cholesteatoma will respond to intensive local treatment without knowledge of the local pathogens. A culture is therefore not always necessary.

Imaging

✓ High resolution CT scans will confirm intracranial pathology. CT can also help to delineate the extent of disease and show local bone erosion.

✗ Cholesteatoma is treated by mastoid surgery in most cases and the extent of the operation is determined by the findings at the time of surgery.

Option 4. Prescribe antibiotics.

CSOM without cholesteatoma

✓ Topical antibiotic/steroid ear drops are effective in the treatment of chronically infected ears. However, they must be combined with aural toilet and microscopic suction. Local dressings on ribbon gauze or expandable sponge may be useful in the early days of treatment.

✓ Dry-mopping alone is a less effective means of treatment. A recent community-based project on the treatment of CSOM in school children in Kenya has shown that a combination of dry-mopping, topical antibiotic-steroid drops and systemic antibiotics was much more effective than dry-mopping alone (Smith *et al.*, 1996).

✗ Local antibiotic sensitivity, particularly to drops containing neomycin or propylene glycol, may occur.

✗ Bacterial resistance is likely with prolonged use of ear drops or systemic antibiotics.

CSOM with cholesteatoma

✓ If acute infection is treated with antibiotics just before surgery, there should be less inflammation, less bleeding and less chance of wound infection. However, attention is not often given to this in practice and mastoid surgery continues to be done on infected ears.

✗ Antibiotic drops may alleviate discharge from CSOM with cholesteatoma but this effect is likely to be temporary.

✗ Topical antibiotic drops are unlikely to give long-term relief or to stop the progressively destructive nature of this condition. The disease is a slow insidious destructive process in which the cholesteatoma permeates the middle ear and eventually extends through the additus to the mastoid bowl.

Mastoid cavity infection

✓ Topical antibiotic drops are useful in treating infections of the mastoid cavity, which is created after mastoid surgery. However, infected cavities usually contain moist debris and underlying pus. Thorough cleaning is therefore essential.

✗ Antibiotic drops can induce local skin sensitivity, and bacterial resistance as described above.

Option 5. Operate.

CSOM without cholesteatoma

✓ If an aural polyp is present, this should be removed surgically.

✓ Infants may occasionally develop an acute mastoid abscess, which requires surgical drainage.

✗ CSOM usually responds to intensive local therapy, which includes thorough aural toilet and topical antibiotic drops. CSOM in children has been shown to respond to intensive medical treatment, aural toilet and removal of granulations, particularly if commenced more than 6 weeks before histopathological middle ear changes have occurred. It has been suggested that mastoid surgery should be considered if otorrhoea recurs after two admissions for i.v. therapy (Kenna *et al.*, 1993).

✗ Mastoid surgery is associated with risks to the integrity of the facial nerve, and with causing vertigo, hearing loss, tinnitus and altered taste perception.

CSOM with cholesteatoma

✓ The treatment for this disease is mastoid surgery. The extent of the surgery is determined by the disease.

✗ Surgery and general anaesthesia do carry unavoidable risks, and if these are high then the disease should be managed conservatively by microscopic suction.

Mastoid cavity infection

✓ Revision mastoidectomy is sometimes the only way of controlling frequent or persistent infection. This may be due to residual osteitis of cancellous bone or poor access and ventilation of the cavity. The goals of revision surgery are to open the external meatus widely, lower the facial ridge, remove residual osteitic bone and block communication with the eustachion tube.

✗ Intensive local treatment can avert the need for revision surgery in many cases.

✗ There is still a risk of intracranial complications arising from an infected mastoid cavity, if left untreated.

✗ The operative risks are the same as described above.

History checklist

• Enquiry should be made regarding the onset of symptoms, whether the patient has undergone previous ear surgery and whether there is any hearing loss, tinnitus or vertigo. CSOM is normally painless and associated chronic headache should alert one to the possibility of intracranial complications.

Examination checklist

• The ear should be cleaned and, if possible, examined with a microscope. The eardrum will usually be perforated in either the tympanic or the attic regions. If there is a defect in the attic, a cholesteatoma should be sought. Facial nerve function should be assessed and an audiogram obtained.

Rituals and myths

• A central perforation is usually associated with tubotympanic inflammatory disease without cholesteatoma. However, this is not always true, and a cholesteatoma may still be present within the middle ear.

Pitfalls

• CSOM with cholesteatoma is usually a slow insidious destructive disease, which is seen most often in adults. However, in children the disease progresses much more quickly.

• Complications usually present as an acute exacerbation in a chronically infected ear. A malodorous discharge is an early sign and usually implies that anaerobes are present. Complications may be extracranial such as mastoiditis, facial paralysis, labyrinthitis and petrositis. Intracranial complications include an extradural, intracerebral or subdural abscess, meningitis, sigmoid sinus thrombophlebitis and otitic hydrocephalus.

Referrals

• Any ear that fails to settle after intensive aural toilet and topical therapy.

• Any ear with a cholesteatoma.

• Any patient with an associated chronic headache in whom an intracranial complication is suspected.

Hints for investigators and prescribers

• Microscopic assessment is essential. This can usually be done in an out-patient clinic but occasionally general anaesthesia is required.

• Most ear drop preparations combine an antibiotic and a steroid to reduce the inflammatory response. The importance of thorough regular aural cleaning cannot be emphasized enough, and without this, the application of topical drops will probably lead to the emergence of resistant bacteria.

• More than one pathogen is present in nearly 60% of patients (average three organisms).

• A foul smell implies that anaerobes are likely to be present. These coexist with aerobes in about 50% of cases (Erkan et al., 1994). No significant differences in bacteriology have been found between children and adults (Vartiainen et al., 1996).

• Intensive aural toilet combined with topical gentamicin is usually effective if there is a persistent discharge due to Pseudomonas spp. but if the infection does not resolve systemic antibiotics may be indicated. Systemic antibiotics have been shown to be more effective than disinfectants (hydrogen peroxide, borax powder) in treating chronically discharging ears (Papastavros et al., 1989). If Pseudomonas spp. are present, a prolonged course of oral ciprofloxacin may be indicated. However, disinfectants are a useful adjunct and treatment should continue for 10 days after the discharge ceases.

- An Otomize spray may be more appropriate for an infected mastoid cavity, where drops may not cover the whole of the mucosa.
- S. aureus is more likely in ears with cholesteatoma, whereas P. aeruginosa is more common when there is chronic ear disease without cholesteatoma (Vartiainen et al., 1996).

Further reading

Arguedas, A.G., Herrera, J.F., Faingezicht, I. and Mohs, E. (1993) Ceftazidime for therapy of children with chronic suppurative otitis media without cholesteatoma. *Pediatr. Infect. Dis. J.* **12**: 246–247.

Erkan, M., Aslan, T., Sevuk, E. and Guney, E. (1994) Bacteriology of chronic suppurative otitis media. *Ann. Otol. Rhinol. Laryngol.* **103**: 771–774.

Fliss, D.M., Dagan, R., Meidan, N. and Leiberman, A. (1992) Aerobic bacteriology of chronic suppurative otitis media without cholesteatoma in children. *Ann. Otol. Rhinol. Laryngol.* **101**: 866–869.

Kenna, M.A. (1994) Treatment of chronic suppurative otitis media. *Otolaryngol. Clin. N. Am.* **27**: 457–472.

Kenna, M.A., Rosane, B.A. and Bluestone, C. (1993) Medical management of chronic suppurative otitis media without cholesteatoma in children – update 1992. *Am. J. Otol.* **14**: 469–473.

Papastavros, T., Giamarellou, H. and Varlejides, S. (1989) Preoperative therapeutic considerations in chronic suppurative otitis media. *Laryngoscope* **99**: 655–659.

Smith, A.W., Hatcher, J., Mackenzie, I.J., Thompson, S., Bal, I., Macharia, I., Mugwe, P., Okoth-Olende, C, Oburra, H. and Wanjohi, Z. (1996) Randomized controlled trial of treatment of chronic suppurative otitis media in Kenyan schoolchildren. *Lancet* **348**: 1128–1133.

Vartiainen, E. and Vartiainen, J. (1996) Effect of aerobic bacteriology on the clinical presentation and treatment results of chronic suppurative otitis media. *J. Laryngol. Otol.* **110**: 315–318.

Chapter 5
EYE INFECTIONS

M.T. Watts

Chapter contents

1 Acute conjunctivitis

Conjunctivitis is simply inflammation of the conjunctival lining of the eye and lids. Often the term is loosely used to imply bacterial infections causing such inflammation and although this is indeed frequently the cause, it is also important to consider other aetiologies.

The nature of discharge is often a helpful clue to the diagnosis; purulent discharges are often representative of true bacterial infections, while stringy mucoid discharge is more suggestive of an allergic process. Although conjunctivitis is uncomfortable, severe pain should prompt a careful search for any coexisting corneal disease or even intraocular inflammation. Even when the diagnosis seems apparent, it is important to examine the ocular adnexae and the eye itself in order to exclude more serious disease, which may require urgent referral.

Management options
1. Do nothing.
2. Treat with a broad-spectrum topical antibiotic.
3. Collect a conjunctival swab and treat with a broad-spectrum topical antibiotic.
4. Collect a conjunctival swab and treat with an appropriate antibiotic if indicated.

Option 1. Do nothing.

Tell the patient that acute conjunctivitis is a benign condition which is often self-limiting.

✓ Many patients will get better without any treatment. Potential adverse reactions to topical treatment are completely avoided, and money saved on prescriptions. If the condition does not resolve, the bacteriology has not been confused by treatment.

✗ Many cases will not resolve spontaneously for some weeks, and some will not resolve on their own at all. The patient and doctor will be troubled by further visits.

✗ The infection may spread to the other eye, or to family members and other close contacts. Recovery will be longer than if treated.

Option 2. Treat with a broad-spectrum topical antibiotic.

✓ Most cases will rapidly resolve completely.

✗ Some patients will develop allergic reactions to the antibiotic or preservative. This may lead to an apparent worsening of the conjunctivitis, whereas in truth there is new pathology.

✗ If the conjunctivitis does not respond, culture of the conjunctiva may be unsuccessful in identifying an organism and its sensitivity. Treatment will need to be stopped before meaningful bacteriology can be achieved.

✗ Many patients will be treated unnecessarily. Many people, and children in particular, find taking drops difficult, inconvenient and unpleasant.

Option 3. Collect a conjunctival swab and treat with a broad-spectrum topical antibiotic.

✓ Most patients will be successfully treated, and appropriate bacteriology will shortly be available for those few who are not.

✗ The vast majority of patients do not need conjunctival swabs, and so many will be exposed to the unnecessary trouble and expense of an inappropriate test.

Option 4. Collect a conjunctival swab and treat with an appropriate antibiotic if indicated.

✓ Only those patients who truly need treatment will receive it, and they will always be treated with an antibiotic to which the organism is sensitive.

✗ Many patients will have unnecessary conjunctival swabs when they would have responded to a broad-spectrum antibiotic anyway.

✗ There will be a delay between taking the conjunctival swab and institution of treatment, during which the conjunctivitis may have progressed.

History checklist

General

- Other than identifying any predisposition to infection in the case of recurrent conjunctivitis, there is no need for general history-taking.
- Any history of contact with infectious disease is helpful in identifying epidemics of disease, which typically occur in viral conjunctivitis.
- In neonates, the onset of the conjunctivitis is particularly relevant, since conjunctivitis present at birth is ophthalmia neonatorum which requires hospitalization and treatment, together with identification of the maternal source of infection.

Specific

- Chronic blepharitis and allergy are often confused with infectious conjunctivitis. The nature of discharge from the eye is helpful in differential diagnosis. Is there discharge from the eye, and what is its nature?

   Copious watery discharge suggests viral infection.

   Purulent discharge suggests bacterial conjunctivitis.

   Stringy mucoid discharge with itching and watering suggests allergy.
- Does the patient wear contact lenses? If yes, this may be the source of the infection, and the lens should be removed immediately to prevent further infection and possible corneal involvement. Culture of the lens, solutions and storage vehicles should be undertaken in severe infection or if the cornea is involved.
- Is there severe pain? If yes, it is unlikely that this is simple conjunctivitis which is uncomfortable but not generally associated with severe pain. Uveitis should be considered.
- Has the patient taken antibiotic drops? If yes, and the 'infection' has persisted, culture of the conjunctiva should be undertaken after 24 hours of treatment. The diagnosis should be reconsidered since conjunctivitis not responsive to broad-spectrum topical antibiotics is relatively uncommon.

Examination checklist

- Is only the conjunctiva red? If yes, and the eye appears otherwise quiet (no abnormality within the anterior chamber), the condition is probably simple conjunctivitis. If no, and there is also swelling of the lids, or fever, or the area below the inner canthus of the eye (the nasolacrimal sac) is swollen and tender, then there is a more significant cellulitis, requiring systemic treatment.
- Is there any associated lid disease? If yes, this may take the form of an infected meibomian gland (chalazion) or more diffuse inflammatory disease of the lid margin (marginal blepharitis). Both these conditions predispose to conjunctivitis, but require treating in their own right, i.e. by incision and curettage of a chalazion, and lid cleansing with cotton buds dipped in weak shampoo solution for marginal blepharitis.
- Is there any preauricular lymphadenopathy? If yes, it is likely that there is either viral or chlamydial infection of the eye. The former is almost always bilateral, and the latter usually unilateral with purulent discharge.
- Is there any associated skin pathology? It is important not to miss coexisting skin diseases, such as infected eczema or herpes simplex virus, which may require specific treatments.
- Is there nasolacrimal reflux on pressure over the nasolacrimal sac? If yes, then it will be necessary to treat this to prevent recurrent attacks. The reflux of copious mucopurulent

material through the puncta at the inner canthus when the nasolacrimal sac area is compressed implies obstruction, and often surgical cure is necessary to prevent more serious infections of the sac itself (dacryocystitis).

Referrals

- Ophthalmia neonatorum should not be discharged from hospital until treated. Other cases of conjunctivitis require referral if failing to respond to conventional treatment, or if there is any question as to the diagnosis.
- Slit lamp examination will usually establish a firm diagnosis and exclude other pathology, such as uveitis.
- The hospital service would be totally incapable of treating every case of conjunctivitis if all were referred indiscriminately.

Rituals and myths

- Eyes should be bathed in a boiled solution of salt water. There is no logical basis to this time-honoured treatment of conjunctivitis, which is often complicated by an irritative conjunctivitis superimposed on the infection when hypertonic solutions are inadvertently created by boiling.
- Children with recurrent conjunctivitis need syringing of the nasolacrimal duct. It is true that delayed patency of the nasolacrimal duct will lead to recurrent conjunctivitis in children. If this persists beyond the age of one year, then surgical rupture of the persistent membrane at the lower end of the nasolacrimal duct may indeed be indicated but resolution is usually spontaneous, and surgery is often complicated by recurrent obstruction.

Pitfalls

- Ophthalmia neonatorum is technically any conjunctivitis occurring within the first 10 days of life. Chlamydial infection is the commonest cause. Not only can this be complicated by severe systemic illness, and in particular pneumonitis, but diagnosis mandates the identification and treatment of any maternal infection and examination of her sexual contacts. Sexually active adults should be counselled.
- Vancomycin solutions, being of pH 3, are irritant to the eye.
- Adenoviruses are the commonest cause of epidemic viral conjunctivitis, and certain strains are highly contagious. They are readily passed on by direct contact with tears, or by nasopharyngeal secretions. If the clinician is not aware of the risks, conjunctivitis can be rapidly spread through a surgery.

Hints for investigators and prescribers

- Conjunctiva swabs are not normally required because empirical antibacterial therapy will cover the most probable infective agents, except Chlamydia spp.
- Chlamydial infection should be suspected, if there is failure to respond to earlier empirical therapy, or because of specific risk factors (for example, ophthalmia neonatorum, or conjunctivitis in an adult who has recently changed their sexual partner). Specific investigation for Chlamydia spp. infections can usually be reserved for cases where conjunctivitis is unresponsive to first-line broad-spectrum antibacterial drops. Conjuctiva swabs should be rubbed vigorously enough to dislodge epithelial cells that may contain Chlamydia spp., but not too vigorously as to cause abrasions. Since there are many laboratory technologies for Chlamydia spp. diagnosis, for example, culture, antigen detection, and polymerase chain reaction, swabs should be placed into the specific transport medium, recommended by your laboratory.
- In all cases, when swabbing the conjunctiva, any discharge should be removed before swabbing the conjunctiva itself – the actual site of the infection. The aim is to avoid collecting extraneous matter and/or overgrown bacterial flora, factors which may impair the interpretation of microbiological results.

- Topical treatment may take the form of eye drops or ointment. Drops must be applied accurately and at least four times a day if they are to be effective. Ointments need only be applied twice a day but tend to blur the vision.
- Any remaining eye drops or ointment must be discarded at the end of a course of treatment, because they are susceptible to extraneous bacterial contamination during use and may, therefore, act as a source of infection if they are used again later on.
- Systemic therapy eliminates the pathogen from all sites and also makes topical therapy redundant.

Further reading

McCulley, J.P., Dougherty, J.M. and Denau, D.G. (1982) Classification of chronic blepharitis. *Ophthalmology* 89: 1173–1180.

Ostler, H.B. (1993) *Diseases of the External Eye and Adnexa.* Williams and Wilkins, Baltimore, MD.

Tabbara, K.F. and Hyndiuk, R.A. (eds) (1986) *Infections of the Eye.* Little Brown, Boston, MA.

Ullman, S., Roussel, T.J. and Forster, R.K. (1987) Gonococcal keratoconjunctivitis. *Surv. Ophthalmol.* 32: 199–208.

2 Bacterial keratitis

Bacterial keratitis is a rare but potentially sight-threatening disease, which requires early recognition and prompt treatment. Some organisms rapidly penetrate the eye and can lead to a perforation of the cornea within 24 hours of initial infection. A high index of suspicion is therefore required, and in any patient with apparent conjunctivitis, a close examination of the cornea should be made. Severe pain or any area of corneal opacity (which may represent intracorneal abscess) should prompt immediate referral to a specialist. Contact lens wear is an increasingly common cause of bacterial keratitis, and the history of this should be sought. Prompt treatment usually leads to cure, but any delay can be disastrous.

Management options
1. Do nothing.
2. Treat with a broad-spectrum topical antibiotic.
3. Collect a corneal scrape and treat with a topical broad-spectrum antibiotic.

Option 1. Do nothing.

✓ There is a small chance that the cornea may improve spontaneously, but this is unlikely.

✗ The patient will very probably develop worsening pain and loss of vision.

✗ There is a high chance that the cornea will perforate, requiring emergency tectonic corneal grafting. Results from this are often poor, and endophthalmitis often supervenes.

✗ Subsequent litigation will be difficult to defend!

Option 2. Treat with a broad-spectrum topical antibiotic.

✓ Many ulcers will be effectively treated without recourse to any painful or invasive procedures, and without hospitalization.

✗ If there is no response to topical therapy, delay will have occurred in isolating the organism and deciding appropriate treatment. Certain organisms are very aggressive and can lead to loss of vision during this period.

✗ Many infections will only respond to fortified strengths of antibiotic, and conventional broad-spectrum topical treatment such as chloramphenicol is inadequate.

Option 3. Collect a corneal scrape and treat with a topical broad-spectrum antibiotic.

✓ This is effective in the large majority of bacterial keratitis cases. Even if initial therapy fails, identification of the organism should soon follow, allowing appropriate changes.

✗ Fortified antibiotics are required. These must be made specially by a pharmacy and have a short shelf-life. Some are toxic to the corneal epithelium, delaying healing. Hospitalization is generally required, and treatment should be half-hourly, including during the night in the early, critical stages.

✗ This treatment is expensive, time-consuming and unpleasant for the patient, and many patients would improve with simpler treatment regimes.

History checklist

General
● Bacterial keratitis is a rare and serious condition, with potential for destruction of the eye. Although most cases are related to specific pathology of the eye, any likely systemic predisposition to infection should be identified. In particular, open wounds that

are infected, systemic immunosuppression, and poor overall nutrition and hygiene are relevant.

Specific
- Does the patient wear contact lenses? If yes, it is important to culture the lens, any solutions used and the storage vessel for the lenses in search of organisms. Acanthamoeba spp. keratitis should be considered in any cases of contact lens-induced keratitis, as an alternative pathogen to bacteria.
- Is there any local eye or lid disease? This may include blepharitis, previous surgery, lacrimal sac infection, etc., all of which predispose to keratitis, and need appropriate management.

Examination checklist
- Is the corneal sensation normal? If no, this may be due either to the keratitis itself, or the cause of it. Recurrent viral keratitis, surgery, or other rare disorders can lead to reduced sensation and secondary bacterial keratitis.
- Is there an associated reaction in the anterior chamber? This may take the form of a fibrinous reaction or frank hypopyon level of pus in the anterior chamber. Either of these implies that the infection is no longer limited to the cornea and must be treated as endophthalmitis.
- Certain bacteria, most notably Pseudomonas spp., will rapidly lead to endophthalmitis and perforation of the cornea.
- Is the ulceration limited to the cornea or does it spread into the sclera? An ulcer which transgresses the limbus, which is the division between cornea and sclera, is likely to be associated with a systemic vasculitis. Although such ulcers can become infected, this appearance is not a simple bacterial keratitis and should be managed by treatment of the underlying disease.
- Is there fluorescein staining over the area of ulceration? If yes, it is most likely that it is truly a bacterial keratitis, particularly in the presence of redness of the conjunctiva and whitish appearance of the ulcer (i.e. abscess). Marginal keratitis can mimic bacterial keratitis by presenting a whitish 'ulcer' at the corneal periphery. It is not usual for this to take up fluorescein stain. If there is any doubt, treat as a bacterial infection.
- Is there any apparent cause for the ulceration? This may include presence of adnexal infection, foreign body within the cornea or underneath the upper lid, or manifestation of previous diseases, such as herpetic keratitis. It is quite unusual for a bacterial keratitis to develop in an entirely healthy cornea which has suffered no previous disease, trauma or contact lens wear.

Referrals
- All patients with bacterial keratitis, or suspected bacterial keratitis, should be referred immediately to an eye clinic, and treatment must be started at once.

Rituals and myths
- Urgent Gram staining of all specimens should be undertaken. This ritual is equally irrelevant to management of bacterial keratitis as it is to management of endophthalmitis, and for the same reasons. It is necessary to cover a broad-spectrum of bacterial infection, prior to formal identification of an organism by culture. Antibiotics should not be omitted on the basis of 'likely pathogen' as identified by Gram stain, particularly since there may be more than one.
- Marginal infiltrates that do not stain with fluorescein can be assumed to be marginal keratitis. It is true that bacterial infection usually leads to loss of the epithelium, and that the condition of marginal keratitis which is a hypersensitivity reaction to previous exposure to bacterial exotoxin normally demonstrates intact epithelium, but it is not safe to

assume that any whitish infiltration of the cornea is anything other than bacterial. Treatment of marginal keratitis is with topical steroid which obviously has catastrophic effects on infectious keratitis.

Pitfalls

- Infection with unusual organisms. Not all apparent (supposed) bacterial keratitis is due to bacterial infection. Failure to respond to treatment, failure to identify an organism, or unusual features, such as severe pain and radial neuritis in the cornea, should prompt investigation for unusual causes of infection (e.g. Acanthamoeba spp., Candida spp.). This may necessitate not only scrape of the cornea but formal biopsy.
- Toxicity of topical treatment. Many topical treatments are toxic to the corneal epithelium in the high doses required for effective treatment. Sometimes this may appear as an apparent failure to respond to treatment when in fact it is the treatment causing the problem.
- Inadequate strength of drops. The standard preparations of topical antibiotic are not sufficiently strong to treat many bacterial infections of the cornea, although they may be sufficient for simple conjunctivitis for which they are designed. Fortified preparations of antibiotic should be prepared for the treatment of bacterial keratitis.

Hints for investigators and prescribers

- Patients with suspected keratitis should be referred immediately to a specialist, who has the expertise to collect the most appropriate diagnostic specimen (notably a corneal scrape) and who can liaise closely with the laboratory. Patients should be asked to take their contact lenses and storage cases to the specialist.
- Prescibers ought to be aware that steroids carry a risk of seriously aggravating infections.
- First line empirical therapy needs to be both appropriate (in bacterial keratitis, Gram-positive and Gram-negative organisms must be covered), and intensive.
- For superficial infections of the eyelid, topical therapy may be appropriate, but ointment, not drops, should be applied.

Further reading

Alfonso, E., Mandelbaum, S., Fox, M.J. and Foster, R.K. (1986) Ulcerative keratitis associated with contact lens wear. *Am. J. Ophthalmol.* **101**: 429–433.

Asbell, P. and Stenson, S. (1982) Ulcerative keratitis. Survey of 30 years' laboratory experience. *Arch. Ophthalmol.* **100**: 77.

Watts, M.T. and Nelson, M.E. (1992) *External Eye Disease: A Colour Atlas.* Churchill Livingstone, London.

3 Endophthalmitis

Endophthalmitis is the most serious and urgent of all eye emergencies. Early and vigorous treatment will often rescue an eye from otherwise certain blindness, and immediate recognition of the problem and referral to a specialist is essential.

Most commonly, endophthalmitis follows an intraocular surgical procedure, but may also occur following trauma, severe corneal infection or, rarely, as a manifestation of systemic sepsis. Although once established, the diagnosis is very obvious, with corneal opacity, pus within the anterior chamber, and loss of red reflex, accompanied by the symptoms of pain and loss of vision, in earlier stages of evolution it may be less easy to diagnose.

Pain in the eye associated with lid oedema is very suggestive of intraocular infection, particularly following recent surgery.

Management options

1. Treat with broad-spectrum topical antibiotics.
2. Treat with topical and systemic antibiotics.
3. Undertake a diagnostic tap of the anterior chamber and inject antibiotic.
4. Undertake single port vitreous biopsy through the pars plana, as well as an anterior chamber tap, and inject antibiotic.
5. Undertake formal vitrectomy, through three ports, remove the infected vitreous and inject intraocular antibiotic.

Option 1. Treat with broad-spectrum topical antibiotics.

✓ Surgery is avoided, and in many cases resolution of the infection will be achieved as long as the infection is with a relatively non-virulent organism, and caught early.

✗ If infection has already become established in the vitreous, an opportunity to treat effectively will be missed. More complex surgery may be required later, and the final visual outcome will be compromised.

✗ Identification of the organism will never be achieved, and if this treatment strategy fails, subsequent antibiotic choice will be difficult to make.

Option 2. Treat with topical and systemic antibiotics.

✓ Surgery is avoided and resolution may be achieved.

✗ Penetration of the eye of systemic antibiotics is generally poor, and it is certainly not possible to guarantee bactericidal doses without intraocular injection.

✗ The usefulness of systemic antibiotics in the management of endophthalmitis is unproven, and the patient is exposed to potential anaphylaxis with no proven benefit.

✗ If the treatment does not work, identification of the organism, and selection of effective treatment, has been compromised.

Option 3. Undertake a diagnostic tap of the anterior chamber and inject antibiotic.

✓ This is an effective treatment strategy for most endophthalmitis in which the infection has not reached the vitreous when the posterior chamber is intact.

✓ If the vitreous is not involved this treatment avoids surgery, and can be undertaken as an out-patient.

✗ It can be impossible to detect whether or not the vitreous is involved at an early stage and therefore the opportunity to effectively treat early vitreous disease is missed.

✗ Injection of the intraocular antibiotic without 'making room' for it by removing some of the vitreous, may itself rupture the posterior capsule.

✗ If the strategy fails, effective treatment is once again delayed and visual outcome is reduced.

Option 4. Undertake single port vitreous biopsy through the pars plana, as well as an anterior chamber tap, and inject antibiotic.

✓ This is the most effective management in all cases in whom the presenting visual acuity is light perception or better.

✓ Even if the treatment is not immediately effective, early identification of the organism allows an effective strategy for further treatment to be planned.

✗ Surgery is involved, which may need to be repeated if not effective within 48 hours.

Option 5. Undertake formal vitrectomy, through three ports, remove the infected vitreous and inject intraocular antibiotic.

✓ This is usually effective in bringing infection under control, although the retinotoxic effects of the organism may still limit ultimate visual recovery.

✓ The likelihood of needing repeat surgery, which may be required if the vitreous is only biopsied, is reduced.

✗ The surgery is complex, and best undertaken by a surgeon experienced in vitreoretinal techniques. General anaesthesia is preferred by many surgeons for this.

✗ If patients present with vision of better than light perception, this technique offers no likely better visual outcome than if the vitreous is simply biopsied.

History checklist

General

- A general history, indicating any predisposition to infection such as diabetes, use of oral steroids, immunosuppression, recent surgery, illness, or presence of sources of infections, such as open wounds, chest infection, should be taken.
- Management of endophthalmitis is principally surgical, and general anaesthesia is preferred in some situations (three-port vitrectomy). Enquiry into fitness for this is appropriate at an early stage.

Specific

- Endophthalmitis most commonly follows surgery to the eye, and usually occurs within a few days of operation.
- Has the patient had eye surgery? If yes, the timing of the surgery should be sought. Although infection is usually early, the presence of sutures, e.g. in corneal graft surgery, or the presence of a thin cystic conjuctival bleb as seen in trabeculectomy surgery for glaucoma, is a continued risk of endophthalmitis. The patient can develop simple conjunctivitis which can progress to infection within the eye via the sutures or thin conjunctival bleb.
- If there is no history of recent surgery, other precipitants should be identified. These include the wearing of contact lenses, presence of lid-margin disease ('blepharitis') and nasolacrimal obstruction. If contact lenses have been worn, the lens, its case and any solutions should be taken for culture.
- A history of epiphora suggests nasolacrimal obstruction, and pressure over the nasolacrimal sac may lead to reflux of mucopurulent material, which should be cultured.
- Has any treatment been given already? If yes, note should be taken of these, as they may confuse the clinical picture. It should be remembered that many topical preparations are available over the counter, and patients may have taken antibacterials without realizing.
- Most patients who have recently had surgery will still be taking topical steroids, and these usually need to be stopped.

Examination checklist

- What is the visual acuity? In established endophthalmitis, the visual acuity is always reduced, although in the early stages it is not necessarily so. Pain is characteristic, and in post-operative patients the combination of pain and reduced vision must be regarded as endophthalmitis until proved otherwise. If the visual acuity is reduced to light perception or worse, a three-port vitrectomy is indicated, but if vision is better than this, a vitreous biopsy through a single port is preferred.
- Is there adnexal infection? The ocular adnexae, which include the lids, nasolacrimal system and lacrimal gland should be examined for source of infection. Pressure over the nasolacrimal sac may lead to reflux of pus through the punctum.
- Is there corneal disease? A corneal abscess is an obvious cause of endophthalmitis. Chronic disease may lead to corneal thinning, and threatened or actual perforation should be considered.
- Is there a hypopyon? A hypopyon is simply a fluid level of pus within the anterior chamber. Although it can be seen as a purely inflammatory reaction, in the presence of pain and lid and conjunctival swelling, it is most suggestive of endophthalmitis.
- Is there a red reflex? If no, the endophthalmitis involves the vitreous. This implies much more extensive infection than when only the anterior chamber is involved, and a much poorer visual prognosis. If there is no red reflex, assessment of the posterior pole should be supplemented by ultrasound B-scan.

Referrals

- Early treatment is often effective. Delay is catastrophic. False diagnosis will waste the patient's and ophthalmologist's time. This is of little importance, since the consequences for all of a missed diagnosis are so serious.

Rituals and myths

- Urgent Gram staining of all specimens should be undertaken. This ritual which involves the trouble and expense of an emergency microbiologist, does not contribute to management of the condition, since in the first 24 hours, broad-spectrum antibiotics should be used whatever the results of Gram stain. Although endophthalmitis is usually the result of infection with a single organism, until culture and sensitivity is available, a policy of eliminating all possible pathogens should be followed.
- Painless hypopyon is 'reactive' and should be treated with topical steroid. It is certainly true that pain is suggestive of endophthalmitis, in the presence of uveitis soon after surgery, but the converse is not true, and if patients who do not have pain are not treated as having infection, then although the minority who have a true purely inflammatory uveitis will improve on steroids, the others will worsen rapidly.
- In established endophthalmitis the prognosis is so poor that treatment is useless. This carried an element of truth about it before the days of aggressive management of endophthalmitis and vitrectomy surgery. It is no longer the case and many patients with very severe endophthalmitis recover a good level of vision.

Pitfalls

- Delay in diagnosis and treatment. Hours matter in the treatment of endophthalmitis. In severe infection, e.g. by Pseudomonas spp., a corneal ulcer may progress to perforation and loss of vision in 24 hours. It is not sufficient to have a 'trial of therapy' overnight and delay sight-saving surgery.
- Failure to respond to treatment. Even if an aggressive management has been undertaken early on, some eyes will not respond to conventional therapy. Repeat surgery to remove further vitreous infection may be needed, and other organisms such as fungi and viruses should be considered.

- Use of retinotoxic agents. Some intraocular antibiotics are extremely retinotoxic, and the final visual outcome may be poor in spite of good recovery from infection and good anatomical result, because of the toxicity of agents such as gentamicin. Many authorities still recommend these agents despite their toxic effects, while they are very rarely indicated.

Hints for investigators and prescribers

- Patients with suspected endophthalmitis should be referred immediately to a specialist for a two-fold surgical intervention: (a) aspiration of aqueous and/or vitreous to provide the samples that are essential for a precise laboratory diagnosis – a prerequisite to specific and effective treatment; (b) intraocular administration of empirical antibiotics.

Further reading

Endophthalmitis Vitrectomy Study Group. (1995) Results of the endophthalmitis vitrectomy study: a randomised trial of immediate vitrectomy and of intravenous antibiotics for the treatment of post-operative bacterial endophthalmitis. *Arch. Ophthalmol.* **113**: 1479–1496.

Roth, D.B. and Flynn, H.W. (1997) Antibiotic selection in the treatment of endophthalmitis: the significance of drug combinations and synergy. *Surv. Ophthalmol.* **41**: 395–401.

Seal, D.V. and Kirkness, C.M. (1997) The criteria for intravitreal antibiotics during surgery for removal of intraocular foreign bodies. *Eye* **6**: 465–468.

4 Periocular infections

Periocular infections are often trivial self-resolving diseases, but their proximity to the eye and potential for a retrograde spread mandate a cautious and meticulous approach to their management. Particularly in children, periocular infection can rapidly develop into life-threatening orbital cellulitis, and delay in treatment may be fatal. It is important to assess the general physical state of the patient as well as the local problem, since septicaemia often supervenes in orbital cellulitis. Early assessment of the sinuses is important in orbital cellulitis, and referral of immediate joint ophthalmic and ear, nose and throat (ENT) management is important.

More commonly, periocular infections are less serious and can be managed by local measures. Recurrent lid margin infections are often managed by patients themselves and education is an important part of the treatment. As with other ocular infections, severe pain is a warning sign of more severe infections and should prompt close examination.

Management options
1. Do nothing.
2. Give broad-spectrum antibiotics orally.
3. Collect appropriate culture samples and administer i.v. antibiotics. Samples may include swabs from the lids, canaliculi, nasopharynx and blood cultures.
4. Undertake surgical drainage of the infection and use antibiotics.

Option 1. Do nothing.

✓ Some mild periocular infections are self-limiting e.g. a stye may discharge itself with complete resolution, untreated.

✗ Resolution may not occur spontaneously, or may take some weeks to occur. Periocular infections can spread retrogradely to the orbit, cavernous sinus and brain, and in severe cases are fatal.

✗ Discharge of infections in some situations may lead to long-term problems, e.g. an infected nasolacrimal sac (dacryocystitis) may resolve itself by discharge through the skin, leading to creation of a permanent fistula from the sac to the skin and constant discharge through it. Early treatment avoids this.

Option 2. Give broad-spectrum antibiotics orally.

✓ Many cases of periocular infection will resolve. The tissues around the eye are well vascularized, and bactericidal levels of antibiotic may be rapidly achieved. Treatment can be as an out-patient.

✗ In children, a pre-septal cellulitis may rapidly spread to the posterior orbit. Simply prescribing antibiotic without addressing an underlying cause for infection, such as infected sinuses, will not lead to resolution. Posterior orbital cellulitis may be fatal. In adults, deterioration is generally less rapid, but the same principles apply that oral antibiotics alone will not suffice in the presence of any abscess or established infection.

✗ If any infection is not rapidly controlled, bacteriology will have been compromised by the use of broad-spectrum treatment.

Option 3. Collect appropriate culture samples and administer i.v. antibiotics. Samples may include swabs from the lids, canaliculi, nasopharynx and blood cultures.

✓ The large majority of periocular infections will resolve using this regimen. It is unusual to have to surgically drain a periocular infection.

✓ If the initial choice of antibiotic is not effective, sensitivity will soon be available to allow appropriate changes to be made.

✗ Intravenous antibiotic treatment requires hospitalization. This is time consuming, expensive and inconvenient to the patient. Fatal anaphylactic reactions can occur to i.v. drugs.

✗ Established sinus infection leading to orbital cellulitis by spread into the orbit through the very thin bony walls of the orbit will not resolve until the sinuses are drained. It is essential to have an early ENT opinion on children with orbital cellulitis who may become very ill very quickly if their sinuses are not treated.

Option 4. Undertake surgical drainage of the infection and use antibiotics.

✓ This will lead to the most rapid resolution of the infection, and in certain situations is the only treatment that will be effective.

✗ Drainage of some periocular structures may lead to damage, e.g. the lacrimal ductules may be damaged by surgical incision of the lacrimal gland leading to a chronic dry eye.

✗ The orbit is relatively inaccessible surgically. Posterior infection may be adjacent to the optic nerve, with obvious associated dangers in surgery.

✗ The associated oedema of tissues with infection will make identification of tissue planes difficult or impossible. Adequate drainage may be difficult to achieve.

History checklist

General

- History of systemic effects that any periocular infection may have led to, is important. In particular, fever in the presence of periocular swelling is suggestive of the presence of orbital cellulitis, which is life-threatening.
- A medical history should include enquiry into any predisposition to infection, e.g. in diabetes the fatal condition of orbital mucormycosis is sometimes seen. A history of alcohol abuse is almost always present in necrotizing fasciitis of the orbit.
- Sinus disease predisposes to orbital infection, particularly in children.
- Trauma may be quite trivial around the orbit, but lead to severe infectious consequences.

Specific

- Have the lids been subject to previous blepharitis? This may simply include symptoms of dry, gritty eyes, but may be more severe with chronic discharge and crusting. Any blepharitis predisposes to local infection.
- Is there a history of epiphora? If yes, this may be indicative of nasolacrimal obstruction, and consequent stasis of secretions within the nasolacrimal system, which is a strong predisposition to orbital cellulitis.
- Has the patient had recent eye surgery? If yes, the apparent periocular infection may be an indicator of endophthalmitis, and careful examination of the eye is required to exclude this.

Examination checklist

- Are the lids swollen? If yes, this is suggestive of orbital cellulitis. If there is also proptosis, pain on eye movement, or reduced pupil constriction to light, there is likely to be infection behind the orbital septum. This is a sinister sign which requires the patient to be admitted to hospital for urgent i.v. antibiotic. Pyrexia is also suggestive of spread of infection to the retroseptal space.
- Is there tenderness over the nasolacrimal sac? If yes, there is likely to be dacryocystitis, or infection within the sac. Often there is a history of epiphora. Compression of the nasolacrimal sac (situated deep to the skin below the inner angle of the eyelids) may lead to reflux of pus or mucopurulent material.

- Is there any obvious focus of infection in the eyelids? If yes, this is the likely cause of the associated lid swelling. A simple stye (hordeolum externum) or meibomian cyst (chalazion) may become infected and lead to an unpleasant cellulitis around it.
- Is the lacrimal gland tender? Dacryoadenitis is quite rare, and not always associated with infection. Lacrimal gland tumours can present with painful swelling which may masquerade as periocular infection. In bilateral lacrimal gland swelling, non-infective aetiologies, e.g. sarcoidosis, should be considered.

Referrals
- All patients with orbital cellulitis associated with proptosis, pyrexia, reduced ocular motility, abnormal pupil reaction or systemic malaise, should be admitted to hospital as an emergency.
- Adults with mild preseptal cellulitis in the absence of these signs can be treated as outpatients as long as they have regular and frequent review.
- Other cases of periocular infection are generally suitably managed in the community, unless unusual features develop which may require investigation, e.g. biopsy.
- Delayed patency of the nasolacrimal duct, which causes babies to have continued epiphora, are not usually treated surgically until the age of 9 months, unless infections are frequent and severe. Referral prior to this age is not usually indicated.

Rituals and myths
- Mucopurulent discharge from the lids should be treated with antibiotic. There is no need to treat such discharge, unless frank infection develops, with associated conjunctivitis. Many children with congenital non-patent nasolacrimal ducts receive multiple courses of topical antibiotic quite unnecessarily, and occasionally develop adverse reactions to such drugs. It is better just to cleanse the lids.
- Use topical antibiotics in adnexal infections. Topical treatment for systemic illness is not helpful, but many practitioners continue to use, for example, chloramphenicol drops in the presence of orbital cellulitis, where the appropriate treatment is administration of parenteral antibiotic. Used alone, topical treatment is dangerous, and used in conjunction with parenteral treatment, is superfluous.

Pitfalls
- Necrotizing fasciitis. This is an unusual necrotic reaction to infection with Streptococcus spp. and often follows minor trauma, particularly in patients with a history of alcohol abuse. Although it may appear as a standard case of orbital cellulitis, the spread along fascial planes is rapidly progressive, and systemic collapse and death may rapidly supervene through septic shock. Treatment is early and complete debridement of all necrotic tissue, with antibiotic. Absence of pin-prick sensation in the skin in cellulitis is suggestive of necrotizing fasciitis.
- Sinus disease. Early ENT opinion is important in all cases of orbital cellulitis, and particularly in children. Underlying sinus disease may not be obvious, but cellulitis secondary to sinus infection will not settle until this is addressed.
- Non-infective periocular inflammation. There are a number of unusual inflammatory diseases affecting the periocular tissues which may appear as infections. Lacrimal gland swelling and tenderness, particularly if bilateral, may be caused by inflammatory processes such as sarcoidosis, for example. Orbital cellulitis is mimicked by orbital pseudotumour, and biopsy is required to confirm this if suspected.
- Although very rare, rhabdomyosarcoma in children may present with an apparent infectious orbital cellulitis, but does not, of course, respond to antibiotic.

Hints for investigators and prescribers

- Collection of blood for culture is mandatory in any patient who is febrile, or with apparent soft tissue inflammation. Such patients, because they are at risk of local or distant septic complications, warrant broad-spectrum systemic antimicrobial therapy as a matter of urgency. Cover against all strains of Streptococcus pneumoniae and Haemophilus influenzae should be included in the chosen empirical regimen.
- For superficial infections of the eyelid, topical therapy may be appropriate, but ointment, not drops, should be applied.

Further reading

Hubert, L. (1937) Orbital infections due to nasal sinusitis. Study of 114 cases. *N. Y. State J. Med.* **37**: 1559–1564.

Israele, V. and Nelson, J.D. (1987) Periorbital and orbital cellulitis. *Paediatr. Infect. Dis. J.* **6**: 404–410.

Scott, G.I. (1960) Orbital cellulitis and cavernous sinus thrombosis. *Trans. Ophthalmol. Soc. UK* **80**: 435–450.

Chapter 6
GASTROINTESTINAL INFECTIONS

J.E. Coia

Chapter contents

1 Gastroenteritis

The symptoms of gastroenteritis may result from a variety of causes, including both infectious and non-infectious aetiologies. Clinical features may be limited primarily to the upper gastrointestinal tract, with nausea, vomiting and upper abdominal pain, or they may be predominantly referable to the lower tract with diarrhoeal features. In some cases there will be a mixture of upper and lower tract symptoms. The precise pattern of symptoms, their duration and onset in relation to possible consumption of incriminated foodstuffs etc., may provide important clues as to the underlying aetiology. A detailed consideration of all the possible causative agents and their potential discriminatory features is beyond the scope of this text, and the reader should refer to a standard microbiology or infectious diseases text.

Management options

1. Do nothing. No investigations or treatment.
2. Prescribe oral rehydration. No investigations.
3. Manage as for Option 2, but prescribe an anti-motility agent if there are diarrhoeal symptoms.
4. Manage as for Option 2, but prescribe an antibiotic active against the commonly isolated gastrointestinal pathogens.
5. Manage as for any of the above options, but send a stool specimen for culture as well.

Option 1. Do nothing. No investigations or treatment.

Advise the patient that most episodes of gastrointestinal upset are self-limiting. Suggest that they should return for further treatment/advice if symptoms persist.

✓ Cheap option which avoids investigation or treatment.
✓ Many trivial gastrointestinal problems will settle with this management.

✗ No specific diagnosis is obtained.
✗ The patient is unlikely to be happy that you are doing nothing to investigate or treat their unpleasant and distressing symptoms.
✗ The patient will be deterred from seeking medical advice in future.
✗ If symptoms are the result of infection with one of the wide range of infectious gastrointestinal pathogens, considerable avoidable morbidity (and even mortality in some cases), will occur.
✗ Outbreaks of infection may not be detected or controlled.

Option 2. Prescribe oral rehydration. No investigations.

Advise the patient that most episodes of gastrointestinal upset are self-limiting. Suggest that they should return for further treatment/advice if symptoms persist.

✓ Ensuring replenishment of lost fluids is often sufficient to manage episodes of gastroenteritis.
✓ No inconvenience or cost of investigation.

✗ No specific diagnosis is obtained.
✗ The patient may be unhappy that you are doing nothing to investigate or relieve their unpleasant and distressing symptoms.
✗ Outbreaks of infection may not be detected or controlled.
✗ Some infections with potentially serious sequelae may not be diagnosed promptly, e.g. verocytotoxigenic Escherichia coli infection.

Option 3. Manage as for Option 2, but prescribe an anti-motility agent if there are diarrhoeal symptoms.

✓ The patient may derive more rapid symptomatic relief.
✓ No inconvenience or cost of investigation.

✗ No specific diagnosis is obtained.
✗ Outbreaks of infection may not be detected or controlled.
✗ Some infections with potentially serious sequelae may not be diagnosed promptly, e.g. verocytotoxigenic E. coli infection.
✗ There is some evidence that anti-motility agents may be contraindicated in certain infections, e.g. patients with E. coli O157 infection are more likely to develop haemolytic uraemic syndrome if they have received these agents.

Option 4. Manage as for Option 2, but prescribe an antibiotic active against the commonly isolated gastrointestinal pathogens.

✓ The patient may derive more rapid symptomatic relief.
✓ No inconvenience or cost of investigation.

✗ No microbiological diagnosis.
✗ Outbreaks of infection may not be detected or controlled.
✗ Some infections with potentially serious sequelae may not be diagnosed promptly e.g. verocytotoxigenic E. coli infection.
✗ There is some evidence that anti-motility agents may be contraindicated in certain infections, e.g. patients with E. coli O157 infection are more likely to develop haemolytic uraemic syndrome if they have received these agents.
✗ A number of studies suggest that antibiotics may paradoxically prolong the duration of symptoms of gastroenteritis.

Option 5. Manage as for any of the above options, but send a stool specimen for culture as well.

✓ Investigation may be particularly useful in the patient whose symptoms do not settle promptly with simple measures, and in whom an infective aetiology cannot be otherwise excluded.
✓ A specific diagnosis may be obtained, which may help in avoiding sequelae of infection, advising on risk of cross infection, and detecting and managing outbreaks.
✓ Urgent investigation may be required in the setting of an ongoing outbreak.
✓ Valuable information about the epidemiology of infectious gastroenteritis may be obtained.
✓ If an antibiotic is thought to be required, a more appropriate agent may be selected in the light of any pathogens isolated.

✗ Inconvenience and expense of investigation.
✗ In many cases will not alter the management of the individual patient.

History checklist

General
- Duration of symptoms. If symptoms have been present for more than 3–4 weeks, an infectious aetiology is much less likely.
- Pattern of symptoms. An attempt should be made to ascertain the precise nature and pattern of symptoms present, e.g. is the problem predominantly nausea and vomiting, or are diarrhoeal symptoms the main feature. The precise frequency and nature of stools passed etc. may provide some useful clues as to aetiology (see Specific history below).

- Travel history. A history of recent foreign travel may increase the potential range of pathogens which should be considered, e.g. visits to areas where typhoid or cholera are endemic.
- Food history. The patient should be asked about consumption of raw or undercooked foods, variations from their usual diet, and, recent meals eaten in restaurants or from 'take away' shops. Specific enquiry about the consumption of unpasteurized dairy products and/or untreated waters should be made.
- Fever. A history of fever should be sought. The patient may complain of night sweats, needing to change pyjamas etc.
- Recent medication. Many drugs may produce gastrointestinal upset, and a history of recent medication, particularly antimicrobial therapy, should be sought.

Specific
- Blood or mucous in stool. The presence of blood or mucus in the stool may suggest dysenteric Campylobacter spp. or verocytotoxigenic E. coli infection.
- Similar symptoms in social/household contacts. The occurrence of similar symptoms in family/social contacts, particularly those who have shared common foodstuffs should suggest the possibility of a food-borne outbreak and/or secondary transmission.
- Animal exposure. Recent close contacts with wild or domestic animals or their excreta should be enquired about.

Rituals and myths
- Salmonella serology is a useful adjunct in the diagnosis of salmonellosis. The value of such serological investigation is doubtful, particularly in the investigation of non-typhoidal salmonellosis.
- Patients with diarrhoea should fast to rest the bowel. Dehydration is one of the most common and important complications of gastroenteritis, particularly in children.
- Antibiotics should never be given for the treatment of diarrhoea. Persistent or invasive infection, e.g. due to Salmonella spp. or Campylobacter spp., may require antibiotic therapy in order to eradicate the organism or control symptoms and avoid sequelae.

Pitfalls
- Anti-motility agents should not be prescribed for patients with verocytotoxigenic *E.coli* infection.
- Altered bowel habit, particularly persisting for more than 3–4 weeks is an important presenting feature of a variety of non-infectious conditions including gastrointestinal tumours and inflammatory bowel disease.
- Systemic spread of food-borne pathogens may result in septicaemic illness, particularly at the extremes of age, or the development of metastatic infection, e.g. Salmonella spp. osteomyelitis.

Hints for investigators and prescribers
- Specific oral rehydration therapy is particularly important in the management of gastroenteritis in children.
- If the history suggests an outbreak of food- or water-borne disease, the need to investigate and to notify the relevant public health authorities should be remembered.
- Although fluoroquinolones are widely used in the empiric management of traveller's diarrhoea, significant resistance among some of the common gastrointestinal pathogens has now been described, and may limit their usefulness in the management of such infections in the future.
- If the patient is pyrexial, immunosuppressed or systemically unwell, blood cultures should be collected.

Further reading

Anon. (1993) Gastrointestinal tract infections. In: *Medical Microbiology* (eds. C.A. Mims, J.H.L. Playfair, I.M. Roitt, D. Wakelin, R. Williams and R.M. Anderson). Mosby, London.

Anon. (1996) The management of infective gastroenteritis in adults. A concensus statement by an expert panel convened by the British Society for the Study of Infection. *J. Infect.* **33**: 143–152.

Guerrant, R.L., Hughes, J.M., Lima, N.L. *et al.* (1990) Microbiology of diarrhoea in developed and developing countries. *Rev. Infect. Dis.* **12**: S41–50.

Tallett, S., MacKenzie, C., Middleton, P. *et al.* (1947) Clinical, laboratory, and epidemiologic features of a viral gastroenteritis in infants and children. *Pediatrics* **60**: 217.

2 Antibiotic-associated diarrhoea

Antibiotic-associated diarrhoea (AAD) is a common complication of antimicrobial chemotherapy. The range and severity of symptoms may vary widely, from a mild self-limiting illness to a severe life-threatening colitis. The underlying pathogenic mechanism is thought to be a perturbation of the normal gut flora as a result of the action of the antibiotic. The more severe manifestations of AAD, which include pseudomembranous colitis (PMC) and the development of associated complications, e.g. toxic megacolon, are thought to be due to overgrowth of endogenously or exogenously acquired Clostridium difficile.

C. difficile may be isolated from the healthy gut in a small proportion of individuals. The isolation rate is increased in the elderly and in hospitalized patients. The normal gut flora usually prevents overgrowth as part of the phenomenon of 'colonization resistance'. The important virulence determinant is thought to be the production of potent cytotoxins. The significance of the isolation of non-toxigenic strains, even in the presence of symptoms, is uncertain.

Management options
1. Do nothing. No investigations or treatment.
2. Stop antibiotics.
3. Manage as for Option 2, but collect a stool specimen for culture and detection of C. difficile toxin.
4. Manage as for Option 3, but if C. difficile toxin is detected, prescribe oral metronidazole or vancomycin, which are active against this organism.
5. Manage as for Option 3, but prescribe oral metronidazole or vancomycin before laboratory results are available.

Option 1. Do nothing. No investigations or treatment.

Advise the patient that symptoms should settle on completion of the course of antibiotics. Tell the patient to return if symptoms persist.

✓ Cheap option which avoids investigation and treatment.
✓ May be effective in mild cases.

✗ If you have made the diagnosis, do you not want to do something about it?
✗ The patient is not likely to thank you for doing nothing about their unpleasant symptoms, particularly if you prescribed the antibiotics.
✗ AAD may progress with development of more severe manifestations.

Option 2. Stop antibiotics.

Advise the patient to return if symptoms persist or recur.

✓ Many patients will settle on this treatment.
✓ Simple and cheap option.

✗ Some patients may develop more severe manifestations.
✗ Specific microbiological diagnosis is not made.
✗ No specific therapy given which is active against C. difficile.

Option 3. Manage as for Option 2, but collect a stool specimen for culture and detection of C. difficile toxin.

✓ Specific microbiological diagnosis may be made.
✓ Presence of faecal cytotoxin may alert you to possible risk of development of more severe complications.

✓ Many patients will respond to this management.
✓ Other infectious cause of diarrhoea may be identified.

✗ Investigation required.
✗ No specific therapy given which is active against C. difficile.

Option 4. Manage as for Option 3, but if C. difficile toxin is detected, prescribe oral metronidazole or vancomycin, which are active against this organism.

✓ Specific therapy active against C. difficile may reduce risk of progression and/or limit duration of symptoms.
✓ The patient may be pleased to receive a prescription for something!

✗ Even if faecal cytotoxin is detected, the patient may not require specific therapy if symptoms are already settling.
✗ Even antibiotics which are active against C. difficile have been associated with causing AAD, so symptoms may be prolonged.
✗ Unnecessary use of antibiotics may promote the emergence of resistant organisms.

Option 5. Manage as for Option 3, but prescribe oral metronidazole or vancomycin before laboratory results are available.

✓ Specific therapy is given which is active against C. difficile.
✓ The patient may be happy to receive a prescription.
✓ Potential risk of development of more severe manifestations may be reduced if the symptoms are due to C. difficile.

✗ Even antibiotics which are active against C. difficile have been associated with causing AAD, so symptoms may be prolonged.
✗ Unnecessary use of antibiotics may promote the emergence of resistant organisms.
✗ Expensive option, as a large numbers of patients will be treated unnecessarily.

History checklist

General
- Diarrhoea. The frequency and nature of the diarrhoea should be assessed in order to gauge the severity of the illness.
- Abdominal pain. This may or may not be a feature of AAD.
- Vomiting. Other features of gastrointestinal intolerance, such as nausea and vomiting may be associated with antibiotics, but such features are not usually the result of C. difficile infection.

Specific
- Recent antibiotic therapy. AAD should be suspected in any patient who is currently receiving antibiotics, or who has had antibiotic therapy in the preceding 2–6 week period.
- Nosocomial acquisition. Any patient who is in or has recently come from a ward in which there have been other cases of C. difficile infection may be at risk, even without current or prior antibiotic therapy.
- Chemotherapy. A number of agents used in cancer chemotherapy may potentiate the risk of AAD as a result of their effects on the normal gut flora.
- Blood or mucus in stool. The presence of blood and/or mucus in the stool should alert the clinician to the possible development of more severe manifestations of AAD.

Rituals and myths

- All cases of AAD are the result of C. difficile infection. The majority of cases of simple AAD are not the result of C. difficile infection.
- It is only broad-spectrum antibiotics which produce AAD. Whilst broad-spectrum agents are more commonly the cause of AAD, virtually all antibiotics have been associated with producing this condition, including those used in the treatment of C. difficile infection!

Pitfalls

- Severe C. difficile infection is potentially life-threatening.
- C. difficile infection has been associated with a number of nosocomial outbreaks, and symptomatic patients should be nursed in source isolation.
- Patients who have had antibiotics recently may still have another infectious or non-infectious cause of diarrhoea.

Hints for investigators and prescribers

- The most useful investigation from a diagnostic standpoint for suspected C. difficile infection is detection of faecal cytotoxin. Although isolation of the organism may be useful from an epidemiological point of view, this may be time consuming, insensitive, and the significance of the isolation of non-toxigenic strains is doubtful.
- AAD arising from C. difficile infection is frequently relapsing in nature, and the possible need for repeated courses of therapy should be borne in mind.

Further reading

Borriello, S.P. (ed.) (1984) *Antibiotic Associated Diarrhoea and Colitis.* Martinus Nijhoff 1, Boston, MA.

Gebhard, R.L., Gerding, D.N., Olson, M.M., *et al.* (1985) Clinical and endoscopic findings in patients early in the course of Clostridium difficile-associated pseudomembranous colitis. *Am. J. Med.* **78**: 45–48.

Gerding, D.N. (1989) Diseases associated with Clostridium difficile infection. *Ann. Intern. Med.* **110**: 255.

Price, A.B. and Davies, D.R. (1977) Pseudomembranous colitis. *J. Clin. Pathol.* **30**: 1–12.

3 Cholecystitis

In over 80% of cases, inflammation of the gall-bladder is associated with the presence of calculi. The pathogenesis of this condition is thought to involve the impaction of these gallstones in the neck of the cystic duct which leads to obstruction. However, it has been increasingly appreciated in recent years that acalculous cholecystitis may arise in around 10% of cases. In studies which have cultured the bile in acute cholecystitis, bacteria have been isolated in 50–70% of cases. In the remainder, the inflammation is thought to derive from a variety of physical and chemical factors. Infection is much more commonly present in association with stones or instrumentation of the gall-bladder than in malignant obstruction.

The organisms involved in acute cholecystitis are most commonly components of the normal gut flora (coliform organisms, anaerobic rods and cocci, and enterococci), either in pure or in mixed culture. Emphysematous cholecystitis is an uncommon form of acute cholecystitis associated with gas formation due to Clostridium spp. If seen most commonly in elderly diabetic men, and is associated with significantly higher mortality than that of acute cholecystitis due to the more frequent occurrence of gangrene and perforation.

If complete or partial obstruction of the septic biliary tree occurs, then the serious complication of ascending cholangitis may develop. This is usually as a result of impacted calculi, although duct strictures, malignant lesions and pancreatitis can all cause this syndrome, characterized by the occurrence of jaundice, fever and rigors. Untreated, the syndrome may progress rapidly to the development of generalized sepsis, shock and the formation of a liver abscess.

Management options
1. Do nothing. No investigations or treatment.
2. Prescribe oral antibiotics. No investigations.
3. Manage as for Option 2, but investigate for the presence of gallstones and/or other obstruction within the biliary tree.
4. Manage as for Option 2, but arrange for urgent surgical referral. If bile is obtained by aspiration or surgical intervention, modify antibiotic therapy according to the sensitivities of any organisms isolated.

Option 1. Do nothing. No investigations or treatment.

Advise the patient to return if symptoms recur.

✓ Cheap option – no expensive investigations or treatment.

✗ No specific diagnosis is obtained.
✗ The patient is unlikely to be happy that you are doing nothing to investigate or treat their unpleasant and distressing symptoms.
✗ The patient will be deterred from seeking medical advice in future.
✗ Symptoms may worsen, and particularly if there is infection within the tract, complications including abscess formation, generalized sepsis and perforation may develop.

Option 2. Prescribe oral antibiotics. No investigations.

Advise the patient to return if symptoms recur.

✓ No expensive investigations.
✓ Mild, uncomplicated cases may settle.

✗ No specific diagnosis is obtained.

✗ The patient may be unhappy that you are doing nothing to investigate their unpleasant and distressing symptoms.

✗ Symptoms may worsen, and particularly if there is infection within the tract, complications including abscess formation, generalized sepsis and perforation may develop.

✗ Although this may be adequate for the management of some mild cases, recurrence may be a problem.

Option 3. Manage as for Option 2, but investigate for the presence of gallstones and/or other obstruction within the biliary tree.

✓ Specific diagnosis may be reached.

✓ If calculi and/or other obstruction are present then referral for subsequent definitive surgical management can be arranged.

✗ Symptoms may worsen, and particularly if there is infection within the tract, complications including abscess formation, generalized sepsis and perforation may develop in the interim.

Option 4. Manage as for Option 2, but arrange for urgent surgical referral. If bile is obtained by aspiration or surgical intervention, modify antibiotic therapy according to the sensitivities of any organisms isolated.

✓ Definitive diagnosis may be obtained.

✓ Development of complications may be more readily detected and/or avoided.

✗ There is much controversy about the nature and timing of appropriate surgical intervention in this condition.

✗ Many patients will not require acute surgical intervention.

History checklist

General
- Pain is typically localized to the right upper quadrant or the epigastrium, but more generalized abdominal pain may occur. The pain is typically severe and of sudden onset, rising quickly to maximum intensity. The pain does not occur in waves like intestinal colic and may typically last for an hour or more.
- Fever may be important in suggesting the possibility of infection in the tract.
- Nausea and vomiting may occur, often in association with the abdominal pain.

Specific
- Jaundice. The occurrence of jaundice should suggest the possibility of obstruction within the biliary tract.
- Recent surgery. Any history of recent surgery or instrumentation involving the biliary tree should be elicited.

Rituals and myths
- Patients with gallstones are fat, fair and fertile. Whilst some patients will undoubtedly find themselves in this category, gallstones can occur in a much wider group of individuals.

Pitfalls
- The development of jaundice without pain should raise the suspicion of underlying malignant disease impinging upon the biliary tree.
- Acute cholecystitis should not be confused with ascending cholangitis which requires urgent acute endoscopic or surgical intervention in combination with broad-spectrum intravenous antibiotics active against the major components of the gut flora. Even with appropriate treatment this condition carries a significant mortality.

Hints for investigators and prescribers

- Antibiotic therapy for cholecystitis should achieve adequate biliary concentration and be active against the main components of the gut flora, including coliform organisms, anaerobic rods and cocci, and enterococci.
- As outlined above, there is a great deal of controversy surrounding the issue of the most appropriate nature and timing of any surgical intervention in the management of cholecystitis.

Further reading

Berk, J.E. and Zinbers, S.S. (1985) Acute cholecystitis: medical aspects. In: *Gastroenterology*, 4th Edn (eds J.E. Berk, W.S. Haubrich, M.H. Kalser *et al.*). WB Saunders, Philadelphia, PA, pp. 3597–3616.

Jarvinen, H.J. and Hastbacka, J. (1980) Early cholecystectomy for acute cholecystitis: a prospective randomized study. *Ann. Surg.* **191**: 501–510.

Truedson, H., Elmros, T. and Holm, S. (1983) The incidence of bacteria in gall bladder bile at acute and elective cholecystectomy. *Acta Chir. Scand.* **149**: 307–313.

4 Liver abscess

Although relatively uncommon, liver abscesses usually arise as a result of the spread of infection from some other intra-abdominal source, most commonly in the biliary tree, to the liver. Haematogenous spread via the portal vein or hepatic artery is also important, but direct extension from an existing focus is not uncommon. Twenty per cent of cases have no evidence of any pre-existing infection. Pyogenic liver abscess is an important complication of liver transplantation.

Given that the majority of these abscesses arise as a result of pre-existing intra-abdominal infection, it is hardly surprising that the majority of organisms recovered from liver abscesses comprise components of the normal gut flora (coliform organisms, anaerobic rods and cocci, and enterococci), either in mixed or in pure culture. Streptococcus milleri and Staphylococcus aureus are important pathogens in liver abscess, and comprise a significant proportion of isolates. Some studies have suggested that anaerobes may play a role in almost half of these infections, frequently as components of mixed infections. Amoebic liver abscess (usually solitary) occurs as a complication of Entamoeba histolytica infection in 5–10% of cases.

As with other intra-abdominal abscesses, the morbidity and mortality which may be associated with untreated liver abscesses is high. The mortality associated with multiple small abscesses continues to be high relative to that with a solitary large abscess. The presentation of liver abscess may be insidious as the clinical features are often non-specific, particularly in the absence of any obvious predisposing cause.

Management options

1. Prescribe broad-spectrum antibiotics active against the main components of the gut flora, staphylococci and streptococci, and anaerobes.
2. Manage as for Option 1, but arrange for investigations to assess extent of abscess as appropriate, e.g. abdominal CT scan or ultrasound.
3. Arrange for investigations to assess extent of abscess as appropriate, e.g. abdominal CT scan or ultrasound, and drain the abscess.
4. Manage as for Option 3, but prescribe antibiotics as for Option 1.
5. Treat as for Option 4, but collect material for culture, and modify antibiotic therapy depending upon the sensitivities of any micro-organisms isolated.
6. Treat as for Option 5, but check amoebic serology if there is any history of previous dysenteric illness, particularly if there is a solitary abscess in the right lobe of the liver.

Option 1. Prescribe broad-spectrum antibiotics active against the main components of the gut flora, staphylococci and streptococci, and anaerobes.

Advise the patient to return if symptoms recur.

✓ Cheap option – no expensive investigations or complicated interventions.
✓ May occasionally be effective in very small abscesses.

✗ Symptomatic relief is likely to be short-lived, or non-existent in the presence of significant disease.
✗ Disease may progress on discontinuation of therapy.
✗ No specific antimicrobial therapy.
✗ Extent of disease is not assessed to confirm diagnosis or monitor outcome of therapy.
✗ Amoebic abscess will be inadequately treated.

Option 2. Manage as for Option 1, but arrange for investigations to assess extent of abscess as appropriate e.g. abdominal CT scan or ultrasound.

Advise the patient to return if symptoms recur.

✓ No complicated interventions.

✓ May occasionally be effective in very small abscesses.

✗ Symptomatic relief is likely to be short-lived, or non-existent in the presence of significant disease.

✗ Disease may progress on discontinuation of therapy.

✗ No specific antimicrobial therapy.

✗ Amoebic abscess will be inadequately treated.

Option 3. Arrange for investigations to assess extent of abscess as appropriate, e.g. abdominal CT scan or ultrasound, and drain the abscess.

Advise the patient to return if symptoms recur after drainage.

✓ Definitive management of underlying pathology.

✗ Disease may recur if residual infection persists.

✗ No specific antimicrobial therapy.

✗ Amoebic abscess will be inadequately treated.

Option 4. Manage as for Option 3, but prescribe antibiotics as for Option 1.

Advise the patient to return if symptoms recur after drainage.

✓ Definitive management of underlying pathology.

✓ Antibiotics should help minimize risk of recurrence.

✗ No microbiological diagnosis.

✗ No specific antimicrobial therapy.

✗ Amoebic abscess will be inadequately treated.

Option 5. Treat as for Option 4, but collect material for culture, and modify antibiotic therapy depending upon the sensitivities of any micro-organisms isolated.

✓ Definitive management of underlying pathology.

✓ Antibiotics should help minimize risk of recurrence.

✓ Specific microbiological diagnosis allows appropriate targeted therapy to be used.

✓ Spectrum of antimicrobials may be narrowed, which should help reduce side-effects.

✗ Costs increased.

✗ Amoebic abscess will be inadequately treated.

Option 6. Treat as for Option 5, but check amoebic serology if there is any history of previous dysenteric illness, particularly if there is a solitary abscess in the right lobe of the liver.

✓ Definitive management of underlying pathology.

✓ Antibiotics should help minimize risk of recurrence.

✓ Specific microbiological diagnosis allows appropriate targeted therapy to be used.

✓ Spectrum of antimicrobials may be narrowed, which should help reduce side-effects.

✓ Possible amoebic abscess is not missed.

✗ Costs increased.

History checklist

General

- Pain. Right upper quadrant pain may be a feature of liver abscess, but more generalized abdominal discomfort and referred pain to other sites may also occur, e.g. shoulder tip pain associated with diaphragmatic irritation.

- Fever, which may show characteristic recurrent spikes, is a frequent finding in patients with liver abscess.
- As with other intra-abdominal abscesses, the patient may complain of night sweats, needing to change pyjamas etc.
- Malaise. Non-specific malaise and lethargy, with or without associated weight loss, may be a feature of liver abscess.

Specific
- Predisposing primary intra-abdominal disease, trauma or recent surgery. Liver abscess should be suspected in any patient with a history of a predisposing lesion, e.g. cholecystitis/cholangitis, appendicitis or recent surgery. This is particularly the case in those patients who have had a stormy post-operative course.
- Nausea and vomiting may occur in association with liver abscess.
- Preceding dysentery. A history of preceding dysenteric illness should be sought, and this may raise the possibility of amoebic abscess.
- Abdominal distension. The patient may complain of abdominal fullness, distension or bloating.
- Respiratory symptoms. Occasionally patients may present with symptoms and signs of respiratory illness as a result of spread of infection through the diaphragm, and/or associated pleural effusion.

Rituals and myths
- Liver abscesses always produce abdominal pain. The symptoms and signs arising from liver abscess may be relatively non-specific, e.g. fever and night sweats.
- Appropriate antibiotic therapy alone, targeted against pathogens isolated from blood cultures or diagnostic aspirates, will always be effective in treating liver abscesses. Although some studies suggest that liver abscess may sometimes be adequately treated by antibiotics alone, most collections will require some form of drainage procedure if a successful prolonged cure is to be attained.

Pitfalls
- If the radiographic or other evidence suggests the possibility of hydatid disease, serologiocal tests for Echinicoccus species must be performed prior to any attempt at diagnostic or therapeutic drainage, as there is a significant risk of intra-abdominal dissemination.
- Untreated, or inadequately treated liver abscess is associated with significant mortality due to secondary bacteraemia, erosion of a major viscus or blood vessel, or the debilitating effects of a chronic inflammatory process.

Hints for investigators and prescribers
- Microbiological investigation of suspected liver abscess should include the collection of blood culture specimens, preferably before antibiotic therapy is instituted. The isolation of S. milleri in several blood cultures from patients with an indolent clinical course, and elevated liver enzymes in the absence of evidence of endocarditis should strongly suggest the diagnosis of liver abscess.
- Resolution of temperature, and monitoring of serial C-reactive protein measurements may be useful in assessing clinical progress. Antibiotic therapy should continue for at least 1 month (4 months for multiple abscesses).
- Additional empiric anti-amoebic therapy should be considered in any patient with a solitary right lobe abscess, even if bacteria are found in the aspirate fluid, because of the possibility of a secondarily infected amoebic abscess.

Further reading
Gerzof, S.G., Johnson, W.C., Robbins, A.H. *et al.* (1985) Intrahepatic pyogenic abscesses: treatment by percutaneous drainage. *Am. J. Surg.* 149: 487–494.

McCorkell, S.J. and Niles, N.C. (1985) Pyogenic liver abscess: another look at medical management. *Lancet* 1: 803–806.

Miedema, B.W. and Dineen, P. (1984) The diagnosis and treatment of pyogenic liver abscesses. *Ann. Surg.* 200: 328–335.

Reynolds, T.B. (1982) Medical treatment of pyogenic liver abscesses. *Ann. Intern. Med.* 96: 373–374.

5 Diverticulitis

As the average age of our population increases, so too do the problems associated with diverticular disease. Almost a third of those over the age of 60 are affected, and this figure rises to 60% in those older than 70. It is estimated that around a quarter of patients with diverticular disease are symptomatic.

Diverticular disease is a disease of the developed world, and is rare in many of the developing countries of Asia and Africa. It is currently believed that this reflects differences in dietary habits, particularly the lack of fibre in modern low-residue diets. This appears to result in increased intraluminal pressure in the colon which can produce herniations of the mucosa through weak points in the underlying musculature to produce a blind-ended sac or diverticulum. Although simple diverticular disease is initially asymptomatic, it is thought that thickening of the bowel wall and associated changes in the surrounding musculature can eventually produce symptoms of abdominal pain, even in the absence of significant inflammation.

Diverticulitis is an inflammatory process which results from perforation of the fundus of a diverticulum. This perforation, which may be large or small results in the development of pericolic inflammation with the formation of a local microabscess. The organisms involved comprise the normal aerobic and anaerobic flora of the large bowel, e.g. coliforms, enterococci and anaerobic rods and cocci. It appears that the majority of such perforations heal spontaneously with the development of associated adjacent fibrosis and granulation, which may in turn yield further symptoms.

Acute diverticulitis may be complicated by the development of an intra-abdominal abscess or even frank peritonitis. Other complications include the formation of associated fistulae or strictures, haemorrhage from erosion of a vessel in the bowel wall, and the development of intestinal obstruction.

The complications associated with acute diverticulitis may include generalized peritonitis, which might require emergency surgical intervention. Consideration of detailed surgical management is beyond the scope of this chapter.

Management options
1. Prescribe simple analgesics.
2. Prescribe simple analgesics, but with additional guidance.
3. Treat as for Option 2, but pay careful attention to fluid intake and diet. In mild cases manage in the community on liquid diet initially, with reintroduction of solids as symptoms improve. In more severe cases admit to hospital on nil by mouth diet with i.v. fluids. Reintroduce liquids then solids as symptoms improve.
4. Treat as for Option 3, but in addition prescribe antibiotics active against the common gut organisms to treat any associated infection. Administer orally in the community or intravenously in hospital. Consider possible requirement for acute surgical intervention.
5. Treat as for Option 4, but in addition arrange investigation such as sigmoidoscopy/colonoscopy, barium enema or even laparotomy when acute symptoms have resolved, to confirm the diagnosis and exclude underlying malignant disease. Consider possible requirement for acute surgical intervention.

Option 1. Prescribe simple analgesics.

Advise the patient to return if symptoms persist.

✓ Cheap option – no expensive drugs or investigations.
✓ May be effective in very mild episodes.

✗ Symptomatic relief is likely to be short-lived, or non-existent in the presence of significant disease.

✗ Alternative/additional pathology is not excluded, e.g. colonic carcinoma.
✗ No advice on helping to avoid further episodes, e.g. by increasing dietary fibre, use of laxatives etc.
✗ No specific antimicrobial therapy.

Option 2. Prescribe simple analgesics, but with additional guidance.

Advise the patient to return if symptoms persist. Advise patient on measures to help prevent further episodes, e.g. by increasing dietary fibre (fruit, vegetables, bran etc.) and avoiding constipation (use of mild laxatives if required).

✓ Cheap option – no expensive drugs or investigations.
✓ May be effective in very mild episodes.
✓ Advice may help to reduce/prevent recurrences.

✗ Symptomatic relief is likely to be short-lived, or non-existent in the presence of significant disease.
✗ Alternative/additional pathology is not excluded, e.g. colonic carcinoma.
✗ No specific antimicrobial therapy.

Option 3. Treat as for Option 2, but pay careful attention to fluid intake and diet. In mild cases manage in the community on liquid diet initially, with reintroduction of solids as symptoms improve. In more severe cases admit to hospital on nil by mouth diet with i.v. fluids. Reintroduce liquids then solids as symptoms improve.

Advise the patient on measures to help prevent further episodes, e.g. by increasing dietary fibre (fruit, vegetables, bran etc.) and avoiding constipation (use of mild laxatives if required).

✓ More effective management of symptoms.
✓ More adequate assessment and opportunity to observe for development of possible complications.
✓ Advice may help to reduce/prevent recurrences.

✗ Alternative/additional pathology is not excluded, e.g. colonic carcinoma.
✗ No specific antimicrobial therapy.

Option 4. Treat as for Option 3, but in addition prescribe antibiotics active against the common gut organisms to treat any associated infection. Administer orally in the community or intravenously in hospital. Consider possible requirement for acute surgical intervention.

✓ More effective management of symptoms.
✓ More adequate assessment and opportunity to observe for development of possible complications.
✓ Advice may help to reduce/prevent recurrences.
✓ Antibiotics may help to resolve acute symptoms and prevent infective complications, e.g. peritonitis and abscess formation.

✗ Alternative/additional pathology is not excluded, e.g. colonic carcinoma.

Option 5. Treat as for Option 4, but in addition arrange investigation such as sigmoidoscopy/colonoscopy, barium enema or even laparotomy when acute symptoms have resolved, to confirm the diagnosis and exclude underlying malignant disease. Consider possible requirement for acute surgical intervention.

✓ More effective management of symptoms.
✓ More adequate assessment and opportunity to observe for development of possible complications.

✓ Advice may help to reduce/prevent recurrences.
✓ Antibiotics may help to resolve acute symptoms and prevent infective complications, e.g. peritonitis and abscess formation.
✓ Alternative/additional pathology is excluded, e.g. colonic carcinoma.
✓ Patient anxiety may be reduced if malignant disease is excluded.

✗ Investigation may be expensive.
✗ Investigations have associated morbidity and mortality.
✗ Investigations are uncomfortable and may increase patient anxiety, even if negative.

History checklist

General
- Alteration of bowel habit. Acute diverticulitis may complicate long-standing diverticular disease which frequently results in episodes of constipation which may alternate with bouts of diarrhoea.
- Acute diverticulitis is commonly accompanied by fever, which is often swinging in nature, and related features should be specifically enquired about, e.g. sweats etc.
- Vomiting may occur, either as part of generalized systemic upset, or due to the presence of some degree of intestinal obstruction.
- Weight loss. Excessive or unplanned weight loss may suggest an alternative diagnosis, e.g. colonic carcinoma.

Specific
- Acute diverticulitis is frequently accompanied by the onset of central abdominal pain which usually shifts to the left iliac fossa (diverticulae are found most commonly in the sigmoid and descending colon and become increasingly rare in passing from the left to right side of the colon).
- Gastrointestinal bleeding. Passage of bright red blood, melaena or mucus may all be associated with diverticular disease.

Rituals and myths
- Diverticulitis always presents as left-sided abdominal pain. Although acute diverticulitis has been referred to as 'left-sided' appendicitis because of the relative frequency with which the descending and sigmoid colon are affected, patients can present with right-sided symptoms.
- The development of peritonitis is always accompanied by fever. The septic elderly patient may not uncommonly be afebrile, or even hypothermic at presentation.

Pitfalls
- Diverticulitis and colonic cancer may present in a very similar manner, and indeed the conditions may coexist. Although barium studies and colonoscopy may be helpful, it may be impossible to make the diagnosis except at laparotomy.
- Large bowel perforation and peritonitis may be rapidly fatal in the elderly patient. If there is any doubt, it is prudent to observe the patient carefully and request a surgical opinion.

Hints for investigators and prescribers
- Antibiotic therapy for acute diverticulitis should be sufficiently broad-spectrum to provide cover for the bulk of the normal faecal flora, including coliforms, anaerobes and enterococci. Harsh laxatives are generally best avoided in the management of constipation related to diverticular disease.

- Surgery is seldom indicated to prevent recurrence after a single uncomplicated episode of diverticulitis, as 70% of patients who have recovered will have no recurrence.
- If opioid medication is required, morphine, which raises intracolonic pressure, is best avoided. Meperidine hydrochloride is a suitable alternative.

Further reading

Chappius, C.W. and Cohn, I. (1988) Acute colonic diverticulitis. *Surg. Clin. N. Am.* **68**: 301.

Rodkey, G.V. (1994) Diverticular disease: diverticulitis, bleeding, and fistula. In: *Oxford Textbook of Surgery* (eds P.J. Morris and R.A. Malt). Oxford University Press, Oxford, pp. 1025–1036.

6 Dyspepsia

The term dyspepsia refers to a variety of clinical symptoms related to the upper gastrointestinal tract. It has formally been defined as 'upper abdominal or retrosternal pain, discomfort, heartburn, nausea, vomiting or other symptoms considered to be referable to the proximal alimentary tract'.

Dyspepsia is one of the most common chronic medical disorders, affecting 40% of the UK population and accounting for 5% of general practice consultations and almost one-third of gastroenterology referrals. Around half of all dyspeptic patients who are examined endoscopically have an underlying lesion. In order of prevalence in the UK these are oesophagitis, duodenal ulcer (DU), gastric ulcer (GU), and gastro-oesophageal malignancy. The remainder have no obvious underlying lesion and the term 'non-ulcer dyspepsia' is commonly used to describe this clinical entity.

The symptomatic management of the dyspeptic patient has been revolutionized over the last 15 years by the advent of agents which can successfully suppress gastric acid secretion. These H_2 receptor antagonist (H2RA) and proton pump inhibitor (PPI) drugs are now among the most widely prescribed medicines in the developed world. More recently the discovery that Helicobacter pylori, a spiral bacterium which is thought to infect the stomach of about half the population, is responsible for most DUs and many benign GUs, has led to the development of treatment strategies for dyspepsia, based upon eradication of the organism. There is also increasing evidence that long-term colonization/infection may result in the development of gastric malignancy.

The following section will consider the management of the dyspeptic patient with particular reference to the possibility of underlying H. pylori infection. It is not intended to provide a detailed account of the medical and/or surgical options for the management of the other non-infectious causes of dyspepsia.

Management options

1. Prescribe simple antacids.
2. Manage as for Option 1. If symptoms persist or recur prescribe an H2RA or PPI drug.
3. Manage as for Option 1. If symptoms persist or recur prescribe eradication therapy (combination of antibiotics and acid-lowering agents as outlined below) for possible H. pylori infection.
4. Manage as for Option 1. If symptoms persist or recur refer the patient for investigation by barium meal or endoscopy and biopsy. If uncomplicated DU, manage as for Option 3. If complicated peptic ulcer (PU) (previous ulcer complication, e.g. bleeding or perforation), manage as Option 3 and confirm eradication by means of urea breath test or repeat endoscopy. If GU then manage as Option 3 and confirm H. pylori eradication and ulcer healing by endoscopy after 8 weeks. If no lesion is found, reassure the patient, manage symptomatically and consider gastroenterology referral.
5. Manage as for Option 1. If symptoms persist or recur and the patient is <45 and has no alarm features (weight loss >3 kg; dysphagia/vomiting; gastrointestinal bleeding; steroid/nonsteroidal anti-inflammatory drug (NSAID) treatment; previous GU or gastric surgery), then manage as for Option 3. If alarm features present or age >45, then manage as for Option 4.
6. Manage as for Option 1. If symptoms persist or recur and the patient is <45 and has no alarm features (see Option 5), then perform an H. pylori serology or urea breath test. If this is positive, manage as for Option 3. If this is negative consider alternative diagnosis and need for possible gastroenterology referral. If alarm features present or age >45 then manage as for Option 4.
7. Manage as for Option 4 or 6, but confirm eradication of H. pylori in all uncomplicated DU cases who are treated.

8. Manage as for Option 4 or 6, but only confirm eradication of H. pylori in uncomplicated DU cases who are treated, but in whom symptoms recur.

Option 1. Prescribe simple antacids.

Advise the patient to avoid known aggravating factors (e.g. spicy food or excessive alcohol consumption). Advise patient to return if symptoms persist.

✓ Cheap option – no expensive drugs or investigations.
✓ Should deal with trivial, non-recurrent symptoms which are not related to underlying upper gastrointestinal pathology.
✓ No costly investigations.

✗ Symptomatic relief is likely to be short-lived if there is significant underlying pathology.
✗ Repeated prescription of agents which relieve symptoms may delay the diagnosis of serious disease e.g. gastric malignancy.
✗ Advice on lifestyle modification (e.g. reducing alcohol intake or avoiding spicy foods etc.) is not infrequently ignored!

Option 2. Manage as for Option 1. If symptoms persist or recur prescribe an H2RA or PPI drug.

Advise the patient that symptoms may recur on discontinuation of therapy.

✓ Very effective gastric acid suppression – will often yield good symptomatic control.
✓ No costly investigations.

✗ Repeated prescription of agents which relieve symptoms may delay the diagnosis of serious disease, e.g. gastric malignancy.
✗ Since the natural history of peptic ulcer is recurrent, long-term repeated prescription of expensive drugs will be required.
✗ Underlying potentially treatable pathology may be ignored (e.g. peptic ulcer or gastric malignancy.

Option 3. Manage as for Option 1. If symptoms persist or recur prescribe eradication therapy (combination of antibiotics and acid-lowering agents as outlined below) for possible H. pylori infection.

Tell the patient that symptoms may persist for several weeks after eradication and that acid-suppressive therapy alone may need to be continued during this period. Advise the patient that antibiotics may produce diarrhoea, and if appropriate that they may interact with the oral contraceptive pill. If metronidazole is included in the eradication regime, warn the patient of disulfram-like side-effects if alcohol is consumed.

✓ Successful eradication of H. pylori in patients with PU (not associated with NSAID therapy) will achieve long-term cure in 85% of cases.
✓ The patient does not require long-term expensive medication.
✓ Complications of chronic and/or severe peptic ulceration are avoided:
✓ Possible long-term sequelae of H. pylori infection are avoided, e.g. gastric malignancy.
✓ No costly investigations.

✗ No proven benefit to those patients who do not have peptic ulceration due to H. pylori.
✗ Repeated prescription of agents which relieve symptoms may delay the diagnosis of serious disease, e.g. gastric malignancy.
✗ Other underlying potentially treatable pathology is ignored.

Option 4. Manage as for Option 1. If symptoms persist or recur refer the patient for investigation by barium meal or endoscopy and biopsy. If uncomplicated DU, manage as for Option 3. If complicated peptic ulcer (PU) (previous ulcer complication, e.g. bleeding or perforation), manage as Option 3 and confirm eradication by means of urea breath test or repeat endoscopy. If GU then manage as Option 3 and confirm H. pylori eradication and ulcer healing by endoscopy after 8 weeks. If no lesion is found, reassure the patient, manage symptomatically and consider gastroenterology referral.

✓ Accurate diagnosis is obtained, particularly if endoscopy and biopsy performed.
✓ Appropriate management can be selected.
✓ Serious pathology can be identified and treated promptly. Complications of chronic and/or severe peptic ulceration are avoided.
✓ Possible long-term sequelae of H. pylori infection are avoided, e.g. gastric malignancy.
✓ Complications of chronic and/or severe peptic ulceration are avoided.
✓ Negative investigation result may be reassuring for the patient.

✗ Prohibitively expensive, impractical and inappropriate to subject all patients to such extensive investigation.
✗ Unnecessary exposure of patients to associated risks of these investigations.
✗ Facilities to investigate all dyspeptic patients in this manner are unlikely to be available, and paradoxically this may result in an increased delay in investigating those who have alarming features in their history.
✗ Patient anxiety about the investigation.
✗ Negative investigation result may be alarming for the patient!

Option 5. Manage as for Option 1. If symptoms persist or recur and the patient is <45 and has no alarm features (weight loss >3kg; dysphagia/vomiting; gastrointestinal bleeding; steroid/non-steroidal anti-inflammatory drug (NSAID) treatment; previous GU or gastric surgery), then manage as for Option 3. If alarm features present or age >45, then manage as for Option 4.

✓ Further investigations with their associated risks, expense and inconvenience are more effectively targeted.
✓ Treatment is better targeted.

✗ Patients who are not infected with H. pylori may inappropriately receive eradication therapy.
✗ A very small minority of patients under 45 who do have sinister underlying pathology may be inappropriately treated/reassured.

Option 6. Manage as for Option 1. If symptoms persist or recur and the patient is <45 and has no alarm features (see Option 5), then perform an H. pylori serology or urea breath test. If this is positive manage as for Option 3. If this is negative consider alternative diagnosis and need for possible gastroenterology referral. If alarm features present or age >45, then manage as for Option 4.

✓ Further investigations with their associated risks, expense and inconvenience are more effectively targeted.
✓ Treatment is better targeted.

✗ A small percentage of false positive and negative serological results will be obtained. Particular care should be taken with kit tests designed for use in the doctors office, to ensure that these are adequately quality controlled and correctly interpreted by the practitioner.
✗ A very small minority of patients <45 who do have sinister underlying pathology may be inappropriately treated/reassured.

Option 7. Manage as for Option 4 or 6, but confirm eradication of H. pylori in all uncomplicated DU cases who are treated.

✓ May reassure the anxious patient.
✓ May reassure the anxious doctor!

✗ In the uncomplicated patient who is treated and becomes asymptomatic there may be little to be gained.
✗ Extra expense.
✗ Extra inconvenience.

Option 8. Manage as for Option 4 or 6, but only confirm eradication of H. pylori in uncomplicated DU cases who are treated, but in whom symptoms recur.

✓ More effectively targets follow up investigation.
✓ Reduces expense compared to Option 7.
✓ Reduces inconvenience compared to Option 7.

✗ May fail to identify some patients with persistent colonization.
✗ Still expensive.

History checklist

General
- Duration of symptoms? Dyspeptic symptoms are extremely common in the general population, and it may be useful at the outset to establish that this is a recurrent and/or ongoing problem. Onset of symptoms at age >45 should alert the clinician to the increased possibility of underlying malignancy.
- Localization of symptoms? Well-localized epigastric pain is classically associated with 'ulcer-like' dyspepsia, whereas more generalized upper abdominal discomfort is thought to be more characteristic of 'dysmotility-like' dyspepsia. Although many experienced clinicians feel that useful aetiological clues may be obtained from this information, it is clear that subsequent endoscopic findings are frequently discordant with the clinical subgrouping.
- Aggravating and relieving factors? The patient should be asked about anything which exacerbates (e.g. spicy food or excessive alcohol consumption) or relieves (e.g. milk or simple antacids) symptoms.

Specific
- Weight loss? Recent weight loss exceeding 3 kg should alert the clinician to the presence of serious underlying pathology.
- Dysphagia and/or vomiting? Features of upper intestinal obstruction suggest more serious and/or complicated disease.
- Gastrointestinal bleeding? Features of gastrointestinal haemorrhage suggest more serious and/or complicated disease.
- Drug therapy? The use of steroids and NSAIDs are important risk factors for the development of peptic ulceration.
- Previously diagnosed PU? The natural history of PU disease is recurrent, and many patients will have been diagnosed in the past, and should specifically be questioned about this.

Referrals
- Even in the uncomplicated patient under 45 years of age, if H. pylori infection persists with recurrent peptic ulceration, referral to a gastroenterologist should be considered to exclude the possibility of upper gastrointestinal malignancy.

- If a pathological lesion other than PU is found on investigation, referral to a gastroenterologist for further appropriate specialist management should be considered.

Rituals and myths
- Dietary advice is particularly important in peptic ulcer disease. There is little clinical evidence that dietary modification plays a major role in this disease.
- Symptoms alone are sufficient to provide an accurate aetiological diagnosis. There may be significant overlap in the clinical features of the various upper gastrointestinal lesions which may present with dyspepsia.

Pitfalls
- Persistent symptoms despite H. pylori eradication should suggest an alternative diagnosis, which may include a range of benign (e.g. gastro-oesophageal reflux disease) and malignant (e.g. gastric cancer) conditions.
- Healing of GUs should be confirmed.

Hints for investigators and prescribers
- A positive H. pylori blood test indicates H. pylori infection at some time. However, blood tests cannot distinguish between previous and current H. pylori infection, as they remain positive for several months after eradication. The urea breath test remains the most suitable non-invasive procedure to confirm eradication of H. pylori.
- If it is proposed to utilize 'near-patient' serological tests in the doctors office environment, these must be adequately quality controlled and properly performed.
- As discussed above, although useful clues as to the true dyspeptic nature of the patient's symptoms may be gleaned from information on aggravating and relieving factors, the subsequent correlation of clinical impression with the underlying pathological lesion may be poor.
- Most eradication regimes which are currently recommended comprise a combination of two antibiotics and a PPI given for 1–2 weeks. Such a regimen should eradicate H. pylori in 85% of cases. Acid-lowering therapy enhances H. pylori eradication. Long-term acid lowering therapy may still be required in those patients with complications, e.g. previous perforation, haemorrhage or ongoing NSAID therapy.
- Endoscopy in patients who have taken PPI drugs in the previous 4 weeks is often normal and cannot reliably exclude peptic ulcer disease.

Further reading

Colin-Jones, D.G., Bloom, B., Bodenar, G. et al. (1988) Management of dyspepsia: report of a working party. Lancet 336: 576–579.

Jones, R.H., Lydeard, S.E., Hobbs, F.D. et al. (1990) Dyspepsia in England and Scotland. Gut 31: 401–405.

Lind, T., Velhuyzen van Zanten, S.J.O., Unge, P. et al. (1995) The Mach 1 study: optimal one-week treatment for H. pylori defined? Gut 37 (suppl. 2): A7.

Patel, D., Khulusi, S., Mendall, M.A., Lloyd, R., Jazrawi, R., Maxwell, J.D. et al. (1995) Prospective screening of dyspeptic patients by Helicobacter pylori serology. Lancet 346: 1315–1318.

Richter, J.E. (1991) Dyspepsia: organic causes and differential characteristics from functional dyspepsia. Scand. J. Gastroenterol. 26 (suppl. 182): 11–16.

Sung, J.J., Chung, S.C., Ling, T.K., Yung, M.Y., Leung, V.K., Ng, E.K.W. et al. (1995) Antibacterial treatment of gastric ulcers associated with Helicobacter pylori. N. Engl. J. Med. 332: 139–142.

The Eurogast Study Group. (1993) An international association between Helicobacter pylori infection and gastric cancer. Lancet 341: 1359–1362.

Weiss, J., Mecca, J., da Silva, E. and Gassner, D. (1994) Comparison of PCR and other diagnostic techniques for detection of Helicobacter pylori infection in dyspeptic patients. J. Clin. Microbiol. 32: 1663–1668.

Chapter 7
GENITAL INFECTIONS

C. O'Mahony

In the UK there is an extensive network of genito-urinary medicine (GUM) clinics that see the majority of sexually transmitted diseases (STDs). Many patients, however, present to primary care and other professionals, so the process of history, investigation and management needs to be understood widely. Sexual history-taking is a delicate process that becomes easier with experience. The majority of these infections, if managed appropriately, have a highly successful outcome. It is when short cuts and exceptions are made that difficulties ensue.

Interpreting the evidence has to begin with considering the possibility that the presenting problem might be sexually acquired. This is a simple assumption that can be readily made within the setting of a GUM clinic, i.e. the patient has attended the clinic specifically for the purpose of discussing an infection which may possibly have been sexually transmitted. However, in primary care and other settings the patient may be totally unaware of this possibility and the history-taking requires even greater delicacy and tact. Even if the likely outcome of the history-taking is a referral to a GUM clinic, clinicians outside such a setting should be able to inform the patient of the likely procedures, investigations, forms of treatment and the high success rate expected.

Effective management of these conditions requires a thorough understanding of the laboratory facilities at one's disposal, and the time-honoured tradition of elucidating and treating the contact(s) is of paramount importance.

Chapter contents

1 Urethral discharge

Inflammation of the urethra is usually accompanied by discharge and dysuria. The commonest causes are STDs and these are best investigated and managed within the free, confidential and easy access GUM clinics in the UK. The most common identifiable causes are Chlamydia trachomatis and Neisseria gonorrhoeae, but commonly the term non-specific urethritis (NSU) is used as no agent is identified.

Management options

1. Prescribe antibiotics that you are fairly sure will eradicate the common causes and ask the patient to come back only if the discharge does not clear.
2. Collect a swab for N. gonorrhoeae, and if you have the facility, collect a swab (or in some parts of the country a urine) for C. trachomatis, and send all specimens to the laboratory. Prescribe an antibiotic likely to cure gonorrhoea, e.g. a quinolone, and ask the patient to return in a week.
3. Do a urethral Gram stain and collect swabs for N. gonorrhoeae and C. trachomatis. If gonococci are noted on the Gram stain, prescribe antibiotics for gonorrhoea and chlamydial infection (quinolone, followed by a tetracycline for 2 weeks). If gonococci are not noted on the Gram stain, just pus cells, then prescribe the tetracycline for 2 weeks.

Option 1. Prescribe antibiotics that you are fairly sure will eradicate the common causes and ask the patient to come back only if the discharge does not clear.

✓ Many patients would like this approach, as there are no swabs and no firm diagnosis is established to label them as having an STD.
✓ This type of management can be done anywhere, as no investigative facilities are needed.
✓ If the infection is sexually transmitted and has been acquired from a recent casual encounter, and the individual has not had sex with their regular partner yet, this can eradicate the problem and the partner will never find out about the incident.

✗ No diagnosis is made, no contact-trace is possible, and sensitivities are not available, should the discharge not respond to the therapy.
✗ If the infection does not clear up, further investigation has been hampered by the early use of antibiotics.
✗ Epidemiological information, useful to society in general, is missed. Incidence and sensitivities of N. gonorrhoeae are important for society's management of this particular STD.

Option 2. Collect a swab for N. gonorrhoeae, and if you have the facility, collect a swab (or in some parts of the country a urine) for C. trachomatis, and send all specimens to the laboratory. Prescribe an antibiotic likely to cure gonorrhoea, e.g. a quinolone, and ask the patient to return in a week.

✓ Results will be available, and if gonorrhoea is confirmed, it will have been treated and the sensitivities checked.
✓ If C. trachomatis is found, it can then be specifically treated.
✓ The diagnosis of the discharge will be firmly established and contacts can be advised accurately.

✗ The patient may not re-attend, and further treatment for chlamydial infection or postgonococcal urethritis would not be initiated.
✗ A further week will have elapsed, and if the patient does have chlamydial infection, infection of new contacts could have occurred.

Option 3. Do a urethral Gram stain and collect swabs for N. gonorrhoeae and C. trachomatis. If gonococci are noted on the Gram stain, prescribe antibiotics for gonorrhoea and chlamydial infection (quinolone, followed by a tetracycline for 2 weeks). If gonococci are not noted on the Gram stain, just pus cells, then prescribe the tetracycline for 2 weeks.

✓ Sensitivities will be available if N. gonorrhoeae is the cause.

✓ A definitive diagnosis will be made, which allows detailed information to be given to the patient about the diagnosis, and helps epidemiological surveillance.

✓ Prescribing for chlamydial infection, as well as gonorrhoea, when a diagnosis of gonorrhoea has been made, eliminates the high incidence of post-gonococcal urethritis, much of which can be C. trachomatis-associated.

✓ If contact-tracing has been successful, the exact nature of the infection allows optional management of the traced contact.

✗ Leads to some overtreatment if post-gonococcal urethritis would not have occurred.

History checklist

- Is there a urethral discharge? Patients must be asked specifically about 'something leaking from the tip of the penis', as it is critical to establish whether there really is a discharge from the urethra. Some patients with simple balanitis can have discharge collecting under the prepuce and this can be mistaken for urethral discharge.
- When does the discharge occur? Most chlamydial and NSU-type urethral discharge tends to be scanty and more noticeable first thing in the morning, prior to passing urine, when there has been no flushing out of the urethra.
- What colour is the discharge? Patients describing a green or yellow discharge always have a significant pathological process, whereas, a clear or mucoid discharge can occasionally be normal.
- Is there dysuria? This can be very significant, as some patients can be unsure about the discharge, but can be quite passionate about the degree of dysuria, describing it as like 'peeing broken glass'.
- Do the symptoms suggest pathology higher up, i.e. frequency, loin pain, fever, blood in the urine? All of these suggest a urinary tract infection (UTI) as the likely cause.
- Are there any other pathological features in the genital area, i.e. any ulcers on the penis? As well as causing ulcers on the shaft, prepuce and glans, herpes simplex virus (HSV) can cause urethral ulcers which would give rise to a discharge.
- Is there a past history of NSU or gonorrhoea, or investigations for urethral discharge? Patients who have had a previous episode are often quite knowledgeable and can be quite adamant that their present symptoms are exactly the same as the last time they were diagnosed with chlamydial infection etc.
- Is the partner well? It is clearly very significant if the partner has recently been diagnosed as having a problem, or if it is a female partner, is she being treated for pelvic inflammatory disease (PID) or vaginal discharge.
- Has there been a recent partner change? Enquiring about the sexual history can be fraught with difficulties, but with experience, becomes easy.
- What is the sexual orientation? The sites of investigation and subsequent management can depend on whether the individual is homo-, hetero- or bisexual. Again, this can be a delicate area to explore, but the opportunity usually arises at some stage during the consultation for these questions to be asked in a non-threatening fashion.
- Has there been a sexual risk abroad? Contacts abroad are often unprotected and carry a higher risk of acquiring a STD. Also, the range of STDs acquired abroad is likely to be wider than in the UK.
- Have any antibiotics been taken recently, prescribed or not? Some patients are embarrassed about the infection and often raid the cupboard at home to see what antibiotics might be left over from a previous episode – this can complicate subsequent investigations.

- Are there any systemic features, such as joint pain or conjunctivitis or has there recently been a significant gastrointestinal infection, e.g. salmonella, shigella, etc? All of these might point to a concomitant reactive arthropathy which is often associated with a urethral discharge which is not infective, but more likely to be immunological.
- How long is it since passing urine? Obviously, if someone has passed urine while out in the waiting room, a scanty urethral discharge would have been washed away and there may be little to find on examination. Most GUM clinics are so aware of this that there is often a notice in the male toilet, advising patients who have not yet been examined, not to pass urine if at all possible!
- Are any other sites in the genital area affected, i.e. is there pain in the testes or suprapubically?

Examination checklist
- Feel the inguinal glands. It is best to examine the inguinal area first rather than pounce straight on the genitalia in an anxious young patient. Significant inguinal adenopathy is noted with genital herpes and syphilis, and some tropical STDs.
- Examine the testes and epididymis. If there is epididymo-orchitis, the scrotum may look inflamed and it may be obvious that there is an enlarged testes or epididymis, unilateral more often than not. If there is no acute problem, it is worth feeling the epididymis to look for cysts or fibrosis.
- Penis. There may be an obvious green or yellow discharge from the urethra. If not, it may be necessary to retract the foreskin somewhat to see the urethral tip. If there is no discharge, it is important to strip the urethra, i.e. hold the penis in one hand and gently stroke a finger underneath the penis along the urethral tract from as far back as can comfortably be reached, drawing fluid down the urethra towards the urethral orifice. The vast majority of urethral discharges are scanty and this procedure is crucial if proper specimens are to be obtained for Gram stain and culture, or enzyme-linked immunosorbent assay tests.
- Penile skin. Examine the prepuce and shaft for other lesions, i.e. ulcers or even a candidal balanitis. If there is extensive inflammation at the head of the penis, it is not unusual to find increased numbers of pus cells in the urethra and this may not, in fact, be urethritis, but more a reflection of the general inflammation. Therefore, Gram stains have to be interpreted cautiously in the presence of other infections of the head of the penis.
- Urine examination. The traditional time-honoured examination of first and second catch urines is not always necessary and, indeed, if there is a significant discharge and adequate swabs are taken, examining first and second catch urines contribute little to the management. Urines are, however, useful when there is some doubt over the presence of a discharge, and other findings are equivocal. It can be useful to fish out a thread from the first catch urine, but the whole tradition of attaching significance to threads in urine can be fraught with difficulty and a pitfall for the unwary. Some patients with absolutely no symptoms of urethritis or any urinary problems can have threads in the urine which may be of no significance. Doctors suddenly attaching great importance to their presence can alarm the patient, and create yet another self-examiner.

Referrals
- If at all possible, urethral discharge should be managed within the exceptionally successful GUM service throughout the UK. Patients can attend these clinics of their own accord, i.e. without being referred by anyone. The telephone numbers are readily available under 'Special Clinics', 'GUM' or 'General Hospital Enquiries'. The clinics are extremely particular about confidentiality and patients will often be less inhibited about discussing their problems with an impartial professional than with their GP whom they may have known for years.
- Many patients will put their GP under pressure to treat them rather than refer to a GUM clinic, but non-specialists should resist this pressure. If a GP is familiar with the location

and personnel of the local GUM clinic, his reassurance to the patient about the quality of the service is more convincing.

Rituals and myths

- GUM/special/venereal disease (VD) clinics are seedy places populated by unsavoury characters and staffed by professionals who could not make it in their original chosen careers. If this is your impression, it is time to revisit your local GUM clinic and savour the atmosphere, which should be that of a modern, well appointed clinic, staffed by kind and sympathetic professionals who chose the specialty because they are good at communication and putting patients at ease.
- All urethral discharges are caused by VD therefore somebody must have been unfaithful and someone is to blame. This is a dangerous assumption and is patently untrue. For example, the urethral discharge that occurs with a Reiter's type syndrome, secondary to salmonella or shigella gastrointestinal infection, is clearly not sexually transmitted.
- Repeated follow-up examinations and test of cures are necessary after treatment for urethral discharge. This is actually contraindicated, as this type of management is likely to unearth a syndrome of recurrent NSU, which can be induced in the patient by inexperienced doctors repeatedly finding evidence of inflammation on urethral Gram stain or religiously analysing first catch specimens in an otherwise healthy and asymptomatic patient.
- Urethral swabs need to be introduced up to 5 cm and rotated several times for valid results. This often quoted myth has little evidence to back it up and patients who have been subjected to this type of over-enthusiastic swabbing, often feel they have been subjected to the famous 'umbrella test'. This is a legacy from ancient times, when an instrument used to be inserted into the urethra, opened slightly and then withdrawn, to give cell scrapings. Many patients coming to GUM clinics have heard of the 'umbrella test' and are adamant that nothing like that should be done to them. However, with experience, a cotton-tipped ENT-type swab can be gently inserted into the urethra, no more than 1–3 cm, with minimal discomfort.

Pitfalls

- The finding of Gram-negative diplococci on Gram staining of urethral discharge almost always indicates gonorrhoea. However, some of these cases can be due to Neisseria meningitidis which, of course, should still be treated. It will respond to the antigonococcal therapy, but a diagnosis of gonorrhoea should not be made and subsequent management of contacts may be different.
- If intracellular Gram-negative diplococci are noted on a Gram stain of the urethral discharge, it is important to swab other sites that may have been affected, i.e. throat. Gay or bisexual men should have anal swabs collected, irrespective of the urethral findings.
- Very occasionally, a UTI may be the cause of urethral discharge and the usual antibiotics used for chlamydial infection would not be appropriate or effective.
- Apparent recurrence of the infection can in fact be a re-infection. It is important to establish, as far as possible, whether re-infection is a possibility.
- Some patients will say their partner would not come to the clinic, but has gone to their GP and has received treatment. It is crucial to find out if this has actually occurred and what treatment the partner has had, as one has no idea what story was given to the GP, or, indeed, whether the GP's choice of antibiotic has been appropriate.
- The opportunity should not be missed to discuss the possibility of having acquired other STDs at the same time, and the opportunity should be taken to screen for other STDs.
- It is questionable whether tests of cure for chlamydial infection are relevant, but they should certainly be done for gonorrhoea, and should include a throat swab if this was omitted originally.

Hints for investigators and prescribers

- Patients can generally be thoroughly reassured about the effective treatments available for urethral discharge, but it is important to convey to them the risk of re-infection from an untreated partner. Advise them of the importance of completing the full course of treatment and, importantly, of not squeezing and checking for discharge.
- Even in the case of a proven chlamydial urethritis, tests of cure have not been shown to be necessary, as chlamydial infection always responds to a proper and thorough course of antibiotics.
- Gonococcal infection is accompanied by a chlamydial infection in up to 40% of cases, and as there is also a high incidence of post-gonococcal urethritis anyway, it is sensible when treating gonorrhoea to simultaneously treat for chlamydial infection.

Further reading

Adler, M.W. (1995) Urethral discharge, diagnosis and management. In: *ABC Sexually Transmitted Diseases*, 3rd Edn. BMJ Publishing Group, London, pp. 4–8.

Bowie, W.R. (1990) Urethritis in males. In: *Sexually Transmitted Diseases*, 2nd Edn (eds K.K. Holmes, P.A. Mardh, P.F. Sparling and P.J. Weisner). McGraw-Hill, New York, NY, pp. 627–639.

2 Epididymo-orchitis

The history, examination and investigation, and management is largely similar to that of urethral discharge. However, urinary tract pathogens are more likely to be significant in this scenario, so greater attention should be paid to symptoms suggestive of current or past UTI. Testicular ultrasound can be useful, but it is still difficult to differentiate torsion from acute epididymo-orchitis and this is a danger area where a surgical opinion should be sought.

3 Vaginal discharge

Vaginal discharge is commonly caused by a simple imbalance of the normal commensal flora in the vagina. However, sexually transmitted agents like N. gonorrhoeae, C. trachomatis, or Trichomonas vaginalis, can also be responsible. The approach to the history, investigations, and management owes as much to intuition and art, as it does to science. Managed badly, irreparable damage can be done either to a young woman's psychosexual development or to a relationship which might otherwise have flourished. Many of the features have a parallel with the investigation and management of urethral discharge in the male, as previously discussed.

Management options

1. If it sounds like candidosis, i.e. an itchy discharge and there is no admitted likelihood of an STD, prescribe an oral antifungal like fluconazole or itraconazole or an antifungal pessary, or advise the patient to purchase one of these at the local chemist. Review in 1 week.
2. Collect urethral, high vaginal and endocervical swabs and request culture or other methods for detection of C. trachomatis, N. gonorrhoeae, T. vaginalis, Gardnerella vaginalis and Candida spp. Review the case in 1 week.
3. Collect urethral, cervical, endocervical and high vaginal swabs. Gram stains as appropriate, and examination of a wet preparation from the high vaginal swab. Based on the wet preparation, Gram stain, and the clinical features, prescribe for the most likely cause and review the patient in 1 week.

Option 1. If it sounds like candidosis, i.e. an itchy discharge and there is no admitted likelihood of an STD, prescribe an oral antifungal like fluconazole or itraconazole or an antifungal pessary, or advise the patient to purchase one of these at the local chemist. Review in 1 week.

✓ As vulvovaginal candidosis is the commonest cause, this strategy is likely to work most of the time.

✓ It is simple, inexpensive and requires no investigations.

✗ If the cause, however, is N. gonorrhoeae or C. trachomatis, there is a risk of the patient developing an ascending infection and subsequent PID.

✗ If the problem recurs, prior treatment may have clouded the issue.

Option 2. Collect urethral, high vaginal and endocervical swabs and request culture or other methods for detection of C. trachomatis, N. gonorrhoeae, T. vaginalis, Gardnerella vaginalis and Candida spp. Review the case in 1 week.

✓ These swabs will allow definitive identification of the problem.

✗ Many patients will be unhappy if no treatment is initiated to relieve their symptoms.

✗ If the cause is an STD, there is a further week in which onward spread of infection to others or ascending infection in the woman causing PID could occur.

Option 3. Collect urethral, cervical, endocervical and high vaginal swabs. Gram stains as appropriate, and examination of a wet preparation from the high vaginal swab. Based on the wet preparation, Gram stain, and the clinical features, prescribe for the most likely cause and review the patient in 1 week.

✓ In the majority of cases, the history, symptoms, and examination can be enough to lead one to a likely diagnosis, and in specialized hands, if coupled with Gram stains and wet preparation, the likelihood of a correct diagnosis is greatly increased.

✓ If, for example, gonococci are found on a Gram stain, the partner can be dealt with accurately and rapidly, rather than awaiting culture, etc.

✓ Correct epidemiological information for the benefit of society as a whole is gathered.

✗ Facilities for identification of C. trachomatis must be available and these are not currently universal.

History checklist

• Establish if there is a pattern, i.e. how long has the problem been present? Is it of recent onset or is this a recurrent problem which has been going on for months or years? A discharge of recent onset is more suggestive of infection than a discharge that appears, say, on a regular basis, linked to a monthly cycle, etc. Ask the patient to describe the type of discharge, e.g. does it have a particular smell, is it worse after sex, is there a bloody discharge, or is there intermenstrual bleeding? Some patients with bacterial vaginosis (G. vaginalis) spontaneously describe the discharge as having a fishy smell, particularly after having intercourse. Bloody discharges are often significant and a description of intermenstrual bleeding demands consideration of genital tract malignancy.

• Has the patient experienced a similar problem before? Patients who suffer recurrent candidosis or bacterial vaginosis are often well aware of the pattern of recurrence and can identify it readily. Also, some patients may have had experience of having chlamydial infection or gonorrhoea, and describe the current problem as very similar to a previous episode.

• Is there a possibility that this problem could be sexually transmitted? Discussion requires tact and delicacy, which is more easily conducted within the setting of a GUM clinic, where patients expect this type of questioning, as opposed to a general practice setting, where the patient may not have even considered the possibility of a sexually transmitted agent. However, asking questions about their current partner, e.g. does he have 'cystitis' or has he had a bladder problem recently, can help to broach the subject in a non-threatening fashion. It is obviously easier to do this in a situation where there is not a stable ongoing relationship, and one can simply enquire about recent sexual encounters.

• Has there been any sexual exposure abroad? A holiday sexual encounter often carries more risk than a local one, and infections acquired abroad can be more difficult to treat and carry a higher risk of concomitant infection. Also, the range of infections can be broader, bringing in infections like chancroid, lymphogranuloma venereum (LGV), granuloma inguinale and syphilis.

• Have any antibiotics been taken recently, prescribed or not? A recent course of antibiotics for a chest infection, for example, can be enough to bring on an episode of vaginal candidosis. A few capsules of an antibiotic might also mask the presence of N. gonorrhoeae, or for that matter, G. vaginalis.

• Are there any associated symptoms, e.g. itching? Vaginal candidosis is frequently associated with vulvovaginal itching, whereas in bacterial vaginosis, it is unusual to find itching as a symptom.

• When was the last cervical smear test done, and what was the result? A woman who has several inflammatory smears could very well have a chronic cervical infection, i.e. chlamydia, and it is not unusual to find that they have already been booked for colposcopy or even that they have already had one without proper investigations.

• When was the last period, and what form of contraception is being used? If the woman's partner(s) *always* use condoms, then the risk of acquiring an STD is remote, as would be the risk of pregnancy. It is important to know if there is a possibility of pregnancy, as this would govern the choice of antibiotic therapy for the discharge.

Referrals

• The free, confidential GUM service throughout the UK is ideal in that it has an immediate and often open access assessment system – if the patient is prepared to attend. Often primary care physicians will make an assessment based on previous knowledge of the patient, their age, demeanour, etc., before deciding whether to initiate treatment or refer to the GUM service.

Examination checklist

- Inspect the vulva and perineal area for obvious signs of genital candidosis, i.e. erythema, fissuring, and satellite lesions of candida on the skin. Also check for obvious ulcers, e.g. an herpetic infection of the vulval area can also give secondary discharge, and a syphilitic lesion (although rare in the UK) could also cause a discharge.
- Examine the cervix. If there is significant vaginal discharge, no additional lubrication is necessary for the speculum. However, if the patient has just removed a tampon, a small amount of KY jelly will allow easy passage of the speculum. Mucopurulent discharge from the endocervical canal and the cervix is indicative of inflammation, and if after swabbing there is contact bleeding, this is also supportive.
- A bimanual examination to feel the cervix, uterus, adnexae and ovarian area is sometimes indicated. This is mandatory if the patient is complaining of lower abdominal pain, iliac fossa pain or dyspareunia.
- Does movement of the cervix mimic or reproduce the pain? Moving the cervix in a bimanual examination can tilt the uterus, and thus move the Fallopian tubes, which if inflamed, can cause pain. This is highly suggestive of PID.

Rituals and myths

- Patients will be outraged and affronted at questions that imply sexual impropriety. Elucidating the sexual history is a skill requiring tact and delicacy, intuition and an ability to empathize. Experience suggests that some patients suspect they might have acquired a STD, but are too embarrassed to initiate such a history and expect the doctor to ask the relevant questions. There are other patients for whom the possibility of acquiring an STD is absolutely unthinkable and may indeed even take exception to even gentle questioning in this direction. Unfortunately, however, they may occasionally be mistaken.
- Vulvovaginal candidosis is an STD. This is patently untrue. A woman who has never had intercourse can still get vulvovaginal candidosis and even suffer recurrences of this. The friction of sexual intercourse can sometimes set off recurrent candidosis, but patients who are prone to this should use adequate lubrication – irrespective of whether they feel they need it or not!
- Bacterial vaginosis is an STD. Bacterial vaginosis has been described in women who have never had intercourse and, indeed, G. vaginalis can be isolated from women who have never had vaginal intercourse. Although it does seem common in women who do have intercourse, this does not make it an STD. Furthermore, no benefit has been shown in treating the male partner.
- The management and treatment of vulvovaginal candidosis is useless, as recurrences are still common. This myth inevitably has to be dealt with when confronted with a patient with recurrent vulvovaginal candidosis. The patients are often frustrated and in despair, as they feel that because they have got a recurrence the treatment has not worked. They must be reassured that the treatment does work, but that recurrences are common, and can be dealt with promptly in a way that should not interfere with normal life or sexual activity.

Pitfalls

- Re-infection because of no or inadequate treatment of the partner is common, particularly when cases are managed outside the usual GUM setting. If a sexually transmitted agent like N. gonorrhoeae, C. trachomatis or T. vaginalis is identified, it is absolutely essential to establish that the partner has been treated simultaneously, or at least that no intercourse has occurred before he is also clear of infection.

- Tests of cure for chlamydial infection are usually unnecessary. However, in certain cases, they are important, i.e. if the patient herself is worried and wants absolute proof that the infection has cleared, then it should be done. Also, if the patient is pregnant, it is important to be absolutely certain and document eradication.
- It is important, however, not to do a test of cure too early, as most tests of cures are now based on antigen detection, and antigen can persist for several weeks after the initiation of therapy. Therefore, tests of cure should be done 4 weeks after completion of therapy, if at all!
- As with male patients and urethral discharge, the opportunity should not be missed to discuss the possibility of having acquired other STDs at the same time. These should be screened for if possible.

Hints for investigators and prescribers
- Even though vulvovaginal candidosis is extremely common, it can also occur in coexistence with chlamydial cervicitis. Chlamydial infection is particularly common in the UK in the age group 16–19 with the current UK incidence given as 500 cases per 100 000 population in this age group. No opportunity should therefore be missed for screening for this infection, as eradication is 100% with the usual effective treatments. (See 'Hints for investigators and prescribers' under 'Urethral discharge', p. 124.)

Further reading
Adler, M.W. (1995) Vaginal discharge, diagnosis and management. In: *ABC Sexually Transmitted Diseases*, 3rd Edn. BMJ Publishing Group, London, pp. 9–13.

Holmes, K.K. (1990) Lower genital tract infection in women: cystitis, urethritis, vulvo-vaginitis and cervicitis. *Sexually Transmitted Diseases*, 2nd Edn (eds K.K. Holmes, P.A. Mardh, P.F. Sparling and P.J. Weisner *et al.*). McGraw-Hill, New York, NY, pp. 527–545.

4 Genital ulcers

Genital ulcers are commonly caused by infection and many of these infections are sexually transmitted. Other causes can be physical, i.e. trauma or autoimmune ulceration and in many cases the aetiology is never fully established. When presented with genital ulceration, it is important to establish, as far as possible, the likely cause, to carry out appropriate investigations and institute therapy as soon as possible. Further follow-up is often necessary, as some diagnoses are only established on the basis of exclusion criteria.

GUM clinics are ideally placed to provide an easy access, full diagnostic service, with treatment and counselling for this group of patients who are often very distressed. In the UK, genital herpes is the most common cause and the clinical presentation can often be readily recognized, as long as examiners are familiar with the typical history and clinical appearance. However, consideration should always be given to the possibility of rare infectious causes like syphilis, chancroid, granuloma inguinale, and LGV.

Management options
1. Genital herpes is the commonest cause in the UK. The history fits, so simply prescribe an antiviral. No need for an embarrassing genital examination, and advise the patient to return if the condition does not respond.
2. Examine the patient, collect a swab for herpes and await the results before treatment.
3. Examine the patient, collect a herpes culture swab, do not wait for results, and initiate antiherpetic treatment.
4. Examine the patient, collect herpes swabs, do a full STD screen (if possible), i.e. collect swabs for N. gonorrhoeae, C. trachomatis, T. vaginalis, G. vaginalis and Candida spp. Do dark-ground microscopy if syphilis is likely. Commence antiherpes treatment, as the most likely cause. Collect a blood sample for syphilis serology, review the patient in 1 week, and consider a second blood test for syphilis serology in 3 months time.

Option 1. Genital herpes is the commonest cause in the UK. The history fits, so simply prescribe an antiviral. No need for an embarrassing genital examination, and advise the patient to return if the condition does not respond.

✓ Herpes being so common, this option is likely to work in the majority of cases.
✓ Many patients do not actually want to be examined, particularly in primary care, and are relieved that their doctor has not suggested it.
✓ If it is herpes, early and prompt treatment speeds clearance, and there is a possibility that prompt, effective, early treatment may lessen the number of virally infected cells that go into latency.

✗ No diagnosis or initial assessment is made, making it difficult to judge if there has been any improvement. If it is herpes, recurrences are possible and the management of these, including the possibility of onward spread of infection, has not been discussed with the patient.
✗ On the rare occasion that it is not herpes, but syphilis or one of the tropical infections, time has been wasted and further complications could develop.

Option 2. Examine the patient, collect a swab for herpes and await the results before treatment.

✓ If it is herpes, the diagnosis is likely to be firmly established.
✗ The condition will continue and new ulcers may develop.

Option 3. Examine the patient, collect a herpes culture swab, do not wait for results, and initiate antiherpetic treatment.

✓ If it is herpes, the diagnosis is likely to be confirmed and your judgement shown to be correct.

✓ The early initiation of treatment will be appreciated by the patient and may possibly reduce the number of viruses going into latency.

✓ Early treatment may also prevent the development of increasing dysuria and the possibility of urinary retention.

✗ Consideration may not have been given to other causes of the ulceration.

Option 4. Examine the patient, collect herpes swabs, do a full STD screen (if possible), i.e. collect swabs for N. gonorrhoeae, C. trachomatis, T. vaginalis, G. vaginalis and Candida spp. Do dark-ground microscopy if syphilis is likely. Commence antiherpes treatment, as the most likely cause. Collect a blood sample for syphilis serology, review the patient in 1 week, and consider a second blood test for syphilis serology in 3 months time.

✓ This comprehensive investigation profile is likely to give a definitive diagnosis.

✓ If the condition does not respond and one is considering autoimmune ulceration, i.e. Behcet's, the initial tranche of investigations have been done, and one is further down the road towards a diagnosis of exclusion.

✓ Rapid initiation of treatment for herpes can speed the resolution and may reduce the number of latent virus-infected cells.

✓ If recurrences develop, the original diagnosis will have been established, and proper counselling can occur.

✓ The management of the partner can be based on a definitive diagnosis.

✗ Swabbing for herpes can be painful.

✗ As syphilis is so rare, the palaver of dark-ground investigation and bloods for syphilis serology could to be a waste of time.

History checklist

• When did the ulcers first appear? Were they blisters initially? Genital herpes typically has an onset of several hours to days, where the patient often describes a tingling, burning, and often notice a red rash that turns into blisters, which rapidly break down, giving the typical shallow ulcers. The patient can usually describe this sequence of events, which helps distinguish it from, say, an ulcer caused by trauma or syphilis.

• Are the ulcers multiple? Painful? Typical herpetic ulcers are multiple and very painful, and there is often intense dysuria if the ulcers are in the introitus and are in contact with the urine when voiding.

• Is this the first time or is this a recurrence? If the present problem is a recurrent herpetic infection patients often remember the first time it happened, although in some cases the initial episode may have been mistaken for vulvovaginal candidosis or, in males, a balanitis.

• Is there a history of orofacial cold sores in the patient or their partner? As an herpetic infection can readily be transmitted through oral sex, it is important to explore this area fully. Even if the partner has not recently had a cold sore, it should be asked whether the individual or their partner has ever had orofacial cold sores or if, for example, they or their partner have had a recent flu which may have brought on a cold sore. Recurrent oral aphthous ulcers could suggest Behcet's.

• Are there any associated symptoms, i.e. flu-like illness, swollen glands in the groin, feeling feverish, or a rash anywhere on the body? With acute herpetic infections, patients often feel just as unwell as if they have an acute systemic viral infection, with chills, tiredness, feverishness and aching joints. Enquiring about recent rashes may lead one towards the possibility of syphilis.

- Has there been any recent sexual exposure that might fit with the acquisition of an STD? As previously discussed, delicacy and tact is required in this type of questioning. It is also important to establish if a contact has been abroad, as this would greatly widen the range of possible infections.
- Has there been a recent change or initiation of medication, particularly drugs that are known to be associated with fixed drug eruptions? Rarely, drugs such as non-steroidal anti-inflammatory drugs, cotrimoxazole, etc., can be associated with dramatic genital ulceration which can progress to full blown Steven's-Johnson syndrome. However, the association is usually very clear if the proper history is taken.
- Has the patient ever donated blood? If female, when was the last pregnancy? Has there been a visit to a GUM clinic before? All of these are occasions when the individual is likely to have had blood tested for syphilis serology, and it can be important to establish that a patient was negative at some time in the past if syphilis is currently under consideration as the diagnosis.

Examination checklist
- Feel the inguinal glands. In acute herpes infections there is almost invariably a tender inguinal adenopathy. In some females, this can be so severe as to affect the gait, resulting in what is known as the 'John Wayne walk' of genital herpes. Inguinal adenopathy, though not painful, is also associated with syphilitic ulceration and with granuloma inguinale and LGV.
- Examine the ulcerated area. Multiple shallow, painful ulcers are typical of a herpetic infection, whereas, larger single ulcers are more typical of syphilis. Syphilitic ulcers have a characteristic indurated feel.
- A screen for the full range of STDs should also be done, if possible. In female patients with acute genital herpes it is often far too painful to do anything other than take a swab of the ulcerated area. It can be impossible and unfair to attempt to pass a speculum. However, it should be kept in mind that a full screen should be done when the ulceration has cleared, i.e. swabs for C. trachomatis and N. gonorrhoeae, and in the case of females, T. vaginalis, G. vaginalis and Candida spp.
- Investigations from the ulcer area itself? It is crucial that a proper swab be sent for virus isolation. This is currently the best way of proving an herpetic infection. It is, however, very important to remove the slough from the ulcer and take a cotton-tipped swab from the base of the ulcer. The patient must be warned that this can be painful, but it is pointless to send an inadequate swab to the lab. If the history and clinical examination are suspicious of syphilis, dark-ground microscopy is mandatory, but usually only available in the GUM service. Examination for more exotic pathogens require specialist consideration, i.e. chancroid, LGV and granuloma inguinale.

Referrals
- As discussed in the previous two sections, the GUM service is the ideal place for the investigation of genital ulcers.

Rituals and myths
- Genital ulcers mean STD. This particular myth causes a great deal of unnecessary distress and anxiety in patients. If the initial consultation suggests sexual transmission, there is often a great deal of repair work and counselling to be done by the follow-up carers, even if the cause is shown to be innocent transmission. For example, in the UK, genital herpes is commonly caused by HSV type 1 and is usually transmitted through oral sex which, of course, can occur in a perfectly stable, monogamous relationship.
- Syphilis is a common cause of genital ulcers. In the UK, primary genital syphilis is uncommon. It was associated with high risk groups of gay men and sexual contacts abroad. Currently, the incidence in gay men has decreased dramatically and most cases

are caused by heterosexual contact in countries where it is still a major problem. There are occasional localized outbreaks, the most recent occurring in Bristol during 1997.

- The difference between herpes and true love is that herpes lasts for ever. The concept of 'forever' and the fact that there is no cure for herpes is often quoted and only encourages anxiety and distress in patients. At the end of the day, an herpetic ulcer is a cold sore, irrespective of whether it is on the orofacial or genital area. Patients must be encouraged to view it in this light and not as a major life-changing infection. The Herpes Association are very helpful in this regard, and produce a newsletter, and excellent information to help patients cope with the diagnosis (Tel: 0171 609 9061).

Pitfalls

- The laboratory isolation of HSV is not fail-safe and there are often occasions when an apparently adequate swab is taken, but the report indicates 'no virus isolated'. It is important to establish whether the patient has already had some antivirals or has applied Zovirax cold sore cream. Even other noxious chemicals that might be transferred with the swab into the transport media, e.g. antiseptic creams or lotions would interfere with the ability of the laboratory to isolate the virus. There is often an opportunity to swab again if there are recurrences.
- In extremely rare cases, the possibility of coexisting infections needs to be considered. It is not unheard of for syphilis and herpes to be acquired simultaneously, and as with all consultations in the field of GUM, the opportunity should be taken to explore this risk.

Hints for investigators and prescribers

- The clinical presentation of genital herpes, particularly in women, can be mistaken for a UTI. Many patients complain initially of intense dysuria which is often cursorily interpreted as cystitis and the patient is prescribed a course of the usual antibiotics. However, a few days later, as the situation worsens, there is vaginal discharge and dysuria. This is often interpreted as antibiotic-induced vulvovaginal candidosis and an anti-fungal pessary is prescribed. Only after a few more days, as the situation becomes unbearable, does it become clear that an herpetic infection is the likely cause. At least a fifth of cases of female primary genital herpes attending our clinic have had prior treatment for 'cystitis' or 'vulvovaginal candidosis'.
- It cannot be over emphasized that suggestions that genital herpes implies partner infidelity are inappropriate. An enormous disservice is done to a couple and their relationship if the process is not managed correctly from the outset.
- Facilities for swabbing for HSV may not be universally available, particularly in primary care, and although isolating the virus and identifying it as type 1 or type 2 is not crucial to the management of genital herpes, this information does make counselling and further management of follow-ups easier. For example, if the virus is isolated, one is secure in the knowledge of the infection one is dealing with, and further advice can be given in the light of the viral type. HSV-1 does not cause recurrences as often as HSV-2, although the primary HSV-1 genital attack may be very severe. In couples with a monogamous relationship, it is reassuring for them to know that the viral isolate is type 1 and that this fits very neatly with the suggested orofacial genital transmission.
- Recent research suggests that prompt and thorough treatment of the primary attack may reduce the number of latently infected viral cells and might have some bearing on the frequency of recurrences and perhaps even the extent of a recurrence. These studies have been carried out in animal models and therefore must be interpreted cautiously. However, there is no doubt that prompt, early treatment of the primary herpes attack greatly reduces the severity, duration and pain of the episode, and can avoid the expensive complication of urinary retention.
- Some patients are distressed by 'herpetic neuralgia'-type pain, i.e. they get sciatica or pain

in the buttock area as they develop a recurrence. These symptoms need to be explained and reassurance given.

- Rarely, some patients are so upset and distressed by frequent occurrences that they need to be put on maintenance therapy. This is a major decision, with implications for the patient's lifestyle. Maintenance therapy is expensive. Why some patients cope with equanimity and others are devastated can depend on how health professionals have managed the primary episode.

Further reading

Adler, M.W. (1995) Genital ulceration; genital herpes. In: *ABC Sexually Transmitted Diseases*, 3rd Edn. BMJ Publishing Group, London, pp. 22–27.

Barton, S.E., Munday, P.E. and Patel, R.J. (1996) A symptomatic shedding of herpes simplex virus from the genital tract: uncertainty and its consequences for patient management. Editorial review. *Int. J. STD AIDS* 7: 229–232.

5 Prostatitis

The mere mention of the word prostatitis can induce a syndrome known as 'heartsink' in health care professionals. The history, investigation and management of the condition is fraught with difficulties and obstacles at every stage. The management is often unsatisfactory for both the professional and the patient, and much shopping around in search of the elusive cure occurs. To avoid many of the pitfalls associated with this condition, the initial investigations and management should be thorough and complete. Patients consult widely and are often seen by GPs, urologists, genito-urinary physicians, pain clinic doctors, homeopathy practitioners and acupuncture specialists, among others.

The condition can generally be divided into acute or chronic prostatitis and these can be further sub-divided into bacterial prostatitis and abacterial prostatitis. The condition known as prostatodynia is often discussed when one is left with chronic prostatic pain of unknown aetiology. The management of prostatitis, particularly acute prostatitis, when the infective agents are isolated and identified, is relatively straightforward, and correct management can bring excellent results. Therefore, a thorough search for responsible pathogens must be part of the initial process.

The presenting symptoms are varied, and can be acute, with fever, rigors, frequency, dysuria, urgency, haematuria and perineal pain. In chronic prostatitis the symptoms are often more subtle. The pain can be suprapubic, perineal or testicular, radiating down the thighs, but occasionally focusing on the urethra and tip of the penis. There can be various urinary irritative complaints, i.e. frequency, dysuria, variation in stream, urgency, a sense of incomplete emptying of the bladder, haematuria and haematospermia.

The aetiology is mixed. Previously, gonorrhoea was a common cause and should still certainly be checked for. Whether other sexually transmitted agents, i.e. C. trachomatis are a significant cause of acute prostatitis is still controversial. In current practice, UTI organisms are likely candidates and a thorough search for urinary tract anomalies is mandatory.

Management options

1. Prescribe a course of antibiotics with a proven track record in prostatitis, i.e. one of the fluoroquinolones, and if symptoms are resolving, continue the course for at least 2 months.
2. Collect a midstream urine (MSU) and then prescribe an antibiotic, as Option 1.
3. Investigate as for urethral discharge, collect urine samples (see 'Examination checklist'), omit prostatic massage if acute prostatitis is suspected, make a general abdominal and renal examination, take a plain radiograph of the pelvic area, looking for calculi, prescribe a prolonged course of a fluoroquinolone, and review the patient in a week. Review again later, and decide on further radiology, if necessary.

Option 1. Prescribe a course of antibiotics with a proven track record in prostatitis, i.e. one of the fluoroquinolones, and if symptoms are resolving, continue the course for at least 2 months.

✓ Resolution of symptoms is likely and the patient will be glad not to have been through the rigours of the investigation procedures.

✗ No pathogen has been looked for; therefore, a definitive diagnosis has not been made. The investigation of recurrence will be complicated because of the prior therapy.

Option 2. Collect a midstream urine (MSU) and then prescribe an antibiotic, as Option 1.

✓ As the majority of cases are caused by urinary tract pathogens, there is some chance of this identifying the infective agent with the minimum of fuss.

✓ The patient has not been subjected to a rectal examination and may avoid developing the common misapprehension that every time the symptoms need to be investigated a prostatic examination is mandatory.

✓ The risk of precipitating septicaemia by palpating an infected prostate has been avoided.

✗ If the condition recurs, further investigations have been prejudiced.

Option 3. Investigate as for urethral discharge, collect urine samples (see 'Examination checklist') omit prostatic massage if acute prostatitis is suspected, make a general abdominal and renal examination, take a plain radiograph of the pelvic area, looking for calculi, prescribe a prolonged course of a fluoroquinolone, and review the patient in a week. Review again later, and decide on further radiology, if necessary.

✓ Every effort has been made to establish the infective agent, if there is one, prior to commencing antibiotics.

✓ Resolution of symptoms is likely and antibiotic choice could be changed in the light of accumulating results.

✗ The investigation process is lengthy and requires an experienced health professional to perform and interpret the results. Consultation time is long.

History checklist

- Is the condition acute or chronic? The symptoms of acute prostatitis are usually fairly dramatic and patients can give an accurate and detailed history. However, with chronic prostatitis there is often a prolonged vague history, requiring definitive probing.
- Are there any clearly defined precipitating events? i.e. urethral discharge, UTI? A urethral discharge would lead one to suspect gonococcal infection and appropriate investigations, as outlined earlier, would follow.
- Have any previous episodes occurred and, if so, what treatments have been used? Most patients with prostatitis, particularly chronic, have already had multiple investigations and treatments. It is crucial to define these, particularly recent antibiotics, as they may influence current investigations.

Examination checklist

- Examine for urethral discharge. Swabs should be collected for N. gonorrhoeae and urethral Gram stain, although, if recent antibiotics have been given, negative results have to be interpreted accordingly.
- General abdominal examination looking for suprapubic pain, renal tenderness or masses. The detection of any abdominal masses would direct further investigations.
- Digital examination of the prostate. Palpation of the prostate is contraindicated in acute prostatitis. Not only would this be extraordinarily painful, but this could precipitate a bacteraemia and further complications. In chronic prostatitis, the time-honoured method of Meares and Stamey entails segmental investigations that allow localization of infection to the urethra, prostate or bladder. In summary, a first catch urine is produced, then a mid-stream urine sample is collected, prostatic massage is undertaken, and any expressed prostatic fluid collected, and finally, a post-massage urine is collected. Analysis and culture of all samples can identify the pathogen and direct management.
- Further investigations can be required encompassing transrectal ultrasonography, CT or MRI scanning, renal tract ultrasound or i.v. pyelography, and prostatic biopsy.

Referrals

- Alarm bells should ring if symptoms of prostatitis are suspected in a primary care setting. The condition is likely to be long-lasting and require frequent consultations and assessment. It is imperative that the aetiology is established in the early stages, prior to clouding the horizon with antibiotic therapy. GUM clinics with their open access system are often attended by these patients and the management can be appropriate if there are personnel within the clinic willing and capable of the long-term management. Referral to a hospital urologist is also appropriate, but there can be some delay before patients are seen. Obviously, acute prostatitis is an emergency and immediate investigation and management is called for.

Rituals and myths

- Patients with chronic prostatitis are difficult, manipulative, distrusting and often psychologically disturbed. Although there can be an element of truth in this myth, patients may end up like this because of the condition itself and the way it has been dealt with by the medical profession. These patients require an inordinate amount of time and effort devoted to their initial investigations and management. Should chronic follow-up be required, they are best dealt with by experienced, rather than junior hospital staff, as the patient's symptoms are likely to last longer than the junior hospital doctor's contract.
- There has to be a cause, and if further investigations are done repeatedly, the cause will be found. In many cases, a cause is never established and repeated prostatic investigations, scans, etc. become an exhausting waste of time and money. Honesty in discussion with the patient is appropriate and onward referral to pain clinics, etc., may be more important than bitterly pursuing an elusive mythical causative agent.
- Recurrent prostatic massage is of value in the management of chronic prostatitis. It is uncertain whether this myth has anything to do with the possibility of income generation, but either way, it is seldom practised today, and there is no evidence-based medicine to suggest that it is of any value.

Pitfalls

- Short courses of antibiotics for prostatitis are inappropriate. Many patients only begin to get relief after 2 months of therapy. Most units prescribe for 3 months, and are quite prepared to extend the course beyond this.
- Urinary tract pathology, i.e. calculi, must be searched for thoroughly.
- Giving the patient the impression that his symptoms may be psychological is damaging to the doctor/patient relationship and usually results in second, third and fourth opinions being sought. A sympathetic consideration of how the problem is affecting the patient psychologically and impinging on their life is of value, and need not convey the impression of a psychological aetiology.

Hints for investigators and prescribers

- The fluoroquinolones are now established as excellent agents in the management of prostatitis and have largely replaced co-trimoxazole for the management of chronic prostatitis. Acute prostatitis requires i.v. therapy and gentamicin and ampicillin have been used effectively.
- It is often the pain of chronic prostatitis or prostatodynia that causes the main difficulty for patients and emphasis on pain relief is important. A variety of procedures are used, either drug or physical therapy, e.g. pelvic floor retraining, local hyperthermia.
- There is little doubt, however, that an open, honest relationship between the patient and the doctor is crucial for long-term satisfactory management.

Further reading

O'Mahony, C. (1998) The diagnosis and management of prostatitis. In: *Current Practice in Genitourinary Medicine* (eds S.E. Barton and P. Hay). Kluwer Academic and Lippincott Raven Publishers, London (in press).

Thin, R.N. (1997) Diagnosis of chronic prostatitis: overview and update. *Int. J. STD AIDS* 8: 475–481.

Chapter 8
JOINT AND BONE INFECTIONS

B.L. Atkins

Bone and joint infections can be difficult to diagnose and manage because the clinical presentation is often not specific for infection. There may be a broad differential diagnosis based on clinical findings, and even when infection is a certainty, there are a range of infecting organisms. Clinical acumen is vital, but the pathology and radiology also need to be interpreted skillfully in order to optimize patient management. This chapter attempts to rationalize the approach to solving problems in orthopaedic infections that present to the hospital or community physician.

Clinical problem-solving must address whether, for example:

- an acutely inflamed joint is due to an infectious or non-infectious aetiology;
- a patient with symptoms or signs of bony pathology has an infectious or non-infectious condition;
- a patient with a bony abnormality on imaging has an infectious or non-infectious aetiology;
- a patient with clinical evidence of sepsis has a bone or joint infection;
- a patient with known bacteraemia has a bone or joint infection;
- a patient needs a surgical procedure;
- to start empiric or specific antibiotics.

Chapter contents

1 Septic arthritis

Septic arthritis is an inflammatory reaction in the joint space and articular tissues due to infection with a micro-organism that is actively multiplying. The infection can be regarded as *acute* (days) or *chronic* (weeks or months). Presentation is usually with pain and swelling in a joint, often with fever and other constitutional symptoms. Differentiation between septic arthritis and other inflammatory arthritides is often not clinically possible and diagnostic joint aspiration plays an important role.

Management options
1. Initiate basic investigations and diagnostic aspirate. Await results.
2. Initiate basic investigations and refer for therapeutic washout.
3. Initiate basic investigations and regular therapeutic aspiration.
4. Initiate basic investigations, observe, and further investigations as necessary.

Option 1. Initiate basic investigations and diagnostic aspirate. Await results.

✓ Allows time to gather information.
✓ Allows highly specific therapy once the diagnosis is clear.
✓ Avoids the use of antibiotics when the aetiology may be non-infectious.
✓ Avoids a potential surgical procedure when the aetiology may be non-infectious.

✗ There will be a delay in surgical treatment. If this is an acute pyogenic arthritis there will be further destruction of the joint space and articular cartilages, and metastatic infection may supervene with or without systemic sepsis.
✗ In a patient with systemic features of sepsis, a delay in treating the source may result in progression, potentially to severe sepsis and multi-organ failure.

Option 2. Initiate basic investigations and refer for therapeutic washout.

Most cases of septic arthritis benefit from a therapeutic drainage procedure. Sometimes this has to be done repeatedly in order to control infection. In some cases repeated aspiration may suffice if there are contraindications to a general anaesthetic.

✓ Allows a potentially therapeutic procedure to be performed early.
✓ Allows early involvement with a speciality which sees a lot of abnormal joints.
✓ Allows further material to be obtained for bacteriological culture.

✗ An unnecessary procedure is performed if the aetiology is non-infectious. The procedure itself can lead (rarely) to infectious complications.

Option 3. Initiate basic investigations and regular therapeutic aspiration.

✓ Avoids a general or regional anaesthetic, particularly in debilitated patients.

✗ May be less successful than a formal washout procedure.

Option 4. Initiate basic investigations, observe, and further investigations as necessary.

✓ This approach is important in the investigation of any chronic inflammatory process. There should be close consultation with a microbiologist to ensure that the most appropriate specimens are collected.
✓ It allows a diagnostic pathway to be followed with further sampling and biopsying as necessary, free of antibiotics or other agents.

✓ Allows highly specific therapy when a positive diagnosis is made.

✓ Avoids antibiotics if the aetiology is non-infectious.

✗ Delay in antibiotics may, in theory, result in further destruction of the joint. In practice, if the duration of history is long, there will be a reasonable amount of time in which to make the diagnosis.

History checklist

- It is often difficult clinically to differentiate septic arthritis from other arthritides. Fever can occur in any inflammatory arthritis. Key features suggesting an infectious aetiology are the occurrence of rigors, recent intra-articular injection or surgery/trauma to the area. Factors indicating a non-infectious cause are a past history of gout or inflammatory joint disease. However, these pathologies also predispose to septic arthritis.
- How and when did symptoms begin? This will tell you whether this is an acute or chronic infection. Acute infections are usually due to pyogenic organisms such as Staphylococcus aureus, β-haemolytic streptococci and Haemophilus influenzae. Chronic infections may be due to Mycobacterium tuberculosis, Brucella spp. or fungi such as Sporothrix schenckii (rare). Prolonged duration of symptoms can also occur with Neisseria infections.
- What is the site(s) of infection? The knee is the most commonly affected site for bacterial arthritis. The hip is the next commonest site, but diagnosis is often delayed. Children have more infections of the ankle and elbow, whereas adults tend to have more involvement of the shoulder and wrist. The sacroiliac and sternoclavicular joints are rarely infected, except in i.v. drug users. The interphalangeal joints are rarely involved except in Neisseria gonorrhoeae, M. tuberculosis and following an animal or human bite. Multiple joints are involved in 10% of cases especially in rheumatoid arthritis or in infectious arthritis of viral aetiology (e.g. rubella).
- Was there any preceding illness? If yes, this may suggest the possibility of a reactive arthritis following an STD (e.g. chlamydial) or gastrointestinal infection.
- Is there a recent history of trauma or bites? A traumatic effusion predisposes to secondary haematogenous infection. A recent human or animal bite may indicate infection with an oral organism or by Pasteurella mulocida. Infection with Streptobacillus moniliformis can occur 2–3 days after a rat bite.
- Has the patient received a recent intra-articular injection? The commonest infective organism after an intra-articular injection is S. aureus. Infections with Candida spp. also occur after steroid injection.
- Is there a history of travel to an endemic area? Infections to be considered, particularly in cases of chronic septic arthritis, are Lyme disease (tick bite), brucellosis (consumption of unpasteurised milk and cheeses) and mycoses (e.g. Coccidiodes immitis, S. schenckii).
- Is there a history of recent sexual contact? If yes, then consider N. gonorrhoeae as a possible infecting organism. Also ask about urethritis.
- Is there a history of conjunctivitis/urethritis? Also think of Reiter's syndrome.
- Is the patient diabetic, in renal failure (particularly if they are on haemodialysis) or on systemic steroids? These all increase the risk of septic arthritis and may also involve less usual organisms, particularly Gram-negative organisms.
- Is there a history of rheumatoid arthritis or systemic lupus erythematosis (SLE)? These can present as inflamed joints due to the underlying disease, but are also more susceptible to secondary bacterial arthritis.
- Is there a history of, or risk factors for, gout or pseudogout? This may suggest a non-infectious aetiology, although the two can coincide.
- Has the patient recently received antibiotics? This is important, as it may explain negative cultures even in an acute pyogenic infection.

Examination checklist

General
- Look for a rash, e.g. gonoccoccal rash, rubella, Reiter's syndrome.
- Also look for pharyngitis (rheumatic fever or post-streptococcal arthritis).
- Look at the hands for stigmata of endocarditis.
- Look at the eyes for conjunctivitis (Reiter's syndrome).

Specific
- Cardiovascular. Murmurs (endocarditis, rheumatic fever).
- Respiratory. Evidence of tuberculosis (TB) or pneumococcal disease.
- Abdomen. Splenomegaly (endocarditis, brucella, haematological malignancy).
- Other joints. Evidence of inflammatory joint disease and any evidence of sepsis in other joints.
- Local. Erythema, swelling/effusion, warmth, tenderness, limitation of movement.

Pitfalls
- Starting antibiotics before appropriate quality microbiological samples have been obtained.
- Delaying therapeutic washout of the joint in the clinically septic patient.

Hints for investigators and prescribers
- Always take blood cultures.
- Aspirate as much fluid/pus as possible into a sterile universal container for Gram stain, crystals and culture.
- Empiric antibiotics for acute pyogenic septic arthritis should cover the common pathogens (S. aureus, Streptococcus spp., H. influenzae, other Gram-negative bacilli, Neisseria spp.). A parenteral second or third generation cephalosporin is appropriate. Once microbiology results are available, more specific therapy should be used.
- The duration of therapy depends on the whole clinical picture. The recommended duration for suppurative arthritis is 2 weeks of parenteral antibiotics for H. influenzae, Streptococcus spp. and Neisseria spp., and 3 weeks for S. aureus or other Gram-negative bacilli. Some treat for shorter periods intravenously, but use a high dose oral regimen (after microbiological consultation). Therapeutic monitoring of antibiotic levels is also advocated by some. For mycobacterial and fungal arthritis, seek specialist advice.

Further reading
Goldenberg, D.L. and Reed, J.I. (1985) Bacterial arthritis. *N. Engl. J. Med.* **312**: 764–771.

Norden, C., Gillespie, W.J. and Nade, S. (1994) Infectious arthritis. In: *Infections in Bones and Joints.* Blackwell Scientific Publications, Oxford, pp. 320–351.

Sharp, J.T., Lidsky, M.D., Duffy, J. and Duncan, M.W. (1979) Infectious arthritis. *Arch. Intern. Med.* **139**: 1125–1130.

Syrogiannopoulos, G.A. and Nelson, J.D. (1988) Duration of antimicrobial therapy for acute suppurative osteoarticular infections. *Lancet* **1**: 37–40.

2 Prosthetic joint infection

Presentation is either *acute* with fever, severe pain, swelling and erythema or *chronic* over months or years with pain and occasionally sinus formation. Organisms may be introduced locally or by the haematogenous route.

Management options

1. Always refer back to orthopaedics for further assessment. This would include C-reactive protein, erythrocyte sedimentation rate, white cell count, plain X-rays and possibly a joint aspirate. Following this the implant may need to be revised. This may be done as a two-stage procedure.
2. As Option 1, but an exchange arthroplasty is done as one procedure. Appropriate parenteral antibiotics are usually given for a period following the procedure.
3. As Option 1, but the prosthesis is removed and not replaced.
4. As Option 1, but the prosthesis is left *in situ* and long-term suppressive antibiotics are given. Irrigation and debridement are usually performed.

Option 1. Always refer back to orthopaedics for further assessment. This would include C-reactive protein, erythrocyte sedimentation rate, white cell count, plain X-rays and possibly a joint aspirate. Following this the implant may need to be revised. This may be done as a two-stage procedure.

✓ Allows radical clearance of all infected material and cement, and an accurate microbiological diagnosis can be made in most cases.

✓ This method is the most successful in eradicating infection (80–90%).

✗ Requires two operations.

✗ Usually requires lengthy parenteral antibiotics, often via a tunnelled central line.

Option 2. As Option 1, but an exchange arthroplasty is done as one procedure. Appropriate parenteral antibiotics are usually given for a period following the procedure.

✓ Requires only one operation.

✗ May be less successful than a two-stage procedure in eradicating infection (70–80%).

Option 3. As Option 1, but the prosthesis is removed and not replaced.

✓ Requires only one operation.

✓ No prosthetic material is reimplanted into the previously infected area.

✓ A useful procedure for patients who only want one procedure, or have poor bone stock or general condition.

✗ The functional results vary and are not as good as a revision.

Option 4. As Option 1, but the prosthesis is left *in situ* and long-term suppressive antibiotics are given. Irrigation and debridement are usually performed.

✓ This approach is useful if the prosthesis is firmly fixed (no loosening) and therefore functional.

✓ This approach is also useful if the patient is unfit for a general anaesthetic.

✗ An accurate microbiological diagnosis may need to be made by other means (such as a joint aspirate) in order to give specific antimicrobials. Some infective agents (e.g. Pseudomonas spp., Candida spp.) may indicate that treatment is likely to fail.

✗ The infection may progress and cause more bone destruction.

✗ Long-term (in theory, indefinite) antibiotics need to be given. The patient may have poor tolerance or complications of antibiotic therapy.

History checklist

- When was the primary implantation? Infection is more likely when it is an early failure (in the first 2 years after implantation).
- How and when did symptoms start? However, it is usually not possible to distinguish pain in a prosthetic joint that is infected, from the pain of 'aseptic failure'.
- Was there a history of post-operative wound infection or haematoma? These increase the risk of infection.
- Has the patient had temperatures, sweats or rigors? These suggest an acute infection, whether in the immediate post-operative period or later, as a result of haematogenous infection.
- Is there a discharging sinus? This is almost unequivocal evidence for a chronically infected joint.
- Has the patient taken antibiotics recently? This will affect microbiological cultures. Antibiotics should be stopped 2 weeks before any diagnostic microbiological tests in a suspected chronic infection.

Examination checklist

- Assess the degree of systemic sepsis, general fitness for surgery and evidence for systemic infections such as endocarditis, TB or staphylococcal disease. Check other joints.
- Examine the joint for erythema, swelling/effusion, warmth and tenderness.
- Examine the wound for erythema, cellulitis, dehiscence or a discharging sinus.

Referrals

- See above.

Pitfalls

- Giving antibiotics before reliable samples are obtained for microbiology.

Hints for investigators and prescribers

- Interpretation of microbiology results can be difficult, as the organisms that infect joints are the same as those that contaminate specimens. If multiple specimens (five) are taken with separate instruments, and two or preferably three are positive with the same organism, then infection is highly likely. Results should be interpreted in conjunction with the clinical picture, intra-operative findings and histology.
- In the acutely septic patient, antibiotics may need to be given empirically after blood cultures and, if possible, a joint aspirate. S. aureus is the commonest pathogen in this situation but others occur. A second generation cephalosporin would be appropriate, plus 24–48 hours of an aminoglycoside. In cases where methicillin-resistant S. aureus is a risk, a glycopeptide should be added.
- In the chronically infected prosthesis, antibiotics should be withheld until a microbiological diagnosis is clear. The commonest pathogens are coagulase-negative staphylococci. When a chronically infected prosthesis is removed it is reasonable to use empiric glycopeptide until culture results are available.
- Further follow-up antibiotics should be given in conjunction with advice from infection specialists.

Further reading

Cuckler, J.M., Star, A.M., Alavi, A. and Noto, R.B. (1991) Diagnosis and management of the infected total joint arthroplasty. *Orthop. Clin. N. Am.* **22**: 523–530.

Garvin, K.L. and Hanssen, A.D. (1995) Current concepts review: infection after total hip arthroplasty. *J. Bone Joint Surg.* **77-A**: 1576–1588.

Norden, C., Gillespie, W.J. and Nade, S. (1994) Infection in total joint replacement. In: *Infections in Bones and Joints.* Blackwell Scientific Publications, Oxford, pp. 291–319.

Rand, J.A., Morrey, B.F. and Bryan, R.S. (1984) Management of the infected total joint arthroplasty. *Orthop. Clin. N. Am.* **15**: 491–504.

Steckelberg, J.M. and Osmon, D.R. (1994) Prosthetic joint infections. In: *Infections Associated with Indwelling Medical Devices,* 2nd Edn (eds A.L. Bisno and F.A. Waldvogel). American Society for Microbiology, Washington, DC, pp. 259–290.

3 Osteomyelitis

Osteomyelitis can be divided into infection by the haematogenous route, from a contiguous site or due to vascular insufficiency. It can also be classified as *acute* or *chronic*.

Acute osteomyelitis can be regarded as having no inert/dead bone present, so eradication of infection is possible without bone removal. Pus may need to be drained. Presentation is usually with bone pain in conjunction with fever and constitutional symptoms.

Chronic osteomyelitis is associated with the presence of inert or dead material (sequestra), so surgical resection is usually necessary to completely eradicate infection. Presentation may be with only a discharging wound or sinus, or there may be chronic pain and sometimes fever with constitutional symptoms when disease flares.

The existing definitions of acute and chronic osteomyelitis vary in terms of the length of history.

Management options

1. Refer to trauma surgeons when metalwork *in situ*.
2. Refer to neuro-/spinal surgeons when there are neurological complications.
3. Refer to spinal surgeons when there is vertebral osteomyelitis.
4. Investigate, then prescribe specific antimicrobial therapy.
5. Investigate, then prescribe suppressive/symptomatic antimicrobial therapy.
6. Investigate and refer to an interventional radiologist for a drainage procedure.
7. Investigate and refer to orthopaedics for resection of bone and reconstructive surgery as needed.

Option 1. Refer to trauma surgeons when metalwork *in situ*.

✓ Allows management under the team who originally operated. A further operative procedure will usually be needed, sometimes with removal of the original metalwork.
✓ Multiple samples with separate instruments can be obtained intra-operatively, preferably before antibiotics, in order to make a specific microbiological diagnosis.

Option 2. Refer to neuro-/spinal surgeons when there are neurological complications.

✓ Pus can be drained and the compression of the cord relieved. This should prevent the progression of neurological complications.

Option 3. Refer to spinal surgeons when there is vertebral osteomyelitis.

✓ An assessment can be made as to the best way to obtain material for microbiology and histology and stabilization can be carried out if needed.

Option 4. Investigate, then prescribe specific antimicrobial therapy.

✓ This approach usually works for acute osteomyelitis and osteomyelitis due to TB.
✓ Surgery is avoided.
✗ It may be that eradication of infection is not possible without surgical intervention, e.g. drainage of pus in the acute situation or resection of dead bone in chronic osteomyelitis.

Option 5. Investigate, then prescribe suppressive/symptomatic antimicrobial therapy.

✓ This approach may be needed when the patient is too debilitated to have surgery or the surgery is too extensive to perform without major reconstruction.
✓ It can also be used to avoid or postpone radical surgery, for example in diabetics who

may in theory need amputation of a periphery to achieve eradication of infection. These patients may only need treatment when they have a flare-up of symptoms.

✗ Failure to resect disease may result in further progression.
✗ The presence of chronic osteomyelitis may lead to long-term complications such as amyloidosis.

Option 6. Investigate and refer to an interventional radiologist for a drainage procedure.

✓ This will be needed if there is a collection of pus, e.g. subperiosteally or extending into the soft tissues. Examples include a psoas or iliacus abscess. This is usually an acute presentation.
✓ This will allow further quality material to be sent for microbiological culture.
✓ This avoids an operative procedure.

✗ There may be incomplete drainage of pus, requiring a repeat procedure or surgery.
✗ Every procedure has a small complication risk (e.g. haemorrhage).

Option 7. Investigate and refer to orthopaedics for resection of bone and reconstructive surgery as needed.

This is a highly specialized and skilled speciality within orthopaedics and requires surgeons experienced in osteomyelitis and bone reconstruction. Any case of chronic osteomyelitis should be assessed carefully by both orthopaedic and infection specialists in order to discuss the therapeutic options available.

History checklist
- How and when did symptoms start? This will help you to decide whether the infection is likely to be acute or chronic.
- What site(s) is involved? Children are more likely to have long bone osteomyelitis but they do also get vertebral discitis that can extend to osteomyelitis. Adults are at risk of vertebral osteomyelitis. The patient may have multi-focal osteomyelitis (rare).
- Have there been systemic features such as fever, sweats and weight loss? Again, this will help in differentiating acute from chronic osteomyelitis. The degree of acute systemic upset will also determine the rapidity of commencing invasive procedures and starting empiric treatment. If the history is chronic then the possibility of TB, brucellosis or fungal osteomyelitis should be considered. In addition, non-infectious causes such as malignancy are possible.
- Is there a past history of osteomyelitis at the same site? Relapses of apparently cured osteomyelitis can occur decades later.
- Is there a history of recent trauma/bites at the site? If so, this may mean there is osteomyelitis related to a contiguous site. Osteomyelitis can occur secondary to bites or open trauma/fractures. Haematogenous seeding of closed injuries can also occur.
- Is there a history of recent metalwork (fixation devices) at the site. Is there still a device *in situ*? If so, the spectrum of 'pathogens' is broadened to include skin flora organisms such as coagulase-negative staphylococci. The management is also more complicated because, in certain circumstances, the metalwork may have to be removed (refer back to orthopaedics).
- Is there a history of a discharging sinus? This is almost unequivocal evidence for chronic osteomyelitis.
- Have there been recent hospitalizations predisposing to bacteraemia? Do they have a long-term indwelling venous catheter (e.g. haemodialysis)? A patient may have had a line-related bacteraemia, e.g. with S. aureus which may or may not be detected at the time. They may present with fever and bacteraemia and have vertebral osteomyelitis. Recognition of this is often delayed.
- Have there been recent skin lesions predisposing to bacteraemia? This may give you a clue as to the original source of bacteraemia leading to haematogenous osteomyelitis.

- Does the patient have diabetes, renal failure, peripheral vascular disease or chronic ulcers? All these increase the likelihood of developing osteomyelitis due to vascular insufficiency.
- Is there a history of malignancy or alcoholism? These increase the risk of osteomyelitis and often make treatment very problematic.
- Does the patient use i.v. drugs? If so, then in addition to the common pathogens (S. aureus, Streptococcus spp., Gram-negative bacteria) infection with P. aeruginosa is more likely. This can occur in less common sites, for example around the sacroiliac joints. Treatment in this group can also be problematic in terms of compliance with therapy.
- Is there a history of recurrent urinary tract infection or an indwelling urinary catheter? This can be the source of infection for lumbar osteomyelitis. Organisms can track back along a venous plexus to the lumbar spine. Infections are usually with Gram-negative bacilli, and frequently polymicrobial.
- Is there a history of travel to certain endemic areas? If so, consider infection with Brucella spp. and fungi.
- Does the patient have sickle-cell disease? Osteomyelitis in these patients can be very difficult to differentiate from aseptic infarcts of bone. When osteomyelitis occurs, it is most commonly due to Salmonella spp.
- Is there a history of TB or contact with TB? This may increase your suspicion of tuberculous disease.
- Does the patient (child) have Gaucher's disease? This can produce a clinical picture indistinguishable from acute osteomyelitis.

Examination checklist

General
- Look at the skin for staphylococcal or streptococcal skin lesions, chronic ulcers, old or current i.v. cannulation sites, trauma and bites.

Specific
- Cardiovascular. In particular, examine peripheral pulses for evidence of vascular insufficiency and murmurs (endocarditis).
- Respiratory. Look for evidence of TB.
- Abdomen. In particular look for splenomegaly (e.g. brucellosis).
- Neurological. Particularly with vertebral osteomyelitis, look for any evidence of cord compression (surgical emergency).
- Other bone and joint sites. Look for evidence of multi-focal disease, particularly in staphylococcal and tuberculous disease.
- Local examination: look for erythema, swelling, warmth and tenderness. Look for evidence of trauma or overlying ulcer. Look for a sinus (indicates chronic osteomyelitis).

Referrals
- See 'Management options'.

Pitfalls
- Starting antibiotics without obtaining material for microbiology and histology.
- Attempting to eradicate infection with antibiotics when a surgical procedure is necessary.

Hints for investigators and prescribers
- Empiric antibiotics are needed in the acutely septic patient. These should preferably be prescribed after samples are obtained for microbiology, and certainly after blood cultures. Empiric regimens should cover the likely organisms. A second generation cephalosporin is a reasonable option. If the patient has a risk factor for a nosocomial infection then antimicrobial agents active against MRSA should be considered, plus a broad-spectrum

agent active against Gram-negative bacteria. An anaerobic agent should be used where there is likely to be necrotic material or deep pus.

- In other situations, antimicrobial agents should be withheld until a specific diagnosis is made. Always discuss specific therapy with the microbiologist/infection specialist.
- The duration of treatment for osteomyelitis is long, often 6 weeks intravenously and 6 weeks orally. Acute osteomyelitis in children is sometimes treated in less time. These treatment regimens often warrant the use of tunnelled central lines and careful monitoring for complications of therapy.

Further reading

Cierny, G. (1990) Classification and treatment of adult osteomyelitis. In: *Surgery of the Musculoskeletal System*, Vol. 5 (ed. C.M. Evarts). Churchill Livingstone, New York, p. 4337.

Haas, D.W. and McAndrew, M.P. (1996) Bacterial osteomyelitis in adults: evolving considerations in diagnosis and treatment. *Am. J. Med.* **101**: 550–561.

Lew, D.P. and Waldvogel, F.A. (1997) Current concepts. Osteomyelitis. *N. Engl. J. Med.* **336**: 999–1007.

Norden, C., Gillespie, W.J. and Nade, S. (1994) *Infections in Bones and Joints*. Blackwell Scientific Publications, Oxford.

Wald, R. (1985) Risk factors for osteomyelitis. *Am. J. Med.* **78**: 206–212

Waldvogel, F.A., Medoff, G. and Swartz, M.N. (1970) Osteomyelitis: a review of clinical features, therapeutic considerations and unusual aspects. *N. Engl. J. Med.* **282**: 198, 260, 316 (3 articles).

Waldvogel, F.A. and Vasey, H. (1980) Osteomyelitis: the past decade. *N. Engl. J. Med.* **303**: 360–370.

Chapter 9
NEEDLESTICK INJURIES

G.W. Smith

Needlestick injuries, that is percutaneous inoculation of blood or body fluids with a needle, scalpel blade, or other sharp instrument, are not just minor physical injuries, but also inflict a psychological wound. The fear of personal infection with HIV or hepatitis B (HBV) or C (HCV) viruses makes the injured feel and act as if they have actually been infected. It is this psychological distress, overt or hidden, that the attending doctor should focus on, as well as the possibility of an infection being manifested at some time in the distant future. Exposure of non-intact skin or mucous membranes, to splashes of blood, or other biological fluids, and human bites are other routes of possible infection. Therefore, the single most important prerequisite in the effective management of the injured, is the reassurance that the risk of infection is small in the overwhelming majority of cases. However, skilful decision-making is needed to identify the exceptional case where action rather than words is imperative.

Hospitals should have an efficient administrative system, which records the circumstances of needlestick injuries and provides direct, instant access of the injured to a clinician expert in dealing with such injuries. The longer the injured has to wait, the deeper the fear of infection grows. The attending clinician should be adept at reassuring and comforting the injured, irrespective of whether he assesses the risk of infection as high or low. An injured colleague is a patient with individual concerns and anxieties, often for their families and partners as well as for themselves. There is also an educational opportunity for the recipient to learn how to avoid having a similar accident again.

Management options
1. Tell the recipient that needlestick injuries are commonplace, and that the risks of infection are very low anyway. As long as they have been vaccinated against HBV, there is nothing to worry about.
2. Tell the recipient you will find out if they have contracted HIV, HBV or HCV. This entails taking a baseline blood sample at the time, followed by further samples up to 6 months after the injury.
3. Tell the recipient they could have been infected with HIV, HBV or HCV and offer post-exposure prophylaxis against HBV and HIV, to be on the safe side.
4. After detailed assessment of circumstances, nature, and severity of a needlestick injury, the risks of infection can be established as negligible. In such cases, reassurance alone is the best course of action.
5. Tell the recipient that you propose to approach the donor and seek their consent to find out if they harbour a blood-borne virus.

Option 1. Tell the recipient that needlestick injuries are commonplace, and that the risks of infection are very low anyway. As long as they have been vaccinated against HBV, there is nothing to worry about.

- ✓ Most recipients will not have been exposed to an infectious agent. Therefore prompt and credible reassurance is what most of them need.
- ✓ There is no need to get involved in what may become a time-consuming and involved process, which usually ends in reassuring the recipient that there is nothing to worry about after all.

✗ Infection may not be prevented in a susceptible recipient who has been contaminated with a blood-borne virus.

✗ Some recipients expect that any reassurance will be backed by convincing scientific reasons. Otherwise, they may seek a second opinion. If the latter is different from the former they will lose confidence in both and worry more.

✗ If they do end up becoming infected, they will have good grounds for litigation.

Option 2. Tell the recipient you will find out if they have contracted HIV, HBV or HCV. This entails taking a baseline blood sample at the time, followed by further samples up to 6 months after the injury.

✓ After 6 months, most recipients can be given proof that they have not caught an infection.

✗ The fact that the doctor advises detailed follow-up will exaggerate the risks in the mind of the recipient, and in some cases may cause morbid anxiety.

✗ The occasional recipient, who is subsequently shown to have become infected, will justifiably ask why nothing was done to prevent the infection.

Option 3. Tell the recipient they could have been infected with HIV, HBV or HCV and offer post-exposure prophylaxis against HBV and HIV, to be on the safe side.

✓ In the event of infection being contracted, everything that could have been done can be seen to have been done – without a time-consuming consultation.

✗ The recipient will need specialized counselling regarding refraining from unprotected sexual intercourse for a least 6 months, or at least until such time as HIV infection has been excluded.

✗ Post-needlestick injury prophylaxis is a very expensive option. Also, recipients will be very worried, and some will be made sick from the toxicity of the antiviral drugs. Litigation may follow.

Option 4. After detailed assessment of circumstances, nature, and severity of a needlestick injury, the risks of infection can be established as negligible. In such cases, reassurance alone is the best course of action.

✓ The recipient will be grateful for your personal attention and care.

✓ Many recipients, particularly health care staff, who have been immunized against HBV, can be assured that the risk of hepatitis is vanishingly small. They can also be assured that the risk of contracting HIV is even smaller, unless they have been inoculated with a relatively large volume of blood .

✗ In some cases, it is not possible from the history alone, to make a reliable assessment of the risk of infection.

Option 5. Tell the recipient that you propose to approach the donor and seek their consent to find out if they harbour a blood-borne virus.

✓ As long as the whole process can be completed within 2–4 hours, you can ascertain whether the recipient has been exposed to any risk of infection. Specific prophylaxis, or reassurance, can then be offered with certainty.

✗ It may be impossible to identify the donor.

History checklist
● Precisely how was the injury sustained and under what circumstances?
  (i) It is not uncommon for an anxious member of staff to report a needlestick injury from a sharp that has not had any clinical contact – in which case reassurance can be made with confidence.

(ii) If the donor cannot be identified, the nature of the injury and whether or not a blood syringe was attached to the needle, will influence the decision to offer post-exposure prophylaxis against HIV.

Examination checklist
- Needlestick injuries are a medical emergency but generally require only a very brief consultation. Physical examination seldom prompts physical treatment, but engenders persuasive reassurance.

Referrals
- In principle, most needlestick injuries can be dealt with effectively by any medically qualified individual, provided that they are familiar with the basic issues surrounding blood-borne viruses in general, and HIV infection in particular. They should have access to local guidelines and relevant educational information on the risks of transmission, and be knowledgeable about the difference between informed consent and counselling, and of the consequences of an HIV test on life insurance.
- If there has been proven exposure to a blood-borne virus, the recipient must be referred for immediate post-exposure prophylaxis.
- If a recipient remains fearful of infection, referral for specialist counselling and support should be made.

Rituals and myths
- Collecting blood for virological tests on recipients after needlestick injuries, as a matter of routine, is of little value, except to satisfy the need to be 'doing something', Medicolegally, health care staff are entitled to compensation for psychological injury and actual infection, though the latter is very rare, without having to prove causality.
- Obtaining informed consent from the donor to test for HIV carriage is straightforward. It does not need to involve counselling to the extent that would be offered, for example, by the specialists in a GUM clinic. An HIV test is performed on the donor in the expectation of a negative result. If there is a suspicion that the donor could test positive, or if the donor is reluctant, or even refuses to consent, exploration of the underlying reasons is indicated for the benefit of the donor, who should then be referred to a specialist in GUM.
- In practice, a negative HIV antibody test on an infectious donor who is seroconverting at the time of the accident is so rare that it should not influence the routine management of needlestick injuries.

Pitfalls
- Failure to consider the risk of tetanus, if an injury was sustained by a discarded needle.
- Protection from HBV is not guaranteed, even if the recipient has received a full course of HBV immunization and has seroconverted. Only a satisfactory antibody concentration against the surface antigen protein of HBV (HBsAg), at the time of the injury, offers a degree of protection. If a protective antibody level at the time of the injury cannot be guaranteed, it must be checked. If this cannot be clarified within 24 hours, a booster dose of HBV vaccine should be given.
- Failure to follow locally agreed policy on needlestick injury management. If a donor is tested without consent, or if the recipient is given unlicensed anti-retroviral post-exposure prophylaxis without informed consent, a law suit could not be defended.
- Absence of e-antigen from the blood of an HBV-positive donor can no longer be taken as an index of low infectivity. Therefore, aggressive post-exposure prophylaxis must be organized for all needlestick recipients exposed to HBV.

Hints for investigators and prescribers
- If the donor is to be tested for blood-borne viruses, the laboratory should be assured that consent has been obtained for HIV testing.

- Clear communication should be established between the recipient, doctor, and laboratory so that positive results prompt immediate post-exposure prophylaxis. The profound therapeutic effect of negative results means that the recipient must always be informed without delay.
- The precise details and manner in which individual needlestick injuries have been managed must be clearly recorded.

Further reading

Easterbrook, P. (1998) Post-exposure prophylaxis for occupational exposures to HIV. *CME Bull. Infect. Dis. Trop. Med.* **1**: 15–19.

Heapy, J., Riordan, T. and Fairchild, Y. (1998) A five year survey of inoculation injuries in Exeter. *Communicable Dis. Public Health* **1**: 61–63.

Sundkvist, T., Hamilton, G.R., Rimmer, D., Evans, B.G. and Teo, C.G. (1998) Fatal outcome of transmission of HBV from an e antigen negative surgeon. *Communicable Dis. Public Health* **1**: 48–50.

Various. (1998) Prophylaxis after occupational exposure to HIV. *Br. Med. J.* **316**: 701–702 (letters).

Chapter 10

ORO-DENTAL INFECTIONS

M.V. Martin

Infections of the oral cavity are common and often perceived as minor. However, they can be serious and potentially life-threatening if not dealt with promptly. Oral infections are often dealt with by both doctors and dentists and it is therefore important that a unified approach to their management is adopted by both groups. It is also important that patients receive definitive curative treatment and not multiple courses of antimicrobials.

Chapter contents

1 Dentoalveolar abscess

This is an infection involving both the tooth, its surrounding tissues and the alveolar bone. It is usually acute, but can also be chronic and long-standing with acute exacerbations. Often patients will not seek help with acute abscesses that drain spontaneously through a sinus and become chronic.

Management options
1. Prescribe antibiotics.
2. Prescribe antibiotics and refer for extraction or drainage.

Option 1. Prescribe antibiotics.

✓ Cheap and easy option.
✓ May restrict the spread of the abscess.
✓ May restrict the metastatic spread of infection to vital organs.

✗ It does not cure the problem, as the cause remains.

Option 2. Prescribe antibiotics and refer for extraction or drainage.

✓ Eradicates the problem.
✓ Should reduce the chance of any serious sequelae.

✗ Often difficult due to 'dental phobia.'

History checklist
- This is often quite simple with the notable feature being severe lancinating, throbbing pain which gets worse when the patient lies down.
- The patient may report pain on closing the teeth together and difficulty in fully opening the mouth (trismus).

Examination checklist
- The most important feature of the examination is to identify the tooth responsible for the abscess and to remove it, or drain the pus formed.
- Identification of the tooth is usually achieved by simple percussion with the handle of a small instrument such as a dental mirror.
- The extent of the swelling must also be defined.
- If there is extensive trismus present, or there is spread below the mandible, then referral to a consultant oral surgeon should be considered.
- Spread of infection below the mandible can lead to involvement of the parapharyngeal space and embarrassment of the airway (Ludwig's angina)
- Trismus can lead to difficulties in gaining access to the mouth.

Hints for investigators and prescribers
- The cause of all dentoalveolar infections should be identified and eradicated.
- Microbiological investigations of dentoalveolar abscesses have shown that the usual cause is a mixture of facultative and obligate anaerobes. The antimicrobial of choice is therefore an aminopenicillin but this is always an adjunct to surgical drainage. In very severe infections with gross diffuse spread, metronidazole can be added to the aminopenicillin. The duration of the antimicrobial is dependent on the response of the patient. If the swelling subsides, the temperature is normal and the cause has been dealt with, then the antibiotics can be discontinued. Often no more than 3 days of antimicrobials are necessary.

- Antibiotics should only be prescribed if there is gross local spread of infection, an elevation in temperature, or there is a real chance of metastatic spread.
- The choice of antimicrobial in patients allergic to penicillin is more problematical. A macrolide remains the first choice, but the ideal dosage and length of treatment has never been fully investigated. Clindamycin is a useful alternative, but care has to be exercised with the potential problems of antibiotic-associated colitis.

Further reading

Fazakerley, M.W., McGowan, P., Hardy, P. and Martin, M.V. (1993) A comparative study of cephradine, amoxycillin and phenoxymethylpenicillin in the treatment of acute dentoalveolar infection. *Br. Dent. J.* **174**: 359–363.

Lewis, M.A.O., McGowan, P., Hardy, P., MacFarlane, T.W. and Lamey, M.-J. (1986) Quantitative bacteriology of acute dentoalveolar abscess. *J. Med. Microbiol.* **21**: 101–104.

Martin, M.V., Longman, L.P., Hill, J.B. and Hardy, P. (1997) Acute dentoalveolar infections: an investigation of the duration of therapy. *Br. Dent. J.* **183**: 135–137.

2 Acute lateral periodontal abscess

This abscess can often be mistaken for a dentoalveolar abscess but arises in the periodontium (the supporting tissues of the teeth). The exact site of the lateral periodontal abscess is in a pocket between tooth and gum. The abscess arises from micro-organisms multiplying in the pocket with anaerobes tending to predominate. Lateral periodontal abscesses tend to arise in patients with pre-existing periodontal disease (periodontitis).

Management options
1. Prescribe antibiotics.
2. Prescribe antibiotics, and refer for further treatment.

Option 1. Prescribe antibiotics.

✓ Cheap non-interventionist option.
✓ Can be effective particularly if metronidazole is used.

✗ Only a short-term remedy. The abscess will recur.

Option 2. Prescribe antibiotics, and refer for further treatment.

✓ Provides definitive treatment.
✓ Prevents the possibility of serious sequelae.

✗ May be difficult due to 'dental phobia'.

History checklist
- This will include some history of periodontal disease, usually bleeding gums, loose teeth or a continuous bad taste in the mouth for a long period of time.
- The pain experienced is usually localized to one tooth, which is painful to percussion and may be continuous or intermittent. The pain can also be dull or sharp.
- There may be an associated systemic malaise with pyrexia and dull continuous pain localized to the affected area.

Examination checklist
- There may be quite extensive swelling in the tissues lateral to the tooth which may elicit pus on gentle pressure. This can extend into the surrounding area and there may be limitation of mouth opening.

Hints for investigators and prescribers
- These lesions usually arise in patients with poor mouth care. Prevention of recurrence depends on good mouth care in the future.
- The prescribing of antibiotics is often not necessary if there is no systemic involvement. Surgery either by extraction, or treatment of the periodontal tissues can eradicate the problem.
- The lesion will recur if the tooth is not extracted, or appropriate periodontal therapy is not carried out.

Further reading
Marsh, P.D. and Martin, M.V. (1992) *Oral Microbiology*, 3rd Edn. Chapman & Hall, London, pp. 171–179.

3 Pericoronitis

This is inflammation around the crowns of erupting teeth. It can occur around any tooth, but is commonly associated with permanent third molar teeth particularly if their eruption is blocked (impaction). When the tooth is impacted, the gum covering it forms a small operculum in which anaerobes can cause a stagnation abscess. Pericoronitis is common in patients aged 17–24 years, as this is the age when third molars are erupting. Pericoronitis may be recurrent until the tooth erupts, or is extracted.

Management options
1. Prescribe antibiotics.
2. Irrigate, and if necessary incise and drain, together with antimicrobials.

Option 1. Prescribe antibiotics.
✓ Simple option that may control the infection.
✓ If metronidazole is used then multiple courses of this antimicrobial can be given if necessary. Resistance to metronidazole by oral anaerobes is rare.
✗ Prescribing antimicrobials does not cure the problem – surgical intervention is necessary.

Option 2. Irrigate, and if necessary incise and drain, together with antimicrobials.
✓ The treatment of choice to resolve the acute phase of the condition.
✓ If surgery is carried out on the impacted tooth after this initial treatment, then resolution will be achieved.
✗ Requires surgical facilities.

History checklist
- There is often a history of initially mild discomfort in the area, which intensifies.
- Often the patient will report continuous dull or sharp pain which can prevent them sleeping.
- The patient will usually be able to localize the painful area precisely.

Examination checklist
- There may be localized or diffuse extraoral swelling and pyrexia.
- Intraorally there is usually swelling on the tissue partially covering the tooth; gentle pressure on this tissue may yield pus.
- The tissue covering the tooth may be traumatized by the opposing tooth.
- There may also be limitation in mouth opening due to trismus.

Hints for investigators and prescribers
- This is an abscess caused by anaerobes infecting a stagnation area under an operculum flap. The initial therapy should be surgical by drainage of the stagnation area. This drainage can usually be achieved by simple irrigation under the flap with fluid. Antimicrobials are really an adjunct to the treatment to prevent gross local and systemic spread.
- The antimicrobial of choice is metronidazole, and usually 3 days therapy is enough to relieve the patients symptoms. The second choice is clindamycin for patients who cannot tolerate metronidazole.
- This condition will reoccur until surgery is done and the impacted tooth extracted.

Further reading

Elliasson, S., Heimdahl, A. and Nordenram, A. (1989) Pathological changes related to long-term impaction of third molars. A radiographic study. *Int. J. Oral Maxillofacial Surg.* **18**: 210–212.

Macgregor, A.J. (1985) *The Impacted Lower Wisdom Tooth.* Oxford University Press, Oxford.

Van der Linden, W., Cleaton-Jones, P. and Lownie, M. (1995) Diseases and lesions associated with third molars. Review of 1001 cases. *Oral Surg. Oral Med. Oral Pathol. Oral Radiol.* **79**: 142–145.

4 'Dry' socket (localized osteitis)

Dry sockets are so-called because they follow extractions of teeth. The socket loses its blood clot and is thought to become infected. There is still debate about the contribution of trauma from the extraction to the aetiology of this condition, but there is agreement that it does play a part.

Management options
The only treatment is to thoroughly clean out the socket and to dress it with some form of sedative dressing. It is therefore best to refer the patient to a dentist as soon as possible.

Antimicrobials will not effect a cure but may help with the management. Metronidazole for 3 days is the best choice of antimicrobial for this condition.

History checklist
- This diagnosis is not difficult to make as there is a history of tooth extraction within the previous 72 hours.

Examination checklist
- There will be development of acute pain, trismus and often facial swelling; the temperature may also be elevated.
- Intraorally there is a tooth socket which contains no blood clot and may be filled with debris.

Further reading
Fazakerley, M., and Field, E.A. (1991) Dry socket: a painful post-extraction complication. A review. *Dent. Update* 18.

5 Actinomycosis

Actinomycosis is classically described as a slow-growing loculated lesion caused by Actinomyces spp. Approximately 90% of actinomycosis cases are cervicofacial in location, with abdominal, thoracic and disseminated lesions accounting for the remaining 10% of reports.

In the last decade it has been recognized that cervicofacial actinomycosis may be of two kinds: the classical slow-growing lesion, and an acute oral infection in which actinomycetes are a coincidental microbiological finding. The latter acute lesions usually resolve without any treatment apart from surgery, and they may represent early actinomycotic lesions which become chronic at a later date. Only chronic actinomycotic lesions will be described.

Management options

There is only one option for this lesion and that is surgery, together with a 4–6 week course of antibiotics. The surgery has to be thorough, with attention to breaking down all the fibrous locules of which the lesion is composed. The antibiotic therapy can be initially i.v., but oral agents can be used when the patient has recovered from surgery.

History checklist

- Patients with actinomycotic lesions most often present with a history of swelling usually in the mandibular molar area. The swelling arises secondary to some kind of trauma to the area, but often patients do not associate the start of the lesion with this event.
- The swelling is often painless and may form sinuses, which release pus.
- Multiple indurated sinuses are not often seen, although this is the description of actinomycosis in some textbooks.

Examination checklist

- There is a firm rubbery lesion of variable size, usually at the angle of the mandible.
- Aspiration will yield pus with granular collections of Gram-positive filaments.

Hints for investigators and prescribers

- Patients may delay seeking help because of fears that the actinomycotic lesions are cancerous.
- This lesion will not resolve without a combination of surgery and long-term antibiotics. The antimicrobial of choice is amoxycillin, usually at least 1 g daily. The end-point of therapy is clinical resolution of the lesion, but this is often difficult to judge as some residual fibrous tissue often remains in the lesional area. Discontinuation of the antibiotics when this residual amount of fibrous tissue is present does not usually result in recrudescence. Patients allergic to penicillin can be given tetracyclines, minocycline being the antibiotic of choice.

Further reading

Martin, M.V. (1984) The use of oral amoxycillin for the treatment of actinomycosis; a clinical and in vitro study. *Br. Dent. J.* **156**: 138–140.

Martin, M.V. (1985) Antibiotic treatment for patients allergic to penicillin; a clinical and in vitro study. *Br. J. Oral Maxillofacial Surg.* **23**: 428–434.

Samuels, R.H.A. and Martin, M.V. (1988) A clinical and microbiological study of actinomycetes in oral and cervicofacial lesions. *Br. J. Oral Maxillofacial Surg.* **26**: 458–463.

Stenhouse, D., MacDonald, D.G. and MacFarlane, T.W. (1975) Cervicofacial and intraoral actinomycosis: a five year retrospective study. *Br. J. Oral Surg.* **13**: 237–240.

6 Angular cheilitis

Angular cheilitis is inflammation and infection at the angles of the mouth. It can be caused by either malabsorption, or by stagnation due to infolding of skin at the corners of the mouth. It is common in elderly patients who wear old dentures and in young women with anaemia.

Management options
1. In the elderly, the dentures need to be remade to eliminate the folding of the skin and to eliminate the stagnation areas. If this is not done, the lesion may become chronic and granulomatous. Referral to a dentist is therefore essential.
2. In young dentate patients, angular cheilitis may be associated with iron, folate or B_{12} deficiency. It can also be an early sign of HIV infection.

History and examination checklist
History is of simple and usually progressive soreness at the corners of the mouth. The examination of the lesion will show inflammation.

Hints for investigators and prescribers
- Angular cheilitis can be difficult to eradicate even with good patient compliance. This may be due to the fact that there is a concomitant intraoral candida infection which may reinfect the angles by salivary contamination. Another reason for lack of resolution is that often the candida are killed but the staphylococci remain.
- It is important to investigate and establish the cause of this condition if it is to be eradicated. The infection is usually caused by a mixture of Candida spp. and staphylococci, and an antifungal drug, combined with an antibacterial is therefore indicated.

Further reading
Samaranayake, L.P. and MacFarlane, T.W. (1990) *Oral Candidosis*. Wright, London, pp. 156–183.
Tyldesley, W.R. and Field, E.A. (1995) *Oral Medicine*, 4th Edn. Oxford University Press, Oxford, pp. 65–66.

7 Oral candidosis

Oral candida infections comprise a heterogeneous group of infections usually caused by C. albicans, but other Candida spp. may also be involved. There have been a number of classifications of oral candidosis but the most useful for clinicians is as follows:

- *Acute pseudomembraneous (thrush).* Occurs in elderly and the young.
- *Acute erythematous.* Found in all areas of the mouth and often associated with broad-spectrum antibiotic use.
- *Chronic plaque-like, chronic nodular.* Hyperplastic lesions that must be biopsied to ensure that they are not neoplastic.
- *Chronic erythematous and pseudomembraneous.* May be secondary to denture wearing but also may be indicative of AIDS.
- *Chronic mucocutaneous.* A rare form of oral candidosis characterized by keratin plaques.

Management options

Oral candidosis can be difficult to manage and is best dealt with by those with experience of this condition. Referral to a consultant in oral medicine is the best course of action.

Further reading

Samaranayake, L.P. and MacFarlane, T.W. (1990) *Oral Candidosis.* Wright, London.

8 Acute (necrotizing) ulcerative gingivitis

Acute (necrotizing) ulcerative gingivitis (ANUG) used to be relatively common in European countries but is apparently decreasing in incidence. The cause of ANUG is still not known but in some cases it is associated with debilitation and poor oral hygiene. It can be seasonal, the highest incidence being in the winter months.

Management options
1. Prescribe antibiotics.
2. Prescribe antibiotics and refer to a dentist for periodontal treatment.

Option 1. Prescribe antibiotics.

✓ Simple option which removes the acute problem.
✓ May help to start resolution.

✗ Does not eradicate the problem and it is likely to recur.

Option 2. Prescribe antibiotics and refer to a dentist for periodontal treatment.

✓ The treatment can eradicate the acute problem.
✓ The problem is unlikely to recur.

✗ To eliminate the gum problem a great deal of patient compliance is necessary.

History checklist
● There is a history of soreness of the gums, bleeding and a bad taste, usually over a 2–3 day period.

Examination checklist
● ANUG can often be diagnosed by the fetid halitosis of the patient.
● Intraorally there is soreness and bleeding of the gums and crater-like ulceration on the gum between the teeth.
● These ulcers spread laterally to involve the whole gum margin, and they may be covered by a white pseudomembrane.

Hints for investigators and prescribers
● The acute phase of ANUG can usually be resolved with 3 days treatment with metronidazole. Topical oral 0.2% (w/v) chlorhexidine can also help in the acute phase to relieve the immediate symptoms. The importance of improving the oral hygiene cannot be overstressed.
● Metronidazole together with periodontal therapy is the only satisfactory option to eliminate this problem.

Further reading
Marsh, P.D. and Martin, M.V. (1992) *Oral Microbiology*, 3rd Edn. Chapman & Hall, London, pp. 167–196.
Tyldesley, W.R. and Field, E.A. (1995) *Oral Medicine*, 4th Edn. Oxford University Press, Oxford, pp. 27–31.

9 Post-operative oroantral communication

This occurs, as the name implies, following extractions of maxillary teeth. A communication between the mouth and the antral cavity occurs. Referral to an oral surgeon for closure is mandatory. Antibiotics must be given prophylactically to avoid sinus infection.

10 Oral viral infections

A large number of viruses affect the oral cavity, particularly in patients that are medically compromised. For details of these infections, the reader is referred to the textbooks of oral medicine in the bibliography to this section. By far the most common oral viral infection is caused by herpes simplex virus type 1 (HSV-1) which is carried by almost 100% of the population. Oral lesions only occur in 30% of the population infected with HSV-1.

There are primary and secondary HSV-1 infections, which may be clinically indistinguishable. Classically, the cold sore that characterizes HSV-1 infection occurs at the junction of the oral and skin epithelium of the lips following exposure to sunlight, menstruation or stress.

Management options
1. Prescribe fluids and warn the patient about the infectious nature of the lesions.
2. Prescribe antivirals and fluids.

Option 1. Prescribe fluids and warn the patient about the infectious nature of the lesions.

✓ Simple inexpensive option.
✓ The lesions usually resolve spontaneously.

✗ Antivirals are effective and can shorten the time the lesion takes to resolve.

Option 2. Prescribe antivirals and fluids.

✓ Can shorten the time for the ulcers to heal.
✓ Absolutely essential in medically compromised patients to avoid further complications.

✗ Expensive.

History checklist
- There is usually a prodromal phase where the patient may have altered sensations to the affected area. These sensations can be felt as burning, itching or just hypersensitivity.
- The vesicles appear a few days later in small collections and eventually burst to leave sore ulcers.
- The ulcers heal uneventfully, usually within 10 days of the start of the prodromal phase.

Examination checklist
- There is usually little difficulty in recognizing the shallow ulcers that occur at the junction of the oral and skin epithelium; they can also occur intraorally.

Hints for investigators and prescribers
- Two antivirals are available: aciclovir and penciclovir. Both are effective, but the latter has been reported to shorten the period of ulceration.
- Systemic medication with aciclovir should be considered, in addition to topical treatment, in medically compromised patients. The use of antivirals is mandatory as they do shorten the time taken for healing.
- Fluids are essential, as patients often find eating very difficult and neglect to take an adequate fluid intake.

Further reading
Scully, C., Flint, S.R. and Porter, S.R. (1996) *Oral Diseases*, 2nd Edn. Martin Dunitz, London, pp. 64–87.
Tyldesley, W.R. and Field, E.A. (1995) *Oral Medicine*, 4th Edn. Oxford University Press, Oxford, pp. 42–52.

Chapter 11
PYREXIA OF UNKNOWN ORIGIN

F.J. Nye

Pyrexia of unknown origin (PUO) has an extremely wide differential diagnosis, but in practice, management and investigations are guided by the individual clinical circumstances of a particular patient. The overall direction in which investigation proceeds will be guided by emerging clues from the results of laboratory tests and imaging, and by what is found on repeat history-taking and physical examination.

For patients with fever presenting in general practice, the important management issues are as follows:

- Has the patient really got a fever?
- Is the fever acute, chronic, or recurrent?
- Is there likely to be a serious or life-threatening cause for the fever?
- What initial investigations, if any, are indicated?
- Is empirical antibiotic therapy justifiable?
- If not, what follow-up arrangements should be made?

For patients in hospital, alternative or additional questions will include:

- Is the observed temperature genuine?
- Have common causes of fever been satisfactorily excluded?
- What are the likely causes of fever given the clinical circumstances (e.g. imported fever, immunosuppression, neutropenia, HIV-related PUO)?
- What investigations are most likely to lead to a successful diagnosis, and in what order should they be carried out?
- At what stage in the diagnostic process is it appropriate to discharge the patient from hospital?
- What is the role of 'therapeutic trials' in the management of PUO?
- What action should be taken if the patient's condition deteriorates, in the absence of a definite diagnosis?
- If exhaustive investigations fail to yield a diagnosis, how should the patient then be managed?

In order to cover the ground as thoroughly as possible, four separate case histories have been selected, each focusing on a different presentation of PUO.

Case 1: PUO investigated in general practice (p. 168)
Case 2: PUO investigated in hospital (p. 173)
Case 3: PUO with a history of recent travel (p. 178)
Case 4: PUO with a history of immunodeficiency (p. 182)

Although the case histories have been selected for their generic nature, the examples relating to recent travel and immunodeficiency in particular, should guide the reader in a particular strategic direction.

Case 1: PUO investigated in general practice

Unexplained fever, present for 1 week, in a 63-year-old woman presenting in general practice.

Management options

1. Refer the patient to hospital.
2. Prescribe a broad-spectrum antibiotic.
3. Do nothing. No investigations or treatment.
4. Recommend antipyretic treatment, and review the patient if symptoms do not improve.
5. Arrange initial investigations and review the patient with the results. Meanwhile, prescribe a broad-spectrum antibiotic.
6. Arrange initial investigations and review the patient with the results. Recommend antipyretics but withhold antibiotics.

Option 1. Refer the patient to hospital.

Tell the patient that you are not sure of the diagnosis and that she needs hospital investigation and treatment.

✓ This may be the best option if the patient looks very ill.
✓ You are trying to establish a diagnosis.
✓ There is a management plan.

✗ For most patients referral will be unnecessary.
✗ Referral will be time-consuming for the patient.
✗ Hospital resources may be used inappropriately.
✗ You will lose the opportunity for effective management in primary care.

Option 2. Prescribe a broad-spectrum antibiotic.

Tell the patient she will get better after a course of antibiotics.

✓ Patients with inapparent bacterial infection, e.g. urinary tract infection (UTI) may well respond to your treatment.

✗ This option does nothing to establish a diagnosis since the fever may settle despite, or because of, antibiotics.
✗ Bacterial sepsis may be masked, with subsequent delay in diagnosis and definitive treatment.
✗ Some patients will delay seeking further help, even if they are becoming more ill, if they believe you have prescribed effective treatment.
✗ You will be needlessly exposing some patients to antibiotic side-effects.
✗ Without any diagnostic information, antibiotic side-effects, such as skin rash, will be difficult to distinguish from features of underlying illness.

Option 3. Do nothing. No investigations or treatment.

Reassure the patient that the fever will get better on its own.

✗ You have done nothing to relieve the patient's symptoms.
✗ This option does nothing to establish a diagnosis.
✗ There is no plan for follow-up or further management.
✗ You will be withholding antibiotic treatment from some patients who might respond.

Option 4. Recommend antipyretic treatment, and review the patient if symptoms do not improve.

Tell the patient she has an infection which you will investigate if she does not improve.

✓ The patient may feel better if the fever responds to antipyretics.
✓ You will not be masking inapparent bacterial sepsis.
✓ There is a plan for further follow-up and management.

✗ An opportunity for initiating investigations will have been missed.
✗ You will be delaying antibiotic treatment for some patients who might benefit.

Option 5. Arrange initial investigations and review the patient with the results. Meanwhile, prescribe a broad-spectrum antibiotic.

Tell the patient she has an infection that should respond to antibiotics, and that you are going to do some tests.

✓ Patients with inapparent bacterial infection (e.g. UTI) may well respond to your treatment.
✓ You are actively seeking a diagnosis.
✓ There is a plan for follow-up and further management.

✗ The results of later bacteriological investigations (e.g. blood cultures) may be compromised.
✗ You will be needlessly exposing some patients to antibiotic side-effects.
✗ The patient will have to be reviewed.

Option 6. Arrange initial investigations and review the patient with the results. Recommend antipyretics but withhold antibiotics.

Tell the patient that she has a probable infection, but that you would like to see the results of tests before prescribing antibiotics.

✓ All management options are still open.
✓ You are actively seeking a diagnosis.
✓ The patient may feel better if the fever responds to antipyretics.
✓ You are not needlessly exposing some patients to antibiotic side-effects.
✓ You will not be masking inapparent bacterial sepsis.
✓ There is a plan for follow-up and further management.

✗ You will be delaying antibiotic treatment for some patients who might respond.
✗ The patient will have to be reviewed.

History checklist

General
- For how long in total has the patient complained of 'fever'? It is helpful to know if the present complaint forms part of a longer illness. Illness present for many months may have an inflammatory cause (e.g. connective tissue disease) but often proves to have no definite organic basis. However, there are many exceptions to this rule and genuine fever, e.g. from malignancy, may persist for a year or longer.
- Is there a history of recurrent fever? Although there is a long list of disorders causing recurrent fever, the cause is often a focus of bacterial infection somewhere below the diaphragm: cholecystitis or cholangitis, intra-abdominal, retroperitoneal or psoas abscess, or UTI (often associated with obstruction and/or calculi). Connective tissue disorders are also fairly high on the list.
- Is there objective evidence of fever? Has the patient, or anyone else, actually taken and

recorded her temperature? If so, are the readings likely to be accurate? If there is no temperature record, keep an open mind (for the time being) on the likelihood of true fever.
- What is the significance of the patient's fever-associated symptoms?

    Rigors. 'Shaking chills' (followed by excessive heat and sweating) are useful clinical markers of a rapid rise in body temperature. Beyond this, little further diagnostic information can be gleaned. Rigors may be associated with a wide range of infections and with some non-infective causes of fever.

    Excessive sweating. Sweating is a common accompaniment of fever: night sweats persisting for several weeks are a classical feature of pulmonary and extrapulmonary TB. Sweating from any cause is, however, usually more noticeable at night and need not necessarily be accompanied by fever. Non-infective causes of sweating include excessive alcohol consumption, anxiety, malignancy and endocrine disorders (thyrotoxicosis, acromegaly and diabetes mellitus).

    Muscle pain. Myalgia is characteristic of virus infections such as influenza and enterovirus infection. However, severe muscle pain can also be a feature of life-threatening illness, particularly overwhelming bacterial sepsis including meningococcal septicaemia. Lumbar myalgia caused by systemic infection may mimic the renal pain of pyelonephritis. Fever and muscle pain are also features of non-infective disorders such as inflammatory myositis and polymyalgia rheumatica.

    Headache. Fever may cause headache, regardless of the underlying diagnosis. Severe headache and photophobia, though characteristic of meningitis, may also be encountered in many other infective processes, e.g. pyelonephritis, pneumonia and bacterial enteritis.

Specific

System review
- Respiratory system. Enquire about nasal discharge, sneezing, sinus pain, sore throat and pain or enlargement of cervical lymph nodes (upper respiratory tract infection). Elicit symptoms of lower respiratory tract infection (cough, sputum production, chest pain and breathlessness).
- Genito-urinary tract. Ask specifically about frequency, dysuria, loin pain and vaginal or urethral discharge (cystitis, pyelonephritis, pelvic inflammatory disease, sexually transmitted disease (STD), etc.).
- Musculoskeletal system. Are there any joint symptoms: pain, swelling, stiffness, limitation of movement? (Rheumatoid arthritis and other connective tissue disorders, pyogenic arthritis, reactive arthritis.)
- Alimentary system. Has there been any abdominal pain, weight loss or diarrhoea? (Malignancy, intra-abdominal sepsis, inflammatory bowel disease.)
- Skin. Has the patient noticed any skin rash? Can she describe it?

Travel abroad
- Has the patient been overseas recently? If so, has she visited any areas where malaria is endemic? Falciparum malaria is a possibility, whatever the symptoms, if she has been in an endemic area within the past 3 months.

Past medical history
- Are there any pointers in the past medical history? Ask particularly about valvular heart disease, TB and previous surgical procedures.

Drugs and alcohol
- Drug fever is uncommon and therefore easily missed. Over 80% of patients with drug fever do not have any accompanying skin rash and only about one in ten will give a history of previous drug allergy. Virtually any drug can cause fever, but a list of the common-

est culprits includes penicillins and cephalosporins, sulphonamides, antituberculosis agents, anticonvulsants (particularly phenytoin) methyldopa and quinidine. Drug fever usually resolves within 72 hours of stopping the agent responsible.
- Alcohol-related disease can be responsible for unexplained fever: alcoholic hepatitis, cirrhosis and primary hepatocellular carcinoma are recognized causes. The patient's long-term alcohol consumption should be assessed and recorded.

Examination checklist
- Take the patient's temperature. This is best taken orally, as the equilibrium time (90 seconds with a mercury thermometer) is less than when the axilla is used.
- Is the patient shivering, hot or sweating excessively?
- Is there any skin rash, jaundice or lymphadenopathy?
- Is there any joint swelling or tenderness?
- Head and neck. Examine the pharynx and mouth and look for evidence of dental sepsis. Is there any tenderness over the paranasal sinuses? Examine the cervical, submandibular and occipital lymph nodes for enlargement (infection or malignancy). Is there any temporal artery tenderness or thickening (temporal arteritis)? Check for neck stiffness (meningitis, meningism, or local disease in the neck).
- Chest and heart. Is there any evidence suggesting lower respiratory tract infection, e.g. tachypnoea, crackles on auscultation, or signs of consolidation or pleural effusion? Are there any heart murmurs?
- Abdomen. Are there any scars from previous surgery? Examine the abdomen, checking particularly for masses, organomegaly and renal tenderness.

Referrals
- Categories of patients who might be considered for referral to hospital include the following:
    The very sick.
    Immunocompromised or immunosuppressed patients.
    Those with indwelling prosthetic devices or grafts.
    Intravenous drug users.
    Patients with valvular heart disease.
    Patients with imported fever.
    Patients who have failed to respond to empirical antibiotic therapy.

Rituals and myths
- Fever means infection. Common exceptions include connective tissue disorders, such as temporal arteritis and polymyalgia rheumatica, inflammatory bowel disease, thromboembolism, hepatic cirrhosis, malignancy and drug reactions. Endocrine causes include thyrotoxicosis, thyroiditis and adrenal insufficiency.
- A therapeutic trial of antibiotics will distinguish bacterial infections from other causes. False negative responses may be caused by bacterial antibiotic resistance, inadequate antibiotic levels at the site of infection or poor patient compliance. False positive responses are usually due to spontaneous resolution of fever. Furthermore, an apparent response to a course of antibiotics may merely represent temporary suppression of infection rather than cure, as in the empirical treatment of patients with undiagnosed endocarditis or deep seated abscess.

Pitfalls
- Feeling hot is not always the same as being hot. Always seek objective evidence of fever.
- Prodromal illnesses are nearly always misdiagnosed as non-specific 'virus infections'. Only days later do the characteristic features of the specific infection emerge (e.g. viral hepatitis, infectious mononucleosis).

- Never assume that the patient will volunteer a history of foreign travel. Only by asking will you avoid missing malaria and other life-threatening infections.
- Bacterial endocarditis is often overlooked, especially when the patient's symptoms are mild. Although most patients will have an audible heart murmur, many will not have any of the peripheral signs of endocarditis. Fever plus a murmur is enough to arouse suspicions.
- Septicaemia in general is notoriously easy to miss: mental confusion, body pain and general 'toxicity' may alert you to the likely diagnosis. Although a haemorrhagic rash is characteristic of meningococcal septicaemia, skin changes may be atypical or absent.

Hints for investigators and prescribers

'Core' investigations for the patient with unexplained fever include the following:

- Midstream urine (MSU) and urinalysis.
- Haemoglobin (Hb).
- White cell count (WCC).
    Neutrophilia. Consider bacterial infection and vasculitis.
    Lymphocytosis. Consider virus infections especially glandular fever.
    Neutropenia. Consider virus infections, drug reactions, malignancy, systemic lupus erythematosus (SLE).
- Platelet count.
    Raised. In inflammatory disorders, e.g. arthropathy and inflammatory bowel disease.
    Lowered. In malaria and some virus infections, and in some patients with SLE.
- Paul-Bunnell test/monospot.
- Erythrocyte sedimentation rate (ESR).
- C-reactive protein (CRP). Levels >100 mg l^{-1} are highly indicative of infection.
- Urea creatinine and electrolytes.
- Liver function tests (LFT).
- A chest X-ray may also be needed. (Consider for patients with pre-existing heart or lung disease, and for those in the risk categories summarized under 'Referrals', p. 171.)

Case 2: PUO investigated in hospital

Pyrexia of unknown origin in a 50-year-old man, investigated in hospital.

Management options

1. Arrange multiple investigations, including invasive procedures such as bone marrow and liver biopsy, as quickly as possible.
2. Carry out investigations in order of increasing complexity and invasiveness. Start with blood tests and progress through imaging techniques to more invasive procedures, including biopsies, until a diagnosis is reached.
3. Adopt a stepwise approach to investigation as in Option 2, but pursue diagnostic clues immediately ('go to where the money is').

Option 1. Arrange multiple investigations, including invasive procedures such as bone marrow and liver biopsy, as quickly as possible.

Tell the patient you are going to make a rapid diagnosis by ordering all the relevant tests straight away.

✓ The patient will be investigated thoroughly.
✓ Time will not be wasted on holding back on diagnostic tests or procedures.

✗ Possible clues from the history, examination or initial tests may be overlooked or ignored.
✗ It is likely that some of the invasive procedures will prove unnecessary, and the patient will therefore be exposed to avoidable discomfort and risks.
✗ The patient will find the full 'shopping list' of tests extremely daunting.
✗ Including every possible test will be very expensive.
✗ The more tests you order, the more likely you are to come up with irrelevant or misleading information.

Option 2. Carry out investigations in order of increasing complexity and invasiveness. Start with blood tests and progress through imaging techniques to more invasive procedures, including biopsies, until a diagnosis is reached.

Tell the patient you will carry out all relevant tests, but will defer the more unpleasant ones for the time being, in the hope that a diagnosis can be reached without them.

✓ The patient will be investigated thoroughly.
✓ He may well be spared some unnecessary invasive procedures.
✓ Investigation will prove less costly than if all possible tests were ordered immediately.

✗ Time may be wasted if a cautious stepwise approach is used.
✗ Possible clues from the history, examination or initial investigations may be overlooked or ignored.

Option 3. Adopt a stepwise approach to investigation as in Option 2, but pursue diagnostic clues immediately ('go to where the money is').

Tell the patient you will carry out all relevant tests but will, if possible, defer more invasive investigations until any diagnostic clues have been followed up.

✓ The patient will be investigated thoroughly.
✓ He may well be spared some invasive investigations.
✓ Investigation will prove less costly than if all possible tests were ordered immediately.
✓ Possible clues from the history, examination or initial investigations will be properly pursued.

✗ Time may be wasted if a cautious stepwise approach is used.

History checklist

General and specific history
For details please refer to Case 1.

- Travel abroad and country of origin. Take a careful history of which countries the patient has visited or lived in during his lifetime. Particular importance should be attached to time spent in sub-Saharan Africa, the Indian subcontinent, the Far East, the Middle East, Oceania, Latin America and the Caribbean. Malaria is the commonest cause (30–40%) of imported fever and should be excluded early in the patient's illness. Second on the list in terms of frequency are respiratory infection, viral hepatitis and dengue. Less common causes (~1% each) include enteric fever, tuberculosis (TB), amoebic liver abscess, typhus, and acute HIV infection. There are a host of rarities: bacterial infections (e.g. brucellosis, relapsing fever, tularaemia), parasitic and protozoal infections (e.g. acute schistosomiasis, visceral leishmaniasis, African trypanosomiasis) and fungal infections (histoplasmosis and coccidioidomycosis).
- Personal and social history. Take a sexual history from the patient. This should include enquiry about possible recent exposure to STDs, as well as an assessment of life-time risk of sexually acquired HIV infection. The patient should be asked whether he has ever used 'street' drugs of any description and particularly whether he has ever injected illicit drugs (HIV, HBV or HCV). He should also be asked about occupational and recreational exposure to birds (psittacosis) or animals (brucellosis, Q fever, toxoplasmosis etc.) and about consumption of unpasteurized milk or milk products (brucellosis and Q fever).

Examination checklist
The list in Case 1 can be used as a basis for the physical examination which must be complete and well documented. It is essential to repeat an initially negative examination every few days in order to pick up emerging physical signs such as the appearance of a heart murmur or of enlarged lymph nodes.

- Factitious fever must be excluded as soon as possible. Clues to the diagnosis include:
  (i) A patient who looks well.
  (ii) Bizzare temperature chart with absence of diurnal variation and/or temperature-related changes in pulse rate.
  (iii) Temperature >41°C.
  (iv) Absence of sweating during defervescence.
  (v) Normal ESR and CRP, despite high fever.
  (vi) Evidence of self-injection or self-harm.
  (vii) Useful methods for establishing the diagnosis of factitious fever include supervised (observed) temperature measurement, and measuring the temperature of freshly voided urine.
- Examination of the skin and nails is particularly important in PUO, searching for skin rashes and nodules, vasculitic lesions and the stigmata of subacute bacterial endocarditis. Nodular skin lesions may represent disseminated fungal infection or metastatic malignancy. Secondaries from colonic, bladder and ovarian tumours are particularly common in the abdominal wall, while breast and bronchial carcinomas often metastasize to the chest wall or scalp. Leukaemia and lymphoma may produce papules, nodules or plaques and a variety of other skin lesions.
- Examination of the eye must include fundoscopy to look for haemorrhages and exudates (vasculitis), Roth's spots (endocarditis), choroidal tubercles, or disseminated fungal lesions. Carcinoma of the breast and bronchus occasionally metastasize to the choroid. A red eye may be a helpful clue to diagnosis: uveitis and/or conjunctivitis may

be encountered in immune complex disorders and reactive arthropathy and conjunctival petechiae may accompany endocarditis. Proptosis, especially if unilateral, suggests possible orbital infiltration by granulomatous tissue or malignancy.

- Examination of the upper airways. Nasal obstruction or bleeding, and sinus pain or swelling may constitute evidence of infection, malignancy or granulomatous disease/vasculitis.
- Rectal examination must be included in order to detect perianal disease (suggestive of inflammatory bowel disease), local sepsis and rectal carcinoma. The prostate should be palpated for evidence of carcinoma or prostatitis. If the prostate is tender or feels 'boggy', prostatic massage can be carried out and the resulting urethral discharge sent to the laboratory for microscopy and culture.

Rituals and myths

- Abnormal liver function tests merit a liver biopsy. Although some conditions involving the liver (e.g. sarcoidosis) will require a tissue diagnosis, many causes of PUO affecting the liver may be elucidated without carrying out a liver biopsy. Raised transaminases should prompt serological screening for hepatitis A, B and C, while elevations of gamma glutamyl transferase and liver alkaline phosphatase may point to metastases or biliary disease (infection or obstruction) as the source of the PUO. A number of infections (cytomegalovirus (CMV), Epstein–Barr virus (EBV), toxoplasma and Q fever) involve the liver as part of a wider systemic process and are usually best diagnosed serologically. Many patients will have non-specific abnormalities of liver function. Misleading tests are particularly common in temporal arteritis (25%), renal carcinoma and primary bone marrow lymphoma.
- A tuberculin skin test is useful for the diagnosis of occult TB (UK). Patients with old inactive TB and those who have received previous Bacillus Calmette-Guérin (BCG) immunization will show skin reactivity to tuberculin purified protein derivative (PPD). Hence, a II to III grade Heaf reaction or a positive Mantoux test (5–14 mm of induration after 10 units of PPD) are consistent with prior immunization, quiescent TB, or active TB. Although strongly positive tuberculin tests may suggest a diagnosis of TB, they are also encountered in patients without active disease who have been repeatedly exposed to mycobacteria e.g. expatriates from tropical areas. A number of factors may suppress the tuberculin reaction:

    Viral infection, particularly infectious mononucleosis.
    Lymphoma and other diseases depressing immunity, including HIV infection.
    Corticosteroids and immunosuppressive therapy.
    Live viral vaccines.

    False negative tuberculin reactions may be found in miliary TB, and in TB of the peritoneum and meninges. Tests can be negative early in the course of acute infection, as in tuberculous erythema nodosum. It may therefore be necessary to repeat an initially negative test after 2 or 3 weeks.
- A normal chest X-ray excludes intrathoracic TB. About 50% of patients with extrapulmonary TB will have a completely normal chest X-ray, although intrathoracic tuberculous lymph nodes often grow larger (for a time) in response to anti-TB therapy and therefore become detectable later. Up to 10% of pulmonary TB is endobronchial and therefore not susceptible to radiological diagnosis. Even with miliary disease the patient may be ill for several weeks before the characteristic X-ray changes occur.

Pitfalls

- Investigating factitious fever. Although factitious fever is an uncommon cause of PUO it should be considered and excluded as early as possible in the management plan. Clues to the presence of factitious fever are given in the section on clinical examination. Time and resources are easily wasted on the investigation of non-existent and self-induced fever. In a report from the National Institutes of Health, of 347 patients admitted to hospital with prolonged fever, 35% had factitious fever or no fever at all.

Hints for investigators and prescribers

- 'Blind' bone marrow biopsy is most useful in disclosing inapparent haematological malignancy, myelodysplasia and TB. It may also lead to a diagnosis of brucellosis, enteric fever, or visceral leishmaniasis. However, the overall yield is low, about 15%, a figure which is likely to be even lower if there are no abnormalities in the peripheral blood. Bone marrow should always be sent for culture as well as microscopy. Liver biopsy carries a higher morbidity than bone marrow biopsy and has a low but appreciable mortality (approximately 0.01%). It has an even lower yield, but will occasionally lead to a diagnosis of TB, lymphoma, or granulomatous disorder including sarcoidosis. Biopsy material should ideally be sent for culture, including TB culture. Liver biopsy is unlikely to be helpful in patients who have normal liver function tests and normal looking liver parenchyma on imaging.

- Temporal artery biopsy should be undertaken in patients over 60 whose ESR is consistently greater than 40 mm h^{-1}. Since arteritis is often patchy, diagnostic yield is increased if a 5 cm section of artery is removed for examination.

Investigation checklists for the management of 'true' PUO are given in the tables below. *Table 1* lists the investigations that should be done in the first week. *Tables 2* and *3* highlight some further non-invasive investigations, and *Table 4* lists invasive procedures and biopsies.

Table 1. Initial investigations (first week) in the management of 'true' PUO

FBC and differential
Erythrocyte sedimentation rate/C-reactive protein
Serum ferritin
Urea, creatinine and electrolytes
Liver function tests and gamma glutamyl transferase
Blood glucose
Creatine phosphokinase
Bone biochemistry
Malaria blood films (if travel history)
Urinalysis
MSU for microscopy and culture
Stool culture
Sputum (if available) for routine microscopy and culture, and microscopy and culture for acid-fast bacilli (AFB)
Blood cultures × 3
Chest X-ray
ECG

Table 2. Serological investigations in the management of 'true' PUO

Viral	Bacterial	Fungal	Protozoan and parasitic
CMV	Brucella	Histoplasma	Toxoplasma
EBV	Q fever	(if travel history)	Amoebiasis
HIV	Chlamydia	Coccidiomycosis	(if travel history)
Hepatitis A, B and C	Mycoplasma	(if travel history)	Schistosomiasis
Parvovirus	Syphilis	Cryptococcus	(if travel history)
Arbovirus	Leptospirosis	(antigen detection)	Visceral leishmaniasis
(if travel history)	Borrelia (Lyme disease)		(if travel history)
	Yersinia		Trypanosomiasis
	Antistreptolysin titre		(if travel history)
	Rickettsia (if travel history)		
	Melioidosis (if travel history)		
	Relapsing fever		
	(if travel history)		
	Bartonella (if travel history)		
	Tularaemia (if travel history)		

Table 3. Further non-invasive investigations in the management of 'true' PUO

Nucleic acid detection (polymerase chain reaction)
    Increasingly used, e.g. for TB, HSV, CMV, parvovirus, dengue, HIV, toxoplasma, Whipples disease
Immunology
    Auto-antibody screen, including anti-double-stranded DNA, antineutrophil cytoplasmic antibody (ANCA)
    Immunoglobulins
    Complement ($C_3 + C_4$) levels
    Cryoglobulins
Tuberculosis screening tests
    Tuberculin (Mantoux) test
    EMSUs ×3 for acid-fast bacilli microscopy and culture
Imaging techniques

Ultrasound abdomen:	Liver tumour or metastases, liver abscess
	Dilated intrahepatic bile ducts
	Renal tumour, abscess or hydronephrosis
	Intra-abdominal/pelvic masses or abscesses
	Ascites
	Enlarged retroperitoneal lymph nodes
Echocardiogram:	Vegetations (note: a normal echocardiogram does not exclude endocarditis)
	Atrial myxoma
	Intracardiac thrombus
CT/MRI scan of thorax and abdomen:	Enlarged lymph nodes
	Organomegaly
	Lung and liver metastases/primary tumours
	Tumours and abscesses
Limited skeletal survey:	Multiple myeloma
	Bone metastases
Isotope bone scan:	Malignancy
	Osteomyelitis/septic arthritis
Labelled white blood cell scan:	Abscesses/focal sepsis
	Inflammatory bowel disease

Table 4. Invasive procedures/biopsies in the management of 'true' PUO

Lumbar puncture
Bronchoscopy/bronchial or transbronchial biopsy/bronchial lavage
Oesophago gastroduodenoscopy
Small bowel meal/enema
Sigmoidoscopy/colonoscopy/barium enema
Laparoscopy
'Blind' biopsies: bone marrow, liver, temporal artery
Biopsies of skin, lymph node, skeletal muscle, kidney

Case 3: PUO with a history of recent travel

A 26-year-old female back packer has recently visited Thailand and West Africa. She is febrile but has no physical signs. Initial investigations: normal chest X-ray, initial malaria blood film negative, WCC $3000 \times 10^9\,l^{-1}$, platelet count $100 \times 10^9\,l^{-1}$.

Management options

1. Make a diagnosis of dengue fever and treat symptomatically.
2. Collect blood, urine and stool cultures and give oral ciprofloxacin for suspected enteric fever.
3. Manage expectantly. Collect blood, urine and stool cultures and repeat the malaria blood film after 24 hours.
4. Collect blood, urine and stool samples. Treat possible malaria, enteric fever and typhus by prescribing oral quinine, ciprofloxacin and tetracycline.
5. Treat as falciparum malaria with oral or i.v. quinine.
6. Treat as falciparum malaria with quinine. Collect blood, urine and stool cultures and add ciprofloxacin if the fever fails to settle. Consider alternative diagnoses and send serum for arbovirus, rickettsial antibodies, etc.

Option 1. Make a diagnosis of dengue fever and treat symptomatically.

Tell the patient that there is no evidence of malaria, and that she has a virus infection which will settle down on its own.

✓ You will not be masking the results of further investigations by giving antibiotics or anti-malarials.

✗ The patient may well have falciparum malaria despite the apparently negative blood film. Untreated falciparum malaria is often rapidly fatal.

✗ Other possible diagnoses, e.g. enteric fever, brucellosis and acute HIV infection, should be considered at this stage and appropriate investigations ordered.

✗ Infections you have overlooked, e.g. typhus and enteric fever, may progress without prompt therapy.

✗ This patient has no specific features of dengue (e.g. rash and myalgia).

✗ Serological confirmation of arbovirus infection takes days to weeks.

Option 2. Collect blood, urine and stool cultures and give oral ciprofloxacin for suspected enteric fever.

Tell the patient she is likely to have 'typhoid' which should respond to your treatment.

✓ You will be treating a common and potentially fatal cause of imported PUO.

✗ The patient may well have falciparum malaria despite the apparently negative blood film. Untreated falciparum malaria is often rapidly fatal.

✗ Other possible diagnoses, e.g. dengue, brucellosis and acute HIV infection, should be considered at this stage and appropriate investigations ordered.

✗ Infections you have overlooked (e.g. typhus) may progress without prompt therapy.

✗ The ciprofloxacin may mask other as yet undiagnosed infections.

Option 3. Manage expectantly. Collect blood, urine and stool cultures and repeat the malaria blood films after 24 hours.

Tell the patient you are not sure of the diagnosis and will wait for the results of further tests.

✓ You will not be masking the results of further investigations by giving antibiotics or anti-malarials.

✓ You are pursuing the most important diagnosis, i.e. malaria, by repeating the blood film.

✗ Untreated malaria may progress suddenly, even within the next 24 hours.
✗ Infections you have overlooked, e.g. typhus, may also progress without prompt therapy.
✗ Other possible diagnoses, e.g. dengue, brucellosis, typhus and acute HIV infection, should be considered at this stage.

Option 4. Collect blood, urine and stool cultures. Treat possible malaria, enteric fever and typhus by prescribing oral quinine, ciprofloxacin and tetracycline.

Tell the patient you are unsure of the diagnosis but that you will give treatment which will cover the main possibilities.

✓ You will be treating several of the likely imported infections in this clinical situation.

✗ Other possible diagnoses, e.g. dengue, brucellosis and acute HIV infection, should be considered at this stage.
✗ You may well miss the chance of diagnosing malaria on subsequent blood films.
✗ Other as yet undiagnosed infections may be masked.
✗ Polypharmacy increases the risks of side-effects.

Option 5. Treat as falciparum malaria with oral or i.v. quinine.

Tell the patient you will start treatment for malaria, which is the most likely diagnosis.

✓ You will be treating the most likely and most dangerous cause of the patient's illness.
✓ You will not be masking other causes of imported fever.

✗ You may well miss the chance of diagnosing malaria on subsequent blood films.
✗ Other possible diagnoses, e.g. typhoid, typhus, brucellosis, dengue and acute HIV infection should be considered at this stage and appropriate investigations ordered.
✗ Infections you have overlooked, e.g. typhoid and typhus, may progress without prompt treatment.

Option 6. Treat as falciparum malaria with quinine. Collect blood, urine and stool cultures and add ciprofloxacin if the fever fails to settle. Consider alternative diagnoses and send serum for arbovirus, rickettsial antibodies, etc.

Tell the patient you will treat her for malaria and will add an antibiotic for typhoid fever if she does not respond.

✓ You will be covering two common and potentially life-threatening causes of imported PUO.

✗ You may well miss the chance of diagnosing malaria on subsequent blood films.
✗ The ciprofloxacin may mask other undiagnosed infections.
✗ Infections such as typhus may progress without prompt and specific treatment.

History checklist
- System review and past medical history as in Case 1.

Travel history
- Take a careful travel history, documenting all countries and areas visited, together with dates of arrival and departure.
- Details of hotels etc. may be important if an environmental infection, e.g. legionellosis or enteric fever is subsequently diagnosed. When did she finally leave the tropics, and on what date did she become ill?
- Ask specifically about visits to rural or bush areas and to game parks (rickettsial infections, trypanosomiasis).

- Has the patient had any contact with hospitals, clinics or refugee camps? (Nosocomial infections, including viral haemorrhagic fever.)
- Has she received any medical treatment while overseas, especially injections or transfusions, and under what circumstances? (Blood-borne viral infections.)
- To what extent has she been exposed to vectors of infection, particularly mosquitoes, ticks and mites?
- What steps has she taken to avoid insect bites?
- Has she had any contact with animals or birds, and has she consumed any unpasteurized milk or milk products (chlamydial infections, brucellosis, Q fever, etc.)?
- Enquire about swimming activities, especially freshwater swimming in areas where schistosomiasis is endemic. Did she notice pruritus after swimming ('swimmers itch') which might indicate cercarial invasion?

Drugs and vaccinations
- What malaria chemoprophylaxis was recommended and what was her compliance with the advice given? Did she have to stop the tablets because of side-effects, gastroenteritis or for some other reason? Did she continue with chemoprophylaxis for 4 weeks after returning home? Ask about pre-travel vaccinations especially typhoid, yellow fever, hepatitis A and B, meningococcal vaccine and BCG.

Personal and social
- Take a sexual history, enquiring particularly about unprotected intercourse with partners from the countries visited.
- Has the patient been treated for any STD or had any symptoms suggesting STD?
- Has the patient injected recreational drugs while overseas? Did she share needles or any other injection equipment?

Examination checklist
- The list in Case 1 can be used as a basis for the physical examination.

General
- Check for the presence of jaundice or pallor. Apart from viral hepatitis, jaundice may be encountered in a number of imported infections including malaria, Q fever, trypanosomiasis and relapsing fever. Haemolytic anaemia is common in severe falciparum malaria. Anaemia is also a well recognized feature of visceral leishmaniasis and trypanosomiasis.
- Examine the skin for evidence of rash, eschars and insect bites. The presence of a generalized maculopapular eruption suggests a differential diagnosis of dengue, typhus or acute HIV infection. A haemorrhagic rash will raise suspicions of meningococcal septicaemia, severe relapsing fever, or viral haemorrhagic fever (VHF) due to arboviruses (e.g. dengue, yellow fever) or transmissible VHF agents (e.g. Lassa fever virus, Ebola virus). 'Rose spots' are characteristic of enteric fever. Only visible on light coloured skins, they are chiefly found on the trunk and fade on pressure.
- The site of entry of insect-borne pathogens may give rise to a characteristic skin lesion. With mite- and tick-borne typhus the lesion consists of a necrotic black papule or 'eschar'. In African trypanosomiasis, the bite of the infected tsetse fly often produces a hot raised inflamed area usually on the extremities, known as the 'trypanosomal chancre'. All these entry-site lesions may be associated with local lymphadenopathy.
- Varying degrees of generalized lymphadenopathy occur in typhus, acute HIV infection, brucellosis, visceral leishmaniasis, trypanosomiasis and relapsing fever.

Examination of the chest
- The presence of chest signs may lead to a diagnosis of pneumonia. Imported pneumonia is often atypical and may be associated with Legionella spp., Rickettsia spp. and Coxiella spp.

infection. Minor chest signs are often encountered in enteric fever, and cough and wheeze are characteristic of acute schistosomiasis (Katayama fever). Dullness at the right lung base from pleural effusion or a raised hemidiaphragm may indicate the presence of an amoebic liver abscess.

Examination of the abdomen

- Liver tenderness is often present in acute viral hepatitis and amoebic liver abscess. With amoebic abscess the tenderness tends to be localized and can often be elicited by pressure over the right lower ribs or intercostal spaces. The pain may be referred to the tip of the shoulder, and there may also be tenderness over the phrenic nerve in the neck.
- There is a long list of imported infections associated with moderate splenomegaly which includes malaria, viral hepatitis, enteric fever, typhus, occult TB, acute HIV infection, acute schistosomiasis, relapsing fever, Q fever and brucellosis. Massive splenomegaly is much less common, but raises suspicions of visceral leishmaniasis or chronic recurrent malaria (tropical splenomegaly syndrome).

Rituals and myths

- A negative blood film excludes malaria. Scanty peripheral parasitaemia is common, particularly when patients have taken chemoprophylaxis, and is easily missed on thin blood films. Examining thick blood films increases diagnostic yield but few routine laboratories have the expertise to use this technique successfully. Repeated thin films should be examined before excluding malaria as a cause of imported fever. Malaria antigen detection techniques such as the 'Parasight-F' should also be employed by the laboratory to increase the chance of detecting low grade parasitaemia, especially in the presence of partial suppression by chemoprophylaxis, or if the laboratory is inexperienced in malaria diagnosis. These tests will only detect falciparum malaria.
- A normal chest X-ray excludes pneumonia as a cause of imported PUO. Atypical pneumonias are often truly atypical in presentation. Radiological signs may appear only after some days of illness.
- Typhoid fever is usually accompanied by relative bradycardia, constipation and splenomegaly. These are all uncommon signs of imported typhoid, which often presents as a 'true' PUO without any specific diagnostic features. Headache and unproductive cough are more characteristic clues which are often overlooked.
- Abnormal liver function tests are important laboratory markers of amoebic liver abscess. Liver function tests are often only minimally abnormal in this condition and are rarely helpful. A neutrophil leucocytosis and an elevated ESR (>50 mm h^{-1}) are more reliable laboratory clues to the diagnosis. Stool microscopy has no predictive value in the diagnosis of amoebic liver abscess.

Pitfalls

- Not considering malaria as a diagnosis. Falciparum malaria is a multisystem infection affecting the gut, brain, kidneys, liver and lungs. Consequently, malaria may present with symptoms in virtually any body system, e.g. with vomiting, diarrhoea, neck stiffness, coma or fits, acute renal failure, jaundice and pulmonary oedema. Not all patients are febrile when first seen. Malaria has to be excluded urgently in any ill traveller returning from an endemic area, whatever the symptomatology.
- Assuming that a 'routine' blood film will exclude malaria. Malaria is a difficult microscopic diagnosis for most laboratories. Unless parasitaemia is very heavy, the routine examination of a blood film for other purposes is very unlikely to yield a diagnosis of malaria. Blood must therefore be submitted with a specific request for malaria parasite examination.
- Assuming that all disease in travellers has an exotic origin. Although imported infections have to be excluded as a cause of illness in returning travellers, common 'Western' diseases are often encountered in this situation. Examples include acute alcoholic hepatitis in patients with jaundice, and inflammatory bowel disease in those complaining of bloody diarrhoea.

Case 4: PUO with a history of immunodeficiency

An HIV-positive man, aged 34, complains of fever, weight loss and loose stools. Apart from wasting there are no positive findings on examination and the optic fundi look normal. Initial investigations include a normal chest X-ray and a CD4 count of $30 \times 10^9 \, l^{-1}$.

Management options
1. Send stool specimens for routine culture and microscopy and start treatment with oral ciprofloxacin and metronidazole.
2. Send stool specimens for routine culture and microscopy and arrange sigmoidoscopy and rectal biopsy. If histology reveals mycobacterium avium-intracellulare complex (MAC) infection, start specific therapy.
3. Send stool specimens for routine culture and microscopy and arrange sigmoidoscopy and rectal biopsy. If histology reveals CMV infection, start treatment with i.v. ganciclovir.
4. Send stool specimens for routine culture and microscopy. Request several blood cultures, to include mycobacterial and fungal isolation, and send serum for cryptococcal antigen detection. Await results.
5. Send stool specimens for culture and microscopy including stains for microsporidia and cryptosporidia. Ask for blood cultures including fungal and MAC isolation and send serum for cryptococcal antigen detection. Arrange both rectal and duodenal biopsies. Treat for MAC if blood cultures are positive and consider adding i.v. ganciclovir if CMV colitis is likely on both clinical and histological evidence.

Option 1. Send stool specimens for routine culture and microscopy and start treatment with oral ciprofloxacin and metronidazole.

Tell the patient he is likely to have a gut infection which will respond to antibiotics.

✓ You may treat an incidental gut infection, e.g. Campylobacter spp. or Giardia lamblia, but these are unlikely to be the only causes of the patient's fever and weight loss.

✗ You have made no attempt to diagnose important causes of fever such as MAC and CMV infection.

✗ The ciprofloxacin may well mask systemic infections, e.g. bacteraemic salmonellosis and MAC infection.

✗ Routine methods will not detect gut infections such as cryptosporidiosis and microsporidiosis.

✗ Undetected gut infection will remain untreated.

Option 2. Send stool specimens for routine culture and microscopy, and arrange sigmoidoscopy and rectal biopsy. If histology reveals specific mycobacterium avium-intracellulare complex (MAC) infection, start specific therapy.

Tell the patient that MAC infection is very likely, and that you will treat it if it is detected on rectal biopsy.

✓ You are seeking a tissue diagnosis which may well reveal evidence of MAC or CMV infection.

✓ If the patient has systemic spread of MAC, he should respond to MAC therapy.

✗ MAC infection may be localized to the rectum: blood cultures are necessary to detect systemic spread.

✗ You have not excluded alternative causes for the patient's fever. If MAC is not the cause, anti-MAC therapy will not improve the patient's symptoms.

✗ The MAC therapy may mask other as yet undiagnosed infections.
✗ Routine methods will not detect gut infections such as cryptosporidiosis and microsporidiosis.
✗ Undetected gut infection will remain untreated.

Option 3. Send stool specimens for routine culture and microscopy and arrange sigmoidoscopy and rectal biopsy. If histology reveals CMV infection, start treatment with i.v. ganciclovir.

Tell the patient that CMV infection is very likely and that you will treat it if diagnosed on rectal biopsy.

✓ You are seeking a tissue diagnosis which may reveal evidence of MAC or CMV infection.
✓ If the patient has CMV colitis he may respond to ganciclovir therapy.

✗ The CMV infection may be relatively localized. In this situation the patient will be exposed to the toxicity and inconvenience of i.v. ganciclovir without any clinical benefit.
✗ You have not excluded alternative causes for the patient's fever.
✗ Routine stool examination will not detect gut infections such as cryptosporidiosis and microsporidiosis.
✗ Undetected gut infections will remain untreated.

Option 4. Send stool specimens for routine culture and microscopy. Request several blood cultures, to include mycobacterial and fungal isolation, and send serum for cryptococcal antigen detection. Await results.

Tell the patient you will look for important infections using blood tests, avoiding endoscopy for the time being.

✓ You will be looking actively for evidence of systemic bacterial, mycobacterial and fungal infection by non-invasive methods.
✓ You will not be masking undiagnosed infection.

✗ Your investigations will miss disorders which require a tissue diagnosis, e.g. CMV infection or gut lymphoma.
✗ Routine methods will not detect gut infections such as cryptosporidiosis and microsporidiosis.

Option 5. Send stool specimens for culture and microscopy including stains for microsporidia and cryptosporidia. Ask for blood cultures including fungal and MAC isolation and send serum for cryptococcal antigen detection. Arrange both rectal and duodenal biopsies. Treat for MAC if blood cultures are positive and consider adding i.v. ganciclovir if CMV colitis is likely on both clinical and histological evidence.

Tell the patient you will investigate for both gut and more generalized infection and that endoscopy will be required.

✓ You will be looking actively for evidence of systemic bacterial, mycobacterial and fungal infection.
✓ You are also seeking a tissue diagnosis which may reveal evidence of CMV or MAC infection. The value of intestinal biopsies is increased if special stains are used, e.g. periodic acid-Schiff reaction for Cryptosporidium spp.
✓ If the patient has systemic MAC infection he should respond to anti-MAC therapy.
✓ If the patient has CMV colitis he may respond to i.v. ganciclovir therapy.
✓ You will not be masking undiagnosed infection.
✓ You are widening the scope of investigations for opportunistic gut infections.

✗ Invasive diagnostic methods are required.

History checklist

General
For guidance on history taking, please see the previous cases.

Specific
A detailed history should be obtained, focusing particularly on medical history (including evidence of previous TB), travel history and drug history.

- Loss of weight is a common complaint in advanced HIV disease. In the context of fever, weight loss is often associated with systemic infection (CMV, MAC or TB) or disseminated malignancy.
- Chest symptoms are non-specific, since many opportunistic infections and malignancies may cause pulmonary damage or infiltration. However, the combination of fever, cough, dyspnoea and central chest discomfort are characteristic of Pneumocystis carinii pneumonia, even when the chest X-ray is normal or shows minimal change.
- Abdominal symptoms such as dysphagia or odynophagia will raise suspicions of Candida spp., CMV or HSV oesophagitis. Abdominal pain is very suggestive of intra-abdominal CMV infection: acalculous cholecystitis from CMV-induced arteritis causes pain localized to the right hypochondrium. CMV may also cause a painful sclerosing cholangitis. Other pathogens implicated in this condition include microsporidia and cryptosporidia. CMV colitis causes abdominal pain and diarrhoea which often contains blood: appendicitis and pancreatitis may also be complications of this infection. MAC gut infection characteristically produces watery diarrhoea associated with fever and weight loss.
- Always ask about visual symptoms such as loss of acuity or increased 'floaters': the latter are characteristic of CMV retinitis. Paraparesis, painful paraesthesiae, or loss of bowel or bladder control will suggest CMV neuropathy or radiculopathy: the differential diagnosis also includes HIV neuropathy/myelopathy and neurosyphilis. A history of headache, dizziness, nausea and vomiting, mental blunting or fits points to the presence of HIV-associated intracranial disease. The commonest diagnoses in this situation are toxoplasma brain abscess, cryptococcal meningitis, CMV encephalitis and primary intracerebral lymphoma.

Examination checklist
The schemes outlined in Cases 1 and 2 can be used as a basis for the clinical examination.

- Skin lesions may give a clue to the cause of fever. Look for cutaneous evidence of Kaposi's sarcoma, lymphoma, cryptococcosis or bacillary angiomatosis (Bartonella henselae infection).
- Examine the oropharynx for evidence of candidosis, oral hairy leukoplakia, HSV infection or Kaposi's sarcoma.
- In the abdominal examination note the presence of any organomegaly or localized tenderness. The latter may suggest a diagnosis of CMV cholecystitis, cholangitis, colitis, appendicitis, or pancreatitis.
- The pupils should be dilated and the optic fundi examined carefully for evidence of papilloedema or retinitis. In the context of PUO, CMV is by far the commonest cause of retinitis. Other pathogens occasionally encountered include toxoplasma, disseminated P. carinii infection, MAC, and cryptococcosis.
- When examining the CNS, pay particular attention to the patient's mental status and level of consciousness. Examine for neck stiffness, but remember that meningism is often absent in HIV-associated intracranial infection. Look for clinical evidence of peripheral nerve damage or radiculopathy, which may suggest a diagnosis of nervous system CMV infection.

Further reading

Bell, D.R. (1995) *Lecture Notes on Tropical Medicine,* 4th Edn. Blackwell Science, Oxford.

Broder, S., Meringan, T.C. Jnr. and Bolognesi, D. (1994) *AIDS Medicine.* Williams and Wilkins, London.

Durack, D.T. (1996) Fever of unknown origin. In: *Oxford Text Book of Medicine* (eds D.J. Weatherall, J.G.C. Ledingham and D.A. Worrell). Oxford University Press, Oxford, pp. 1015–1019.

Mandell, G.L., Bennett, J.E. and Dolin, R. (1995) *Principle and Practice of Infectious Diseases.* Churchill Livingstone, Edinburgh.

Chapter 12
RESPIRATORY INFECTIONS

M.J. Walshaw and M.J. Ledson

Respiratory tract infection implies the presence of organisms multiplying within the respiratory tract that are provoking an inflammatory response and causing respiratory symptoms. Local symptoms caused by such infection include breathlessness, cough, sputum or chest pain.

Sputum production is not necessarily a sign of respiratory infection, even in an individual who usually has no respiratory symptoms. It is merely a feature of excessive bronchial secretion, which commonly occurs in asthma and also in response to inhaled bronchial irritants. In patients with chronic bronchitis it is a sign of ongoing bronchial inflammation. In those with bronchiectasis, it is a sign of mucus pooling and excess secretion.

Sputum colour is not a sign of infection, but merely represents the length of time the sputum has been in the bronchial tree. However, it is unusual for sputum to be in the respiratory tract for long enough to become discoloured unless there is underlying infection. The exceptions to this are asthma, where the sputum may be yellow or green due to the presence of eosinophils, and bronchiectasis, where the rule is for the sputum to be discoloured even when there is no infection. Conversely, patients with acute bronchitis can have bacterial infection even when the sputum is not discoloured.

Orientation
This chapter is laid out in several subsections, illustrating the different clinical conditions in which infection can occur in the respiratory tract.

The commonest infections are those which cause bronchitis, either in previously well individuals or in those with pre-existing chronic bronchitis. Examples are used here to demonstrate the treatment options, and the fact that antibiotics are often not required for what are usually viral causes.

Bronchiectasis is a chronic condition in which it can be difficult to decide whether there is acute pathology. The case history cited is designed to help elucidate this.

Pneumonia is a common subgroup, where the infection usually has more serious consequences. A number of different examples have been cited to illustrate the various aetiologies of pneumonia and the varying treatment options.

Lung abscess and empyema are uncommon conditions, but have similar aetiologies and treatment patterns.

Infections in obstructive airways disease are another common subgroup in which it can be difficult to decide whether antibiotics are necessary. The examples used are designed to highlight these issues.

Finally, tuberculosis (TB) is an uncommon but serious respiratory disease that requires expert treatment. The example given demonstrates the various treatment options.

Chapter contents

1 Acute bronchitis

Acute bronchitis is defined as an acute inflammation of the bronchial mucosa usually due to a viral infection, but also due to bacteria and inhaled chemical agents. It is self-limiting in most cases but recurrent bouts can result in chronic disease (chronic bronchitis).

Clinical case

History
A 25-year-old woman with an unremarkable previous respiratory history presents during the winter months with a 2-day history of dry throat, dysphagia, malaise, and a cough increasingly productive of white sputum. The cough prevents her sleeping at night. She is a non-smoker. Two members of her family have had similar symptoms within the preceding week.

Examination
Pyrexial 37.6°C. Fauces reddened, tonsils OK, no pus, cervical glands not enlarged. Auscultation of chest normal.

Management options
1. Reassure the patient that she merely has acute bronchitis, which is almost certainly viral in nature and should settle on its own within a few days.
2. Explain to the patient that she has bronchitis, but probably does not need an antibiotic. However, you will send off sputum to check and the result will be ready in 2 or 3 days.
3. Reassure the patient that she probably has a self-limiting viral bronchitis and prescribe agents to control her pyrexia and cough.
4. Tell the patient she has bronchitis and prescribe an antibiotic in case it is bacterial in origin.
5. Tell the patient she probably has a viral bronchitis, but you are sending off a sputum sample. Give her antitussive and anti-inflammatory agents.
6. Tell the patient she probably has a viral bronchitis and send off sputum for culture. Prescribe her symptomatic treatment and a broad-spectrum antibiotic to cover any likely potential bacterial pathogen.
7. Tell the patient she has acute bronchitis and prescribe symptomatic medications and also an antibiotic.
8. Tell the patient she has acute bronchitis and that you are sending off a sputum sample in case it is due to a bacterial infection. The patient should return for antibiotic if indicated.
9. Tell the patient she has acute bronchitis which is probably viral in nature but you are sending off a sputum sample in any case. Prescribe symptomatic medication and tell her to return (for an antibiotic) if the symptoms do not settle.

Option 1. Reassure the patient that she merely has acute bronchitis, which is almost certainly viral in nature and should settle on its own within a few days.

✓ Most cases of bronchitis in otherwise healthy patients are viral in origin and will recover without any intervention.

✗ The patient has troublesome symptoms which, while they may be self-limiting, have caused her to seek medical attention. If nothing is offered, she may feel she is being 'fobbed off', damaging the doctor/patient relationship.

✗ The symptoms may cause the patient to return, thus increasing your workload.

✗ The opportunity to investigate and treat what may be a potentially bacterial infection at an early stage has been missed.

✗ You will never find out what is going wrong with your patients.

Option 2. Explain to the patient that she has bronchitis, but probably does not need an antibiotic. However, you will send off sputum to check and the result will be ready in 2 or 3 days.

✓ This is technically correct, and should there be evidence of bacterial infection you will be in a position to start her on the most appropriate antibiotic if necessary.

✗ She is still left with her symptoms which are very troublesome.

✗ She may expect you to give her some sort of therapy at the outset.

✗ The sputum test (which will probably be negative) adds to the cost of the consultation.

Option 3. Reassure the patient that she probably has a self-limiting viral bronchitis and prescribe agents to control her pyrexia and cough.

✓ This diagnosis is technically correct.

✓ The medicines will relieve her inflammatory symptoms and satisfy her need not to leave the consultation without some form of prescription.

✓ You have saved the cost of a sputum culture.

✗ Should the infection turn out to be bacterial after all, the opportunity to discover this and administer an antibiotic at an early stage will have been missed.

✗ You will never find out what is going wrong with your patients.

Option 4. Tell the patient she has bronchitis and prescribe an antibiotic in case it is bacterial in origin.

✓ This will probably treat any bacterial cause of the bronchitis.

✓ She will be happy because she perceives you are doing your job correctly by giving her an antibiotic.

✓ She will probably not need to re-attend for the current problem because even if the bronchitis is bacterial it will have been treated.

✓ You are saving on the cost of a sputum test.

✗ The chances are that the antibiotic is unnecessary and may therefore waste money, increase the potential for antibiotic resistance, and cause side-effects.

✗ You will still have left her with the immediate inflammatory symptoms, which the antibiotic will not alter should she have a viral infection.

✗ By failing to send a sputum sample you will never know if the antibiotic was necessary or even correct.

✗ You will never find out what is going wrong with your patients.

Option 5. Tell the patient she probably has a viral bronchitis, but you are sending off a sputum sample. Give her antitussive and anti-inflammatory agents.

✓ You are treating the patient's symptoms.

✓ You are covering the possibility that the bronchitis may have a bacterial cause.

✗ She may have to return for an antibiotic which will increase your workload.

✗ The sputum test (which will probably be negative) adds to the cost of the consultation.

Option 6. Tell the patient she probably has a viral bronchitis and send off sputum for culture. Prescribe her symptomatic treatment and a broad-spectrum antibiotic to cover any likely potential bacterial pathogen.

✓ You are covering all options.

✓ It is unlikely she will have to come back for review.

✗ The antibiotic is probably unnecessary, thus increasing costs, potentiating side-effects and increasing the risk of possible antibiotic resistance.

✗ The sputum test adds an additional cost to the consultation.

Option 7. Tell the patient she has acute bronchitis and prescribe symptomatic medications and also an antibiotic.

✓ You are covering a bacterial infection.

✓ You are treating her symptoms so she is unlikely to need to return.

✓ You are saving on the cost of a sputum test.

✗ You are treating her with an antibiotic which is most likely to be unnecessary, thus increasing expense and the risk of side-effects and antibiotic resistance.

✗ Because you did not culture her sputum you will never know if she did have a bacterial infection and so you will not find out what is going wrong with your patients.

Option 8. Tell the patient she has acute bronchitis and that you are sending off a sputum sample in case it is due to a bacterial infection. The patient should return for antibiotic if indicated.

✓ This will prevent the unnecessary treatment of a viral bronchitis with an antibiotic, and allow you to choose a relevant antibiotic should there be bacteria present.

✗ You have not treated her symptoms; she may not be happy with your treatment.

✗ She may need to return for an antibiotic if necessary, thus increasing your workload.

✗ The sputum test adds to the cost of the consultation.

Option 9. Tell the patient she has acute bronchitis which is probably viral in nature but you are sending off a sputum sample in any case. Prescribe symptomatic medication and tell her to return (for an antibiotic) if the symptoms do not settle.

✓ You are covering all options and she will be happy because her symptoms should settle on the medication you have given her even if the infection is viral.

✓ By sending off a sputum sample you are allowing for the possibility that this is a bacterial infection.

✓ You will find out what is going wrong with your patients.

✗ She may need to re-attend for an antibiotic if her symptoms do not settle.

✗ The saving you make by not giving her an antibiotic at the start may be offset by the cost of the sputum test.

History checklist

General
- A general history will reveal whether the patient is predisposed to respiratory infections, e.g. diabetic, immunosuppressed or a smoker.
- Smokers and the elderly in particular are more likely to develop bronchitis.

Specific
- Duration of symptoms? By definition, the onset is acute with a short history. A longer history indicates other pathology.

- Prodromal features? Viral infections often have these.
- Cluster of cases? Other family members may be involved, and this is a useful clue when looking for causes of viral bronchitis.
- Specific chest symptoms? Cough, sputum, sore throat, myalgia – all these can occur with viral bronchitis.

Examination checklist
- Examine for general signs of infection, taking the patient's temperature and pulse.
- Examine the throat and cervical glands, looking for inflammation and swelling.
- Examine the chest, looking for signs of consolidation, crackles and wheeze. Bronchitis may cause the latter two, but if the former is present then the diagnosis is not simply bronchitis.

Referrals
- Recurrent bronchitis in an otherwise healthy person should provoke referral to a chest physician.

Rituals and myths
- Discoloured sputum is always infected.

Pitfalls
- While haemoptysis is always possible with acute bronchitis, in a smoker aged >45 years this should always provoke a chest X-ray and referral to a chest physician.
- Wheezy bronchitis may indicate underlying mild asthma, particularly if recurrent.

Further reading
Murray, J.F. and Hadel, J.A. (eds) (1989) *Textbook of Respiratory Medicine.* Saunders, Philadelphia, PA, pp. 708–742.

Sande, M.A., Hudson, L.D. and Root, R.K. (1986) Management of acute and chronic bronchitis. In: *Respiratory Infections. Contemporary Issues in Infectious Diseases* Churchill Livingstone, New York, pp. 149–157.

2 Acute-on-chronic bronchitis

Chronic bronchitis is defined as the production of sputum every day for 2 months or more in 2 consecutive years. In practice, most patients with chronic bronchitis produce sputum on a daily basis. It is due to chronic irritation of the bronchial mucosa and is very common in smokers, older patients and those who have worked with irritant dusts. It is often associated with chronic obstructive airways disease, which is dealt with later. Most patients with chronic bronchitis will develop acute infections (acute-on-chronic bronchitis). These have a different aetiology and clinical features from simple acute bronchitis.

Clinical case

History
A 58-year-old ex-coalminer who smokes 20 cigarettes per day has had a cough productive of grey sputum for the last 3 years. He develops a pyrexial illness associated with breathlessness, a tight chest and increased volumes of green sputum.

Examination
Pyrexial 38°C. In the chest: there are coarse crackles which clear on coughing, as well as scattered wheezes.

Management options
1. Reassure the patient that he merely has acute bronchitis which will probably settle in a few days.
2. Reassure the patient that he probably has an overlying viral acute bronchitis which should settle, but send off a sputum sample in case this shows a bacterial cause.
3. Reassure the patient that he probably has viral bronchitis, but that you are prescribing an antibiotic as a precaution.
4. Reassure the patient that he probably has viral bronchitis but that you are prescribing some symptomatic treatment.
5. Reassure the patient that he has a viral bronchitis, but prescribe a bronchodilator inhaler to relieve his wheezy symptoms.
6. Reassure the patient that he probably has a viral infection, but prescribe an antibiotic and send off sputum in case it is a bacterial infection.
7. Tell the patient he probably has a viral infection, but that you are sending off a sputum sample and prescribing an antibiotic in case it is bacterial. Prescribe antitussives, antipyretics and a bronchodilator to treat his symptoms.
8. Tell the patient he probably has a viral infection, but that you are prescribing an antibiotic in case it is bacterial. Prescribe him antitussives, antipyretics and a bronchodilator to treat his symptoms.
9. Tell the patient he has a viral bronchitis and that you are prescribing antipyretic and antitussive agents and a bronchodilator to treat his symptoms.

Option 1. Reassure the patient that he merely has acute bronchitis which will probably settle in a few days.

✓ Most cases of acute bronchitis, even in patients with preceding chronic bronchitis, are viral in nature and will settle in a few days without any specific treatment.

✓ This approach will cut down on the cost of investigations and treatment in most patients.

✗ The patient has troublesome symptoms which have caused a consultation and if nothing other than reassurance is offered, the patient may lose confidence in you.

✗ Because the patient has chronic bronchitis, a bacterial infection is likely to be the cause of his acute symptoms. He is thus likely to develop complications if you do not treat at an early stage.

✗ The opportunity to obtain an early sputum sample for culture will have been lost.

✗ If the patient's symptoms persist, he will return, thus increasing your workload.

✗ You will never learn more about your patients!

Option 2. Reassure the patient that he probably has an overlying viral acute bronchitis which should settle, but send off a sputum sample in case this shows a bacterial cause.

✓ This is technically correct.

✓ You will find out more about your patients.

✗ If he has to return for an antibiotic when the result arrives, you will have increased your workload.

✗ You have not treated the patient's symptoms and he may not be happy with this.

✗ The sputum test will add to your costs.

Option 3. Reassure the patient that he probably has viral bronchitis, but that you are prescribing an antibiotic as a precaution.

✓ You are covering the possibility of an underlying bacterial cause.

✓ He will probably be satisfied that he has received some treatment from the consultation.

✗ You are increasing your costs by providing a probably unnecessary antibiotic.

✗ You are potentially increasing bacterial resistance patterns by using antibiotics unnecessarily.

✗ You have not treated any of his symptoms.

✗ By not investigating him, you will never learn more about your patients!

Option 4. Reassure the patient that he probably has viral bronchitis but that you are prescribing some symptomatic treatment.

✓ Most patients require symptomatic treatment only.

✓ He has received a prescription from the consultation and will therefore probably be happy.

✓ You have limited your costs by providing him with cheap, symptomatic treatment.

✗ By not prescribing an antibiotic, you have missed the opportunity to treat a potentially bacterial infection early.

✗ By not sending off a sputum sample, you have missed the opportunity to detect a bacterial infection early.

✗ By not investigating patients, you will never learn more about them!

Option 5. Reassure the patient that he has a viral bronchitis, but prescribe a bronchodilator inhaler to relieve his wheezy symptoms.

✓ You are relieving one of his distressing symptoms and he will probably be happy with this.

✓ You are limiting the cost of the consultation by providing him with a cheap treatment.

✗ Because you are not treating his toxic symptoms he may return later, thus increasing your workload.

✗ By not prescribing an antibiotic, you have missed the opportunity to treat a potentially bacterial infection early.

✗ By not sending off a sputum sample, you have missed the opportunity to detect a bacterial infection early.

✗ By not investigating patients, you will never learn more about them!

Option 6. Reassure the patient that he probably has a viral infection, but prescribe an antibiotic and send off sputum in case it is a bacterial infection.

✓ You are treating any potentially serious cause, and backing this up with a sputum culture.
✓ He will probably be happy, because he will see that you are attending to his illness.
✓ By investigating him, you will learn more about your patients.

✗ As you have not treated any of his symptoms, he may return at a later stage, thus increasing your workload.
✗ By prescribing antibiotics and sending off sputum, you have substantially increased the cost of the consultation.
✗ You are potentially increasing bacterial resistance patterns by using antibiotics unnecessarily.

Option 7. Tell the patient he probably has a viral infection, but that you are sending off a sputum sample and prescribing an antibiotic in case it is bacterial. Prescribe antitussives, antipyretics and a bronchodilator to treat his symptoms.

✓ This belt and braces approach will cover all the possibilities!
✓ He will probably be very happy that you are paying so much attention to his needs.
✓ By investigating, you will learn more about your patient.

✗ You are maximizing the cost of the consultation.
✗ You are potentially increasing bacterial resistance patterns by using antibiotics unnecessarily.

Option 8. Tell the patient he probably has a viral infection, but that you are prescribing an antibiotic in case it is bacterial. Prescribe antitussives, antipyretics and a bronchodilator to treat his symptoms.

✓ You are treating his symptoms and covering any possible bacterial infection.
✓ He will probably be very happy that you are paying so much attention to his needs.

✗ You are increasing the cost of the consultation.
✗ You are potentially increasing bacterial resistance patterns by using antibiotics unnecessarily.
✗ By not investigating patients, you will never learn more about them!

Option 9. Tell the patient he has a viral bronchitis and that you are prescribing antipyretic and antitussive agents and a bronchodilator to treat his symptoms.

✓ Since you are treating his symptoms, he will probably be happy with the consultation.
✓ You are reducing your costs by giving him cheap treatments.

✗ By not prescribing an antibiotic, you have missed the opportunity to treat a potentially bacterial infection early.
✗ By not sending off a sputum sample, you have missed the opportunity to detect a bacterial infection early.
✗ By not investigating patients, you will never learn more about them!

History checklist

General
- This will reveal whether the patient is predisposed to respiratory tract disease, e.g. a diabetic or immunosuppressed.

Specific
- Length of symptoms? Do they fulfil the definition of chronic bronchitis?
- Smoking history? The vast majority will have a significant smoking history.
- Occupational exposure? More common in those working in the coalmining industry and those chronically exposed to irritant inhalational chemicals and fibrogenic dusts.
- Specific chest symptoms? Chronic cough and sputum production; features suggestive of acute infection (increased sputum production or discoloration, malaise and breathlessness).

Examination checklist
- Examine for general signs of infection, including temperature, pulse and blood pressure.
- Examine the fingers for clubbing.
- Examine the chest for signs of consolidation, wheeze, lobar collapse and crackles.
- Examine the fauces and cervical glands for inflammation and swelling.

Referrals
- Patients with persistent symptoms, haemoptysis, finger clubbing or recurrent attacks of acute-on-chronic bronchitis should be referred to a chest physician.

Rituals and myths
- Discoloured sputum is always infected.
- Well patients with chronic bronchitis do not usually have organisms in their sputum.
- Chronic bronchitis is *not* a cause of finger clubbing.

Pitfalls
- Haemoptysis in a patient with chronic bronchitis should always be taken seriously.
- Recurrent episodes of wheezy bronchitis may indicate underlying asthma.
- Persistent breathlessness is a sign of respiratory disease other than chronic bronchitis.
- You should have a low threshold for arranging a chest X-ray in these patients.

Further reading
Murray, J.F. and Hadel, J.A. (eds) (1989) *Textbook of Respiratory Medicine.* Saunders, Philadelphia, PA, pp. 708–742.

Sande, M.A., Hudson, L.D. and Root, R.K. (1986) Management of acute and chronic bronchitis. In: *Respiratory Infections. Contemporary Issues in Infectious Diseases.* Churchill Livingstone, New York, pp. 149–157.

3 Bronchiectasis

Bronchiectasis is a morphological description of chronic dilatation of one or more bronchi. It is usually due to poorly treated major respiratory infections, TB, or bronchial obstruction. Cystic fibrosis as a cause of bronchiectasis is not considered here. Most patients will give a history of chronic sputum production, punctuated with acute infections. Physical examination may reveal chest crackles, finger clubbing and wheeze. Dilated bronchi may be visible on plain chest X-ray or CT scan.

Clinical case

History
A 56-year-old man presents with a long history of gradually increasing breathlessness, associated with a cough productive of a cup full of green sputum per day. His symptoms go back to childhood, when he was ill for months with pneumonia and subsequently went to a special school. Over the last 8 days he has become increasingly breathless, with wheeze, malaise, sweating spells and an increased volume of sputum which is sometimes bloodstained. Several members of his family have had viral respiratory illnesses recently.

Examination
Pyrexial 38.3°C. Fauces OK, tonsils OK, no pus, cervical glands not enlarged. In the chest there is a scattered wheeze and coarse crackles. There is finger clubbing.

Management options
1. Reassure the patient that he merely has a viral respiratory tract illness and prescribe antipyretic agents.
2. Explain to the patient that he probably has a viral respiratory infection and that you are prescribing agents to control his coughing, temperature and wheeze.
3. Reassure the patient that he has a viral infection, and that as well as controlling his symptoms, you are sending off sputum to test for bacterial infection.
4. Tell the patient he has a chest infection, that you will investigate this and that you are treating him to control his symptoms and combat any possible bacterial infection.

Option 1. Reassure the patient that he merely has a viral respiratory tract illness and prescribe antipyretic agents.

✓ This is a cheap option!

✓ Antipyretics will control the fever.

✗ Despite the fact that the predisposing factor may well have been a viral infection, in view of the underlying chronic respiratory disease it is highly likely that he has an overlying bacterial infection which you are not treating.

✗ The symptoms will almost certainly cause the patient to return, thus increasing your workload.

✗ The opportunity to investigate and treat what may potentially be a bacterial infection at an early stage has been missed.

✗ You will never learn what has been going wrong with your patients.

Option 2. Explain to the patient that he probably has a viral respiratory infection and that you are prescribing agents to control his coughing, temperature and wheeze.

✓ This is another cheap option!

✗ Antitussive agents are contraindicated in these circumstances, since they will interfere with the clearance of infected sputum.

✗ Despite the fact that the predisposing factor may well have been a viral infection, in view of the underlying chronic respiratory disease it is highly likely that he has an overlying bacterial infection which you are not treating.

✗ The untreated infection will probably cause him to return at a later date, increasing your workload.

✗ If his symptoms persist, he may lose confidence in your abilities.

✗ You will never learn what has been going wrong with your patients.

Option 3. Reassure the patient that he has a viral infection, and that as well as controlling his symptoms, you are sending off sputum to test for bacterial infection.

✓ This procedure is technically correct.

✓ The medicines given to him will help the inflammatory symptoms and satisfy his need not to leave the consultation without some form of prescription.

✓ Should there be a bacterial infection, you will be able to use the most appropriate antibiotic.

✓ By investigating them, you will learn more about your patients.

✗ Should the infection turn out to be bacterial, the opportunity to administer an antibiotic at the earliest stage will have been missed.

✗ A sputum culture increases your costs.

✗ He will need to return at a later date for the result of the sputum culture and an antibiotic.

Option 4. Tell the patient he has a chest infection, that you will investigate this and that you are treating him to control his symptoms and combat any possible bacterial infection.

✓ You are covering most possibilities, and treating any possible bacterial infection as early as possible.

✓ He will be happy because he perceives you are doing your job correctly by giving him an antibiotic.

✓ He will probably not need to re-attend for the current problem because it is likely that any overlying bacterial infection will have been treated.

✓ By investigating, you will learn more about your patients.

✗ The tests and antibiotics add to your costs.

✗ Do you really need to send off sputum if you are going to give an antibiotic anyway?

History checklist

General

A general history will reveal whether the patient is predisposed to respiratory infections, e.g. diabetic, immunosuppressed or a smoker. These groups will be predisposed to developing persistent chest disease, which may end up as bronchiectasis.

Specific

- Length of symptoms? By definition, patients will have had the symptoms for many years.
- Previous history? There is often a history of serious respiratory illness (e.g. TB or childhood pneumonia), after which persistent respiratory symptoms developed.
- Specific chest symptoms? Chronic cough productive of variable volumes of discoloured sputum, haemoptysis, increasing breathlessness and wheeze are typical of bronchiectasis, although in rare cases, 'dry' bronchiectasis can develop.

Examination checklist

- Examine for general signs of acute infection, taking the patient's temperature and pulse.
- Examine the throat and cervical glands, looking for inflammation and swelling.

- Examine the chest, looking for signs of consolidation, crackles and wheeze. All these can be present in a patient with bronchiectasis.
- Examine the hands, looking for anaemia, carbon dioxide retention and clubbing.

Referrals
- Patients with established and persistent bronchiectasis should be under the care of a chest physician.

Rituals and myths
- Discoloured sputum is always infected.
- Haemoptysis in bronchiectasis is always a sign of overlying infection.

Pitfalls
- While haemoptysis is always possible in patients with bronchiectasis (with or without an acute infection), in a smoker aged > 45 years this should always provoke a chest X-ray and referral to a chest physician.
- Many patients with bronchiectasis develop asthma, which requires treatment in its own right.
- Bronchiectasis should always be investigated, to establish the underlying cause.
- While chronic sputum production is a hallmark of bronchiectasis, some patients are not productive ('dry' bronchiectasis).
- The presence of organisms in the sputum of a patient with bronchiectasis does not imply infection, merely colonization, and is not therefore an indication for antibiotic treatment. Antibiotic treatment should depend upon clinical features of infection.

Hints for investigators and prescribers
- The use of regular sputum clearance techniques can play an important part in preventing deterioration in these patients.
- Patients with bronchiectasis often become colonized by respiratory pathogens which are usually the agent responsible during an acute exacerbation. This may help to target appropriate antibiotic therapy before current sputum culture is available.

Further reading
Axford, J. (ed.) (1996) *Chest Disease in Medicine*. Blackwell Scientific Publications, London.
Brewis, R.A.L. (ed.) (1991) *Lecture Notes on Respiratory Disease*, 4th Edn. Blackwell Scientific Publications, London.

4 Pneumonia

An acute lower respiratory tract infection associated with recently developed radiological signs.

Classification of pneumonia
- Community-acquired, typical and atypical
- Hospital-acquired (nosocomial)
- In the immunocompromised

4.1 Community-acquired pneumonia

'Typical' pneumonia

Often has an acute toxic onset with florid lower respiratory tract features. The main causal organisms are Streptococcus pneumoniae (the worst common cause, classic lobar pneumonia, frequent epidemics in the spring); Haemophilus influenzae (infects those with existing respiratory tract disease); Staphylococcus aureus (may follow a bout of influenza, often in the spring); and Klebsiella pneumoniae (florid upper lobe pneumonia).

'Atypical' pneumonia

Often has a more 'atypical' presentation with frequent non-respiratory symptoms. The main organisms are Legionella pneumophila (autumn epidemics, may colonize the water of poorly maintained air conditioning and bathing systems, and cause outbreaks in institutions via aerosol spread in those with pre-existing respiratory tract disease); Mycoplasma pneumoniae (winter epidemics every 4 years, children and young adults); Chlamydia spp.; and Coxiella burnettii. There is an increased incidence of systemic complications, including haemolysis (M. pneumoniae) and myocarditis (C. burnettii and M. pneumoniae).

Clinical case one

History

A 44-year-old male with no significant respiratory past history presents in the spring with a 4-day history of right lower chest pain, increasing shortness of breath, and a cough productive of rust-coloured sputum.

Examination

Pyrexial 38.4°C. Pulse rate (PR) 100 beats per minute (bpm), blood pressure (BP) 140/80 mmHg, respiratory rate 18 per min. Labial herpes simplex virus (HSV). Diminished expansion right hemithorax, with consolidation and a pleural rub.

Management options

1. Prescribe appropriate antibiotics (amoxycillin + erythromycin, or cefaclor + erythromycin if penicillin allergic), which will treat what is clinically a community-acquired pneumonia.
2. Explain to the patient that he has pneumonia and that by collecting sputum for culture you will be able to determine whether you have chosen the right antibiotic for him.
3. Explain to the patient that he has pneumonia and that you are starting antibiotics and arranging a chest X-ray.
4. Explain to the patient that he has pneumonia and that he should be examined in hospital and possibly admitted.
5. Explain to the patient that he has pneumonia, send sputum for culture, start antibiotics and organize a chest X-ray.

6. Explain to the patient that he has pneumonia, send sputum for culture, start antibiotics, take blood for FBC and urea and electrolytes (U&E), and organize a chest X-ray.

Option 1. Prescribe appropriate antibiotics (amoxycillin + erythromycin, or cefaclor + erythromycin if penicillin allergic), which will treat what is clinically a community-acquired pneumonia.

✓ Most cases of community-acquired pneumonia are caused by S. pneumoniae: the presence of this organism is supported by the rust-coloured sputum, herpes labialis, and the relatively young age of the patient.

✗ The patient will need to be reviewed and may not settle.

✗ The patient is systemically unwell and may need more complicated treatment, such as i.v. antibiotics and supplemental oxygen.

✗ Once antibiotics have been commenced, any future sputum culture may be negative, even if the patient remains unwell.

✗ Without a baseline chest X-ray, any follow-up X-rays may be difficult to interpret.

✗ By not investigating your patients, you will never learn more about them.

Option 2. Explain to the patient that he has pneumonia and that by collecting sputum for culture you will be able to determine whether you have chosen the right antibiotic for him.

✓ Your initial antibiotic choice will be correct in most cases, but by culturing sputum you can modify this when the sensitivities are known.

✓ The chance of getting a positive culture is increased by sending off sputum as antibiotics are commenced.

✗ You will need to review more frequently, thus increasing your workload.

✗ The patient is systemically unwell and may need more intensive treatment than you have given him.

✗ Without a baseline chest X-ray, future films may be difficult to interpret.

✗ The sputum culture will add to your costs.

Option 3. Explain to the patient that he has pneumonia and that you are starting antibiotics and arranging a chest X-ray.

✓ Early antibiotics will treat the pneumonia effectively.

✓ A chest X-ray will help define the severity of the pneumonia, and make follow-up films easier to interpret.

✗ The patient may need more intensive treatment than you have given him.

✗ The patient is ill and yet will have to travel to the X-ray department.

✗ By not culturing sputum, you will not know the causative organism, making further antibiotic choices difficult if the patient fails to improve.

✗ By not investigating you patients, you will never learn more about them.

Option 4. Explain to the patient that he has pneumonia and that he should be examined in hospital and possibly admitted.

✓ This is a safe option, in a patient who is unwell with a potentially serious illness.

✓ All the patient's investigations can be performed quickly and together.

✓ Hospital review can quickly establish the seriousness of the patient's condition and whether he needs to remain in hospital.

✗ The patient may have recovered equally well at home, and thus you are wasting resources.

✗ This is a very expensive treatment option!

✗ By handing over care at an early stage, you will never learn more about your patients.

Option 5. Explain to the patient that he has pneumonia, send sputum for culture, start antibiotics and organize a chest X-ray.

✓ The patient will probably improve on this therapy.

✓ Taking sputum for culture as antibiotics are started will increase the chances of growing an organism and also allow you to change antibiotics at an early stage if necessary.

✓ A baseline chest X-ray will be available.

✓ By investigating your patients, you will learn more about them.

✗ This is an expensive option.

✗ The patient may require more intensive treatment, which you are delaying.

Option 6. Explain to the patient that he has pneumonia, send sputum for culture, start antibiotics, take blood for FBC and urea and electrolytes (U&E), and organize a chest X-ray.

✓ The patient will probably improve on this therapy.

✓ Taking sputum for culture as antibiotics are started will increase the chances of growing an organism and also allow you to change antibiotics at an early stage if necessary.

✓ A baseline chest X-ray will be available.

✓ The severity of the pneumonia can be assessed. Factors associated with an increased mortality include age >60, respiratory rate >30 min^{-1}, diastolic BP <60 mmHg, new atrial fibrillation, and urea >7 mmol l^{-1}.

✓ By investigating your patients, you will learn more about them.

✗ This is an expensive option.

✗ The patient may require more intensive treatment, which you are delaying.

Clinical case two

History

A 28-year-old woman with two young children presents with a 14-day history of dry cough, vomiting, diarrhoea and myalgia, 5 days after her husband had been admitted to hospital with pneumonia.

Examination

Pyrexial 37.6°C. Mildly dehydrated, pale. PR 105 bpm. Signs of right lower lobe consolidation. Abdomen normal. Circular erythematous lesions with central blisters on the lower limbs.

Management options

1. Explain to the patient that she has an atypical pneumonia and treat with oral erythromycin 500 mg four times per day.
2. Explain to the patient that she has an atypical pneumonia and that you are prescribing two antibiotics (oral erythromycin and amoxycillin) to ensure that all organisms are treated.
3. Prescribe antibiotics as in Option 2, take blood for FBC, U&E, atypical serology, and organize a chest X-ray.
4. Prescribe antibiotics as in Option 2 and perform the investigations as in Option 3, but also prescribe antiemetics and push oral fluids.
5. Arrange urgent admission to hospital.

Option 1. Explain to the patient that she has an atypical pneumonia and treat with oral erythromycin 500 mg four times per day.

✓ The diagnosis and treatment are probably correct.

✗ The severity of the pneumonia has not been established.
✗ Her gastrointestinal symptoms may prevent oral therapy from working.
✗ She may not be able to cope with her young family without her partner.
✗ By not investigating your patients, you will never learn more about them.

Option 2. Explain to the patient that she has an atypical pneumonia and that you are prescribing two antibiotics (oral erythromycin and amoxycillin) to ensure that all organisms are treated.

✓ You have treated the majority of organisms which are likely to be causing her pneumonia.

✗ The severity of the pneumonia has not been established.
✗ Her gastrointestinal symptoms may prevent oral therapy from working.
✗ She may not be able to cope with her young family without her partner.
✗ By not investigating your patients, you will never learn more about them.

Option 3. Prescribe antibiotics as in Option 2, take blood for FBC, U&E, atypical serology, and organize a chest X-ray.

✓ Appropriate antibiotic treatment has been given.
✓ Some indication of the severity of the pneumonia has been obtained.
✓ You may discover the causative organism, and therefore learn more about your patients.

✗ These tests add to your costs.
✗ The patient is unwell but will have to travel to hospital for the chest X-ray.
✗ Her gastrointestinal symptoms may prevent oral therapy from working.
✗ She may not be able to cope with her young family without her partner.

Option 4. Prescribe antibiotics as in Option 2 and perform the investigations as in Option 3, but also prescribe antiemetics and push oral fluids.

✓ Appropriate antibiotic treatment has been given.
✓ Some indication of the severity of the pneumonia has been obtained.
✓ You may discover the causative organism, and therefore learn more about your patients.
✓ Antiemetics may help her tolerate the oral antibiotics.

✗ These tests add to your costs.
✗ The patient is unwell but will have to travel to hospital for the chest X-ray.
✗ Her gastrointestinal symptoms may prevent oral therapy from working.
✗ She may not be able to cope with her young family without her partner.

Option 5. Arrange urgent admission to hospital.

✓ Her atypical pneumonia may be severe, and she may require early hospitalization (as did her husband).
✓ All the investigations can be performed quickly and easily in hospital.
✓ Any complications can be quickly sorted out.

✗ This is the most expensive option.
✗ Her children will require care.
✗ By handing over care of your patients at an early stage, you will learn less about their illnesses.

Clinical case three

History

A 63-year-old woman with well-controlled maturity onset diabetes has been unwell for 2 weeks with a flu-like illness which has affected several of the members of her family. However, unlike her relatives, over the last 4 days she has had a resurgence of her pyrexia, with increasing breathlessness and a cough productive of yellow sputum.

Examination

Pyrexial 37.3°C. Respiratory rate 18 per min, PR 95 bpm, regular. Crackles widespread in the chest. No wheeze or clinical signs of consolidation in the chest.

Management options

1. Reassure her that she merely has a bug like the rest of her family and that she is just taking longer to get over it.
2. Diagnose a secondary bacterial infection and prescribe appropriate antibiotics.
3. Diagnose a secondary bacterial infection and prescribe appropriate antibiotics. Send off sputum for culture.
4. Diagnose a secondary bacterial infection and prescribe appropriate antibiotics, send off sputum for culture, and arrange a chest X-ray.
5. Diagnose a secondary bacterial infection and prescribe appropriate antibiotics, send off sputum for culture, arrange a chest X-ray, and take blood samples for sugar, U&E and FBC.
6. Send her to hospital.

Option 1. Reassure her that she merely has a bug like the rest of her family and that she is just taking longer to get over it.

✓ This is a cheap option!

✗ You will have to review her, increasing your workload.

✗ If you are wrong, then you will be delaying early treatment of a potentially life-threatening disease.

✗ You will never learn more about your patients if you do not investigate them.

Option 2. Diagnose a secondary bacterial infection and prescribe appropriate antibiotics.

✓ It is likely that she has developed an overlying secondary bacterial infection (probably S. aureus pneumonia) and you are covering this by giving her an appropriate antibiotic.

✓ This is still a fairly cheap option.

✗ By not taking sputum for culture at the earliest possible stage, you may not be able to grow the causal organism, making a change of antibiotic later difficult to judge.

✗ By not arranging further tests, you will not be able to assess the severity of her pneumonia.

✗ The pneumonia may have sent her diabetes out of control – you are not assessing this.

✗ You will never learn more about your patients if you do not investigate them.

Option 3. Diagnose a secondary bacterial infection and prescribe appropriate antibiotics. Send off sputum for culture.

✓ It is likely that she has developed an overlying secondary bacterial infection (probably S. aureus pneumonia) and you are covering this by prescribing an appropriate antibiotic.

✓ This is still a fairly cheap option.

✓ By taking sputum for culture at an early stage, you are increasing the chances of growing the causal organism, making a change of antibiotic easier to arrange should it prove necessary.

✗ By not arranging further tests, you will not be able to assess the severity of her pneumonia.
✗ The pneumonia may have sent her diabetes out of control – you are not assessing this.
✗ You will never learn more about your patients if you do not investigate them.

Option 4. Diagnose a secondary bacterial infection and prescribe appropriate antibiotics, send off sputum for culture, and arrange a chest X-ray.

✓ It is likely that she has developed an overlying secondary bacterial infection (probably S. aureus pneumonia) and you are covering this by prescribing an appropriate antibiotic.
✓ This is still a fairly cheap option.
✓ By collecting sputum for culture at an early stage, you are increasing the chances of growing the causal organism, making a change of antibiotic easier to arrange should it prove necessary.
✓ By arranging a chest X-ray, you are ascertaining the extent of the pneumonia.

✗ She is ill, but will have to travel to hospital for the X-ray to be taken.
✗ The chest X-ray will add considerably to your costs.
✗ By not arranging serological tests, you will not be able to fully assess the severity of her pneumonia.
✗ The pneumonia may have sent her diabetes out of control – you are not assessing this.

Option 5. Diagnose a secondary bacterial infection and prescribe appropriate antibiotics, send off sputum for culture, arrange a chest X-ray, and take blood samples for sugar, U&E and FBC.

✓ It is likely that she has developed an overlying secondary bacterial infection (probably S. aureus pneumonia) and you are covering this by prescribing an appropriate antibiotic.
✓ By taking sputum for culture at an early stage, you are increasing the chances of growing the causal organism, making a change of antibiotic easier to arrange should it prove necessary.
✓ By arranging a chest X-ray, you are ascertaining the extent of the pneumonia.
✓ By collecting blood samples, you are fully assessing the severity of her pneumonia and also checking up on her diabetes.
✓ By fully investigating your patients, you will learn more about them.

✗ All these tests add to your costs!
✗ She is ill, and yet still has to attend hospital for the chest X-ray to be taken.

Option 6. Send her to hospital

✓ This is a safe option!

✗ It is a very expensive option.
✗ She may not be ill enough to justify hospital admission, and be discharged back to your care.
✗ By not investigating your patients, you will never learn more about them.

4.2 Hospital-acquired (nosocomial) pneumonia

The incubation period varies widely and so it is difficult to be certain that a patient has acquired the infection in hospital. A practical working diagnosis is therefore 'a pneumonia developing 2 or more days after admission and not apparent at the time of admission'. Risk factors include being ventilated, post-operative and immobility. Gram-negative organisms and S. aureus are more common than in community-acquired pneumonia.

Clinical case

History
A 70-year-old male smoker is recovering well after undergoing a general anaesthetic for haemorrhoidectomy. On the evening of the third post-operative day he becomes confused.

Examination

Afebrile, PR 98 bpm, sinus rhythm. Respiratory rate 23 per min. Clinical signs of consolidation at the right base. Calves normal.

Management options

1. Diagnose a hospital-acquired pneumonia, obtain a chest X-ray, maintain hydration, and prescribe i.v. cefuroxime 750 mg three times per day.
2. Diagnose a hospital-acquired pneumonia, obtain a chest X-ray, FBC, U&E, and prescribe antibiotics as in Option 1.
3. Diagnose a hospital-acquired pneumonia, obtain a chest X-ray, FBC, U&E, arterial blood gases and blood cultures, and prescribe controlled supplemental oxygen and antibiotics as in Option 1.
4. Manage as for Option 3, but nurse in a well lit side-room and arrange chest physiotherapy.

Option 1. Diagnose a hospital-acquired pneumonia, obtain a chest X-ray, maintain hydration, and prescribe i.v. cefuroxime 750 mg three times per day.

✓ The diagnosis and antibiotic treatment are probably correct.

✗ The severity of the pneumonia has not been assessed.
✗ You have not managed his acute confusional state.
✗ It is difficult to assess supplemental oxygen needs in a smoker who may have overlying obstructive airways disease without assessing arterial oxygen tensions.
✗ No attempt has been made at assisting sputum clearance.

Option 2. Diagnose a hospital-acquired pneumonia, obtain a chest X-ray, FBC, U&E, and prescribe antibiotics as in Option 1.

✓ The diagnosis and antibiotic treatment are probably correct.
✓ Some markers of the severity of the pneumonia have now been determined.

✗ You have not managed his acute confusional state.
✗ It is difficult to assess supplemental oxygen needs in a smoker who may have overlying obstructive airways disease without assessing arterial oxygen tensions.
✗ No attempt has been made at assisting sputum clearance.

Option 3. Diagnose a hospital-acquired pneumonia, obtain a chest X-ray, FBC, U&E, arterial blood gases and blood cultures, and prescribe controlled supplemental oxygen and antibiotics as in Option 1.

✓ The diagnosis and antibiotic treatment are probably correct.
✓ Markers of the severity of the pneumonia have now been determined.
✓ Appropriate supplemental oxygen can be prescribed, when necessary.

✗ You have not managed his acute confusional state.
✗ No attempt has been made at assisting sputum clearance.

Option 4. Manage as for Option 3, but nurse in a well lit side-room and arrange chest physiotherapy.

✓ The diagnosis and antibiotic treatment are probably correct.
✓ Markers of the severity of the pneumonia have now been determined.
✓ Appropriate supplemental oxygen can be given, when necessary.
✓ You have managed his acute confusional state.
✓ Chest physiotherapy will improve his depth of breathing and may aid sputum clearance.

4.3 Pneumonia in the immunocompromised

The causes of immunodeficiency are numerous and include malnutrition, diabetes, uraemia, alcoholism, the primary immunodeficiency syndromes, HIV infection, and the use of chemotherapeutic or immunosuppressive drugs.

Any of the common respiratory pathogens can affect the immunocompromised, but organisms which are not usually pathogenic can also cause infections. These include bacteria, mycobacteria (both typical and atypical), viruses (CMV, HSV, herpes zoster, and measles virus), fungi (Aspergillus fumigatus, Candida albicans), and Pneumocystis carinii.

Clinical case

History
You are called to the haematology ward to review a 38-year-old male patient with acute myeloid leukaemia. He is 3 weeks post his second course of chemotherapy and is in isolation. For 2 days he has become increasingly breathless, particularly during any exertion. He also has a dry cough and a sense of chest discomfort.

Examination
Pyrexial 38.1 °C. Respiratory rate 28 per min. Chest percussion and auscultation unremarkable.

Investigations
Chest X-ray normal. ECG normal. Arterial blood gases: hypoxaemia with a mild hypocapnia. Hb 14, white cell count (WCC) zero, platelets 12. Viral serology awaited.

Management options
1. Induce sputum by giving inhalational hypertonic saline with the assistance of the physiotherapist following careful mouth toilet. Prescribe supplemental oxygen.
2. Perform bronchoscopy and lavage under platelet cover. Prescribe supplemental oxygen.
3. Manage as for Option 2, but also perform a transbronchial biopsy.
4. Try to confirm the diagnosis by either inducing sputum or performing a bronchoalveolar lavage. Prescribe supplemental oxygen and high dose co-trimoxazole, gentamicin, and cefuroxime until further bacteriological results are available.

Option 1. Induce sputum by giving inhalational hypertonic saline with the assistance of the physiotherapist following careful mouth toilet. Prescribe supplemental oxygen.

✓ Sputum obtained by this method can be used to look for bacteria, fungi and viruses by antigen immunofluorescence.
✓ By obtaining good samples for microbiological analysis, you are helping to avoid unnecessary treatment.
✓ The patient's symptoms will be eased by the supplemental oxygen.
✓ You are avoiding the dangers of a bronchoscopy.
✗ The patient is unwell and requires urgent antibiotics.

Option 2. Perform bronchoscopy and lavage under platelet cover. Prescribe supplemental oxygen.

✓ The diagnosis rate for P. carinii is 40–90% by this method.
✓ The patient's symptoms will be eased by the supplemental oxygen.
✓ By obtaining good samples for microbiological analysis, you are helping to avoid unnecessary treatment.

✗ The bronchoscopy can be an unpleasant test for someone in respiratory distress.

✗ You are delaying urgent antibiotic treatment which the patient needs by waiting for samples obtained at bronchoscopy.

Option 3. Manage as for Option 2, but also perform a transbronchial biopsy.

✓ The addition of transbronchial biopsy increase the chances of diagnosing P. carinii to >90%.

✓ The patient's symptoms will be eased by the supplemental oxygen.

✗ Transbronchial biopsy carries a significant risk of pneumothorax in a patient who is already in respiratory distress.

✗ Transbronchial biopsy carries a significant risk of bleeding in a patient who is thrombocytopaenic, despite platelet cover.

✗ You are delaying urgent antibiotic treatment which the patient needs by waiting for samples obtained at bronchoscopy.

Option 4. Try to confirm the diagnosis by either inducing sputum or performing a bronchoalveolar lavage. Prescribe supplemental oxygen and high dose co-trimoxazole, gentamicin, and cefuroxime until further bacteriological results are available.

✓ Either of these ways of obtaining samples are reasonably safe and efficient in this patient.

✓ The patient's symptoms will be eased by the supplemental oxygen.

✓ You are covering most pathogens with your therapy, the most likely of which is P. carinii.

The following sections in this topic refer to all presentations of pneumonia.

History checklist

General

- A general history will reveal whether the patient is predisposed to respiratory infections e.g. diabetic, immune suppressed, or a smoker.
- If the patient is hospitalized, then the infecting organisms may be different, and this will have an influence on therapy.

Specific

- Duration of symptoms? By definition, there will only be a short history. A longer history should prompt suspicion of a more chronic disease, e.g. TB or lung cancer.
- Prodromal features? Viral and atypical pneumonias often have these.
- Cluster of cases? Other cases in the family or area suggest an outbreak of viral or atypical pneumonia. Clusters of cases in institutions suggest legionnaires' disease.
- Seasonal variation? Different infecting organisms cause disease at different times of the year.
- Contact with animals? The organism may have been passed from infected animals, e.g. Chlamydia psittacci from diseased birds (psittacosis).

Examination checklist

- Look for general signs of infection (temperature, pulse, blood pressure). These features can be particularly important in defining the severity of the pneumonia.
- Examine the throat and cervical lymph glands.
- Examine the chest, looking specifically for wheeze, crackles and signs of lobar consolidation.
- Examine the hands, looking for anaemia, finger clubbing and carbon dioxide retention.

Referrals

- Have a low index of suspicion for referring patients to hospital when you diagnose pneumonia.
- Factors associated with an increased mortality include age over 60, respiratory rate >30 min^{-1}, diastolic BP <60 mmHg, new atrial fibrillation, and urea >7 mmol l^{-1}. Any of these should prompt urgent referral to hospital, or if the patient is already hospitalized, aggressive treatment and monitoring.
- Anyone suffering recurrent bouts of pneumonia should be referred to a chest physician for further investigation.

Rituals and myths

- Pneumonia is a trivial illness.
- If the patient has no sputum, they do not have a serious respiratory infection.

Pitfalls

- Recurrent episodes of pneumonia may indicate underlying disease, e.g. bronchial carcinoma.
- While pneumococcal pneumonia is most common, most other organisms can mimic the classic lobar pneumonia.
- Watch out for staphylococcal pneumonia overlying influenza, particularly in the frail and immunocompromised.
- Poorly treated pneumonia is a cause of great long-term morbidity.

Further reading

Finch, R., Macfarlane, J.T., Selkon, J.D. *et al.* (1993) Guidelines for the management of community acquired pneumonia in adults admitted to hospital. The British Thoracic Society. *Br. J. Hosp. Med.* **49**: 346.

Woodhead, M.A. (1992) Management of pneumonia. *Respir. Med.* **86**: 459.

5 Lung abscess

Lung abscess is a localized suppurative lesion of the lung parenchyma. It is usually caused by aspiration, bronchial obstruction, tumour, embolic infection, or following pneumonia (particularly when of staphylococcal or Klebsiella sp. aetiology). There is often a mixed flora, although anaerobes are found in up to 70% of cases.

Clinical case

History
A 54-year-old woman presents with a 6-week history of cough, which has been increasingly productive of purulent bloodstained sputum, and general malaise. She tells you she had visited the dentist and had a filling replaced 1 week prior to her symptoms starting.

Examination and investigations
Pyrexial 39°C. PR 110 bpm, tachycardia. Crackles and dullness to percussion at the right base posteriorly. Chest X-ray shows a cavitating lesion with an air-fluid level in the apical segment of the right lower lobe.

Management options
1. Prescribe appropriate antibiotics to cover both anaerobic and aerobic organisms. Explain to the patient that she has a lung abscess and arrange to review her in 1 week.
2. Collect sputum for culture. Prescribe appropriate antibiotics to cover both anaerobic and aerobic organisms. Explain to the patient that she has a lung abscess and arrange to review her in 1 week.
3. Explain to the patient that she has a lung abscess and that you are organizing immediate admission to hospital.
4. Manage as for Option 1 and refer urgently as an out-patient to a chest physician.

Option 1. Prescribe appropriate antibiotics to cover both anaerobic and aerobic organisms. Explain to the patient that she has a lung abscess and arrange to review her in 1 week.

✓ The antibiotics you have prescribed will cover the majority of organisms found in a lung abscess.

✗ The patient is systemically unwell and may require hospital treatment.
✗ You may not be able to define the organism at a future date if you do not culture the sputum.
✗ You are not looking for TB.
✗ You will need to review the patient.
✗ By not investigating your patients, you will never learn more about them.
✗ You have not defined the aetiology of the infection.

Option 2. Collect sputum for culture. Prescribe appropriate antibiotics to cover both anaerobic and aerobic organisms. Explain to the patient that she has a lung abscess and arrange to review her in 1 week.

✓ The antibiotics you have prescribed will cover the majority of organisms found in a lung abscess.
✓ Sputum culture will probably identify the causal organism(s) and rule out TB.

✗ The patient is systemically unwell and may require hospital treatment.

✗ You are not looking for TB.
✗ You have not defined the aetiology of the infection.
✗ You will need to review the patient.
✗ By not investigating your patients, you will never learn more about them.

Option 3. Explain to the patient that she has a lung abscess and that you are organizing immediate admission to hospital.

✓ The patient is systemically unwell and may require in-patient treatment.
✓ Additional tests such as sputum and blood cultures can be easily done.
✓ If the patient does not settle, bronchoscopy can be performed to look for a foreign body (especially important after the recent dental work).

✗ This is an expensive option.
✗ The patient may well have recovered at home.
✗ By not investigating your patients, you will never learn more about them.

Option 4. Manage as for Option 1 and refer urgently as an out-patient to a chest physician.

✓ The patient may well respond to the appropriate antibiotics.
✓ If the patient does not settle, bronchoscopy can be performed on review at the hospital.

✗ The patient is systemically unwell and may require in-patient treatment.
✗ The patient may have recovered by the time she is seen in the out-patient department.
✗ By not investigating your patients, you will never learn more about them.

History checklist

General
- This will reveal whether the patient is predisposed to respiratory infections e.g. diabetic, immunosuppressed, smoker, pre-existing chest disease.
- Diabetics, in particular, are prone to developing lung abscesses.

Specific
- Length of symptoms? For lung abscess, the symptoms will last for several weeks at least. Patients with lung abscess will often have indolent symptoms, with a gradual onset of weight loss, malaise and respiratory symptoms.
- Precipitating event? For lung abscess, there may have been a single event that has provoked the abscess which the patient may remember, e.g. a visit to the dentist or a choking bout while eating.

Examination checklist
- Examine for general signs of infection, taking the patient's temperature and pulse.
- Examine the throat and cervical glands, looking for inflammation and swelling.
- Examine the chest, looking for signs of consolidation, crackles and wheeze.
- Examine for signs of general good health – the patient may have lost weight and look generally ill.

Referrals
- Lung abscess is unusual in otherwise healthy individuals and should provoke a search for an underlying cause. Referral to a chest physician should be made unless the cause is obvious.

Pitfalls
- An inhaled foreign body will not show on a chest X-ray unless it is radio-opaque, and even then it may be hidden by the heart shadow on a plain film.

- A lung abscess in a smoker may well be due to an obstructing bronchial tumour and this should be actively excluded.
- Lung abscesses will require antibiotics for several weeks to be sure of complete resolution.
- Poor dental hygiene may be a cause of lung abscess, due to inhalation of organisms.

Further reading

Kumar, P.J. and Clark, M.L. (eds) (1990) *Clinical Medicine*, 2nd Edn. Bailliere Tindall, London, p. 677.
Nield, J.E., Eykyn, S.I. and Phillips, J. (1985) Lung abscess and empyema. *Q. J. Med.* **57**: 875.

6 Respiratory infections in obstructive airways disease

Obstructive airways disease is defined as limitation to airflow such that the forced expired volume in 1 second/forced vital capacity (FEV_1/FVC) ratio is <70%. Such patients have an increased risk of susceptibility to organisms which can infect the respiratory tract. In practice, these patients fall into two groups: those with reversible airflow obstruction (asthma) and that group in which there is little or no reversibility (chronic obstructive pulmonary disease or COPD).

6.1 Asthma

This is defined as reversible airflow obstruction. It is a very common disease, particularly among children. Most asthma attacks are not provoked by infection, and even in those where infection is a trigger, viral agents are usually reponsible.

Clinical case

History
A 16-year-old girl presents with a 4-day history of increasing nocturnal cough, a tight chest and exertional wheezing. This was preceded by a feverish illness which had also affected several members of her family. She is producing a small volume of yellow sputum and feels unwell. She was diagnosed as suffering from asthma 4 years ago and although she has required two courses of oral steroids during this time, her asthmatic symptoms are usually well controlled on moderate doses of inhaled steroids and bronchodilators.

Examination
Pyrexial 37.3°C. Respiratory rate 19 min^{-1}. No cyanosis, chest auscultation reveals scattered wheezes but no crackles. Peak expiratory flow rate 220 l min^{-1} (normal range 430–470).

Management options
1. Reassure the patient that she has a viral infection and prescribe antipyretics.
2. Reassure the patient that she has a viral infection, prescribe antipyretics, and collect sputum in case there is an underlying bacterial infection.
3. Reassure the patient that she has a viral infection and prescribe antipyretics, collect sputum in case there is an underlying bacterial infection, and prescribe an antibiotic just in case.
4. Reassure the patient that she probably has a viral infection, prescribe antipyretics and an antibiotic in case it is bacterial.
5. Reassure the patient that she has a viral infection and prescribe antipyretics, collect sputum in case there is an underlying bacterial infection, and prescribe an antibiotic and a course of steroids to cover other problems.
6. Reassure the patient that she has a viral infection and prescribe antipyretics, collect sputum in case there is an underlying bacterial infection, and prescribe an antibiotic and a course of steroids to cover other problems. Tell her to monitor her peak flow measurement – if it falls below 100, she should go to hospital.
7. Refer the patient to hospital.

Option 1. Reassure the patient that she has a viral infection and prescribe antipyretics.
✓ This will treat some of her acute symptoms and make her feel better.
✓ It does not cost you much money.

✓ In most cases, the patient will improve with this therapy: most acute infective respiratory symptoms in asthmatics are due to viruses.

✗ You have not treated her increased asthmatic symptoms.
✗ You have not ruled out the possibility of there being an underlying bacterial infection.
✗ You have not put in place any mechanisms for treating her asthma, should it worsen.
✗ By not investigating your patients, you will never learn more about them.

Option 2. Reassure the patient that she has a viral infection, prescribe antipyretics, and collect sputum in case there is an underlying bacterial infection.

✓ This will treat some of her acute symptoms and make her feel better.
✓ In most cases, the patient will improve with this therapy: most acute infective respiratory symptoms in asthmatics are due to viruses.
✓ You will be able to prescribe an appropriate antibiotic should a bacterial infection be apparent.

✗ She will need to re-attend, increasing your workload.
✗ You have not treated her increased asthmatic symptoms.
✗ You have not put in place any mechanisms for treating her asthma, should it worsen.

Option 3. Reassure the patient that she has a viral infection and prescribe antipyretics, collect sputum in case there is an underlying bacterial infection, and prescribe an antibiotic just in case.

✓ This will treat some of her acute symptoms and make her feel better.
✓ You will be able to change to a more appropriate antibiotic should this be necessary.

✗ You have not treated her increased asthmatic symptoms.
✗ You have not put in place any mechanisms for treating her asthma, should it worsen.

Option 4. Reassure the patient that she probably has a viral infection, prescribe antipyretics and an antibiotic in case it is bacterial.

✓ This will treat some of her acute symptoms and make her feel better.

✗ The speculative antibiotic is probably unnecessary.
✗ You have not treated her increased asthmatic symptoms.
✗ You have not put in place any mechanisms for treating her asthma, should it worsen.
✗ By not investigating your patients, you will never learn more about them.

Option 5. Reassure the patient that she has a viral infection and prescribe antipyretics, collect sputum in case there is an underlying bacterial infection, and prescribe an antibiotic and a course of steroids to cover other problems.

✓ This option covers most possibilities!
✓ This will treat some of her acute symptoms and make her feel better.
✓ You have treated her acute asthmatic symptoms.

✗ The speculative antibiotic is probably unnecessary.
✗ You have not put in place any mechanisms for treating her asthma, should it worsen.

Option 6. Reassure the patient that she has a viral infection and prescribe antipyretics, collect sputum in case there is an underlying bacterial infection, and prescribe an antibiotic and a course of steroids to cover other problems. Tell her to monitor her peak flow measurement – if it falls below 100, she should go to hospital.

✓ This option covers most possibilities!

✓ This will treat some of her acute symptoms and make her feel better.

✓ You have treated her acute asthmatic symptoms.

✓ You have put in place a plan for coping with her asthma, should it worsen further.

✗ The speculative antibiotic is probably unnecessary.

Option 7. Refer the patient to hospital.

✓ This will cover all possibilities.

✓ Any further management (e.g. chest X-ray, blood tests, nebulized bronchodilators) can be easily carried out.

✗ It is a very expensive option.

✗ She is probably not ill enough to require hospital admission.

✗ She may be discharged back to your care if she is deemed not ill enough to remain in hospital.

✗ You will never learn more about your patients if you do not investigate them.

History checklist

General
A general history will reveal whether the patient is predisposed to respiratory infections, e.g. diabetic, immunosuppressed or a smoker.

Specific
- That of asthma should be apparent. There may be other features of atopy.
- Length of symptoms? Although the asthmatic symptoms will have been present for some time, those of the acute infection should only be short-lived.
- Family history? Asthma is frequently an inherited condition.
- Prodromal features? Viral infections may have these.
- Specific chest symptoms? Productive cough, increasing wheeze and breathlessness, a tight chest.

Examination checklist
- Examine for general signs of infection, taking the patient's temperature and pulse.
- Examine the throat and cervical glands, looking for inflammation and swelling.
- Examine the chest, looking for signs of consolidation, crackles and wheeze.
- A peak flow measurement may be helpful.

Further reading
Anon. (1997) The British guidelines on asthma management. *Thorax* **52**: 51.
Barnes, P.J., Rodger, I.W. and Thompson, N.C. (1988) *Asthma: Basic Mechanisms and Clinical Management*. Academic Press, London.

6.2 Chronic obstructive pulmonary disease (COPD)

This is defined as largely reversible airflow obstruction. It is very common amongst those who are elderly or who have smoked cigarettes. In addition, a number of asthmatic patients may develop irreversible airways disease as they become older. Like asthma, most acute infective episodes are provoked by viral rather than bacterial infections. However, many patients with severe COPD will have constant breathlessness, which may merely worsen when there is an overlying infection.

Clinical case

History

A 64-year-old ex-miner who still smokes ten cigarettes per day has had COPD for the last 10 years. He is normally limited in his exercise tolerance to 50 yards and needs to take nebulized bronchodilators twice a day: for the last 18 months he has been taking 5 mg prednisolone per day. He has had two previous hospital admissions for infections in the last 3 years, and usually gets several exacerbations of his breathlessness each year. Over the past 4 days he has had increasing breathlessness and his normally white sputum has become discoloured.

Examination

Pyrexial 37.7°C. Respiratory rate 18 min⁻¹. Lip pursing. No cyanosis, chest auscultation reveals scattered wheeze and a few crackles.

Management options

1. Tell the patient he has a chest infection which is probably viral and prescribe antipyretics.
2. Tell the patient he has a chest infection which is probably viral, prescribe antipyretics and arrange for sputum to be cultured.
3. Tell the patient he has a chest infection which is probably viral, prescribe antipyretics, arrange for sputum to be cultured, and prescribe an antibiotic speculatively.
4. Tell the patient he has a chest infection which is probably viral, prescribe antipyretics, arrange for sputum to be cultured, prescribe an antibiotic speculatively and a short course of oral steroids to treat his breathlessness.
5. Tell the patient he has a chest infection which is probably viral, prescribe antipyretics, arrange for sputum to be cultured, prescribe an antibiotic speculatively and a short course of oral steroids to treat his breathlessness, and arrange a chest X-ray.
6. Send the patient to hospital.

Option 1. Tell the patient he has a chest infection which is probably viral and prescribe antipyretics.

✓ It is likely that his infection is viral in nature and will settle.
✓ This limits your costs.

✗ He is very symptomatic and may feel he needs more treatment.
✗ You are not treating any potential bacterial infection.
✗ You are not looking for any potential bacterial infection.
✗ You have not treated his increased breathlessness.
✗ By not investigating your patients, you will never learn more about them.

Option 2. Tell the patient he has a chest infection which is probably viral, prescribe antipyretics and arrange for sputum to be cultured.

✓ It is likely that his infection is viral in nature and will settle.
✓ You are looking for any bacterial infection.

✗ He is very symptomatic and may feel he needs more treatment.
✗ You are not treating any potential bacterial infection.
✗ You have not treated his increased breathlessness.

Option 3. Tell the patient he has a chest infection which is probably viral, prescribe antipyretics, arrange for sputum to be cultured, and prescribe an antibiotic speculatively.

✓ It is likely that his infection is viral in nature and it will settle.

✓ You are looking for any bacterial infection.
✓ You are treating any potential bacterial infection.

✗ The antibiotic is probably unnecessary.
✗ He is very symptomatic and may feel he needs more treatment.
✗ You have not treated his increased breathlessness.

Option 4. Tell the patient he has a chest infection which is probably viral, prescribe antipyretics, arrange for sputum to be cultured, prescribe an antibiotic speculatively and a short course of oral steroids to treat his breathlessness.

✓ It is likely that his infection is viral in nature and will settle.
✓ You are looking for any bacterial infection.
✓ You are treating any potential bacterial infection.
✓ You have given him a number of treatments which should make him feel you are taking his symptoms seriously.
✓ The steroids are probably necessary, in view of his chronic use of prednisolone.

✗ The antibiotic is probably unnecessary.

Option 5. Tell the patient he has a chest infection which is probably viral, prescribe antipyretics, arrange for sputum to be cultured, prescribe an antibiotic speculatively and a short course of oral steroids to treat his breathlessness, and arrange a chest X-ray.

✓ It is likely that his infection is viral in nature and will settle.
✓ You are looking for any bacterial infection.
✓ You are treating any potential bacterial infection.
✓ You have given him a number of treatments which should make him feel you are taking his symptoms seriously.
✓ The steroids are probably necessary, in view of his chronic use of prednisolone.

✗ The antibiotic is probably unnecessary.
✗ In terms of his acute illness, the chest X-ray will probably add little unless his condition deteriorates.
✗ He will have to travel to hospital for the chest X-ray.

Option 6. Send the patient to hospital.

✓ He will feel safer in hospital.
✓ It will be easier to perform any necessary tests in hospital.
✓ The hospital doctors will not know him as well as you and will therefore not be able to judge how much of his symptomatology is due to his chronic disease.
✓ This is a very expensive option!
✓ He may well be discharged from the accident and emergency (A&E) department back into your care, thus re-presenting to you with the problem

✗ By not investigating your patients, you will never learn more about them.

History checklist

General
This will reveal whether the patient is predisposed to respiratory infections, e.g. diabetic, immunosuppressed or a smoker.

Specific
• Most COPD patients will have chronic symptoms that are readily apparent.

- Duration of symptoms? If the increased breathlessness has been present for some time, it is unlikely that it is due to an acute overlying infection.
- Prodromal features? Viral infections will often have these.
- Specific chest symptoms? These are often merely an increase in the patients usual symptoms.

Examination checklist
- Examine for general signs of infection, taking the patient's temperature and pulse. These can be very helpful in deciding whether the patient has overlying infection, or merely worsening COPD.
- Examine the throat and cervical glands, looking for inflammation and swelling.
- Examine the chest, looking for signs of consolidation, crackles and wheeze.
- A peak flow measurement may be helpful.

Referrals
- Have a low threshold for referring patients with obstructive airways disease to a chest physician.
- Patients with persistent symptoms should always be referred to a chest physician.
- Recurrent 'chest infections' in a patient with COPD should provoke a chest X-ray.

Rituals and myths
- Discoloured sputum is a sign of infection.

Pitfalls
- Patients who have previously required oral steroids during infections will probably need them on this occasion.
- Patients who are on long-term oral steroids should have a short-term boost when infected.
- Always arrange an acute treatment plan for patients with asthma.

Further reading
Anon. (1997) BTS guidelines for the management of chronic obstructive pulmonary disease. *Thorax* **52**: 55.

7 Empyema

This is defined as the presence of pus within the pleural cavity. It can arise after severe pneumonia, rupture of a lung abscess, after thoracic surgery or, rarely, due to rupture of the oesophagus.

Clinical case

History
A 68-year-old male is admitted via the A&E department with a 3-month history of weight loss, lethargy, sweats and shortness of breath. He had an episode of pneumonia 10 weeks before presentation that was treated with a short course of antibiotics in the community.

Examination and investigations
Finger clubbing. PR 110 bpm, sinus rhythm. BP 110/80 mmHg. Pyrexial 37.9°C. Poor skin turgor. The A&E team have performed a chest X-ray which reveals a large left pleural effusion. However, an attempted pleural tap only manages to aspirate a small amount of thick pus. Plaster covering attempted left pleural aspiration site. Diminished expansion left chest. Stony dull to percussion left chest, with absent breath sounds. Chest X-ray shows a large left pleural effusion. Hb 9.8, platelets 620, WCC 34 800.

Management options
1. Commence appropriate i.v. antibiotics and give i.v. fluids.
2. Commence appropriate i.v. antibiotics, give i.v. fluids and repeat the pleural tap to obtain a specimen for culture.
3. Commence appropriate i.v. antibiotics, give i.v. fluids, repeat the pleural tap to obtain a specimen for culture and insert a large bore chest drain to remove the pus.
4. Commence appropriate i.v. antibiotics, give i.v. fluids, repeat the pleural tap to obtain a specimen for culture and insert a large bore chest drain to remove the pus. Explain to the patient that some of the symptoms are due to anaemia and arrange for them to have a blood transfusion (2 units).

Option 1. Commence appropriate i.v. antibiotics and give i.v. fluids.

✓ The patient is dehydrated and febrile and requires i.v. fluids.
✓ There is an undoubted empyema which requires treatment with i.v. antibiotics.

✗ You have done nothing to ascertain what the infecting organisms are, thus selecting the best antibiotics will be difficult.
✗ The patient will not recover if the large volume of pus is left in the chest.
✗ The patient is very unwell and you have not attempted to correct his anaemia.

Option 2. Commence appropriate i.v. antibiotics, give i.v. fluids and repeat the pleural tap to obtain a specimen for culture.

✓ The patient is dehydrated and febrile and requires i.v. fluids.
✓ There is an undoubted empyema which requires treatment with i.v. antibiotics.
✓ You will be able to select the most appropriate antibiotics when the results of the culture are known.

✗ The patient will not recover if the large volume of pus is left in the chest.
✗ The patient is very unwell and you have not attempted to correct his anaemia.

Option 3. Commence appropriate i.v. antibiotics, give i.v. fluids, repeat the pleural tap to obtain a specimen for culture and insert a large bore chest drain to remove the pus.

✓ The patient is dehydrated and febrile and requires i.v. fluids.

✓ There is an undoubted empyema which requires treatment with i.v. antibiotics.

✓ You will be able to select the most appropriate antibiotics when the results of the culture are known.

✓ By draining the pus, you will allow the empyema to resolve.

✗ The patient is very unwell and you have not attempted to correct his anaemia.

Option 4. Commence appropriate i.v. antibiotics, give i.v. fluids, repeat the pleural tap to obtain a specimen for culture and insert a large bore chest drain to remove the pus. Explain to the patient that some of the symptoms are due to anaemia and arrange for them to have a blood transfusion (2 units).

✓ The patient is dehydrated and febrile and requires i.v. fluids.

✓ There is an undoubted empyema which requires treatment with i.v. antibiotics.

✓ You will be able to select the most appropriate antibiotics when the results of the culture are known.

✓ By draining the pus, you will allow the empyema to resolve.

✓ By giving a blood transfusion, you will improve the patient's chronic symptoms.

✗ Because the anaemia is due to the chronic infection and not an acute bleed, a blood transfusion is not essential and merely exposes the patient to the risks associated with the use of blood products.

History checklist

General
- A general history will reveal whether the patient is predisposed to respiratory infections, e.g. diabetic, immunosuppressed or a smoker.
- Diabetics and other patients with chronic immunosuppression are particularly prone to developing empyema.

Specific
- Duration of symptoms? Empyema is a chronic condition, so the patient is likely to have had worsening symptoms for several weeks at least. Patients will usually have symptoms of chronic progressive disease, with lethargy, malaise, sweats and weight loss.
- Precipitating event? There may have been an acute inflammatory episode that started the empyema off, e.g. an episode of pneumonia.
- Specific chest symptoms? Increasing breathlessness, chest pain, chronic productive cough. In empyema, general constitutional symptoms (malaise, weight loss) are often very evident.

Examination checklist
- Examine for general signs of infection, taking the patient's temperature and pulse.
- Examine the throat and cervical glands, looking for inflammation and swelling.
- Examine the chest, looking for signs of consolidation, crackles and wheeze.
- Examine the hands, looking for anaemia, carbon dioxide retention and clubbing.
- Perform a general examination, looking for signs of weight loss and general demeanour.

Referrals
- Empyema is a serious respiratory disease and should be referred to a chest physician for treatment.

- Loculated empyemas should be referred to a thoracic surgeon for thoracoscopic lavage and possible rib resection.

Rituals and myths
- Empyema can be treated with antibiotics alone.
- A short course of antibiotics is all that is required once the empyema cavity has been drained.

Pitfalls
- Poorly treated empyemas can be a cause of long-term morbidity and in the frail and elderly can be life-threatening.
- Almost all empyemas will require at least intercostal tube drainage: simple aspiration is usually insufficient.

Further reading
Nield, J.E., Eykyn, S.I. and Phillips, J. (1985) Lung abscess and empyema. Q. J. Med. **57**: 875.

8 Tuberculosis

Tuberculosis (TB) is an infection caused by Mycobacterium tuberculosis. The lung is the commonest organ involved. Infection can be primary (first exposure), post-primary, or miliary. Post-primary disease is the commonest type seen in the UK, where the commonest sites involved are the apices of the lungs. In the UK, notification rates vary between ethnic groups, e.g. 5:100 000 for Caucasians and 150:100 000 for Asians. While most strains are still sensitive to the combination chemotherapy regimes in use, the incidence of multidrug-resistant M. tuberculosis is increasing.

Clinical case

History
A 78-year-old retired medical professor presents with a 6-month history of weight loss, sweats, and a chronic cough productive of white sputum which on three occasions recently has been bloodstained. He has lost 1 stone in weight over this period and has been feeling increasingly unwell. He is a lifelong non-smoker, and has had no known previous TB contact.

Examination and investigations
Afebrile. PR 78 bpm. BP 140/80 mmHg. Percussion note is dull anteriorly in the right upper chest, with associated crackles on auscultation. Evidence of recent weight loss. Chest X-ray has been reported as 'right upper lobe consolidation – consider TB'.

Management options
1. Commence anti-TB chemotherapy after explaining to the patient that he probably has TB.
2. Commence anti-TB chemotherapy after explaining to the patient that he probably has TB, and collect three specimens of sputum for culture and staining for acid-fast bacilli (AFB).
3. Collect sputum for analysis. Arrange an urgent referral to a chest physician after explaining to the patient that he probably has TB.
4. Explain to the patient that he may have TB and refer him as an emergency to hospital.

Option 1. Commence anti-TB chemotherapy after explaining to the patient that he probably has TB.

✓ The diagnosis is probably correct and in a Caucasian male this treatment will probably be effective.

✗ As you have not arranged for the sputum to be cultured for TB, you will not be able to confirm the diagnosis or change antibiotics easily at a later date. Furthermore, you will not know whether the patient is infectious, and this will hamper contact-screening.

✗ All anti-TB drugs are toxic and it is necessary to monitor liver function. You have not obtained any baseline liver function tests (LFT).

✗ The many possible side-effects of anti-TB therapy have not been explained to the patient.

✗ You have not notified the patient to the authorities, so that contact-tracing can occur.

✗ The patient will require chest physician review.

✗ You will never learn more about your patients by not investigating them.

Option 2. Commence anti-TB chemotherapy after explaining to the patient that he probably has tuberculosis, and collect three specimens of sputum for culture and staining for acid-fast bacilli (AFB).

✓ The diagnosis is probably correct and in a Caucasian male this treatment will probably be effective.

✓ You have arranged for sputum culture which will confirm the diagnosis and enable the best therapy to be given should complications arise.

✗ All anti-TB drugs are toxic and it is necessary to monitor liver function. You have not obtained any baseline LFTs.

✗ The many possible side-effects of anti-TB therapy have not been explained to the patient.

✗ You have not notified the patient to the authorities, so that contact-tracing can occur.

✗ The patient will require chest physician review.

Option 3. Collect sputum for analysis. Arrange an urgent referral to a chest physician after explaining to the patient that he probably has TB.

✓ Sputum analysis may well confirm the diagnosis of TB by the time he sees the chest physician.

✓ If sputum culture is negative, then additional tests (e.g. bronchoscopy, induced sputum) can quickly be arranged.

✓ Baseline investigations can be quickly and easily confirmed.

✓ Appropriate treatment can be commenced and the necessary notification and contact-tracing put in place by the chest physician.

✗ There may be a delay before he is seen at the chest clinic.

✗ You will never learn more about your patients by not investigating them.

Option 4. Explain to the patient that he may have TB and refer him as an emergency to hospital.

✓ Your diagnosis is probably correct.

✓ All the necessary investigations can be performed by the team which assesses him in hospital.

✓ The necessary therapy can be started.

✗ If he is admitted, then this is a very expensive option.

✗ He probably does not require admission to hospital.

✗ You will never learn more about your patients by not investigating them.

History checklist

General
A general history will reveal whether the patient is predisposed to respiratory infections, e.g. diabetic, immunosuppressed, or a smoker. It will also reveal whether the patient has been in contact with a case of TB, or whether there is a preceding history of the disease.

Specific
- Duration of symptoms? TB is an insidious disease, and the patient will often have had symptoms for several months.
- Previous history? There may be history of previous TB (often in childhood) or a close family member with the disease.
- Specific chest symptoms? Chronic cough productive of variable volumes of discoloured sputum, and perhaps haemoptysis. The patient will often complain of night sweats, malaise and weight loss.

Examination checklist
- Examine for general signs of infection, taking the patient's temperature and pulse.
- Examine the throat and cervical glands, looking for inflammation and swelling.
- Examine the chest, looking for signs of consolidation, crackles and wheeze.
- Examine the hands, looking for anaemia, carbon dioxide retention and clubbing.
- Look for signs of chronic infection, e.g. weight loss, general ill health.

Referrals

- Cases of TB should be referred to a chest physician.
- Cases of drug-resistant or atypical disease are best referred to a chest physician with a special interest in TB.

Rituals and myths

- The presence of organisms on sputum microscopy in patients undergoing treatment indicates active infection.
- All patients with pulmonary TB are infectious.
- Casual contact with patients with TB carries a significant risk of infection.

Pitfalls

- TB is a potent cause of long-term lung damage, even if treated correctly.
- All TB chemotherapy is relatively toxic, but most reactions occur in the elderly, when drug dosages may need to be reduced.
- Careful monitoring is required during treatment for TB.

Further reading

Davis, P.D.O. (ed.) (1998) *Clinical Tuberculosis*, 2nd Edn. Chapman & Hall, London.

Ross, J.D. and Horne, N.W. (1983) *Modern Drug Treatment in Tuberculosis*, 6th Edn. Chest, Heart and Stroke Association, London.

Chapter 13
SKIN INFECTIONS

W.S. Robles

The normal human skin is colonized by a variety of bacteria that live as commensals on its surface and within the hair follicles. The human skin becomes colonized from birth. Overgrowth of these resident organisms may cause minor disease. Bacteria not normally considered as resident may sometimes colonize the skin in modest numbers. There is evidence that the type of flora varies with age and that males carry higher numbers of bacteria than females.

The main role of the normal flora is probably defence against bacterial infection throughout bacterial interference. Some areas of skin have specific floras, e.g. nasal vestibule, in which it has been demonstrated that Staphylococcus aureus is present in about 35% of healthy individuals. Other areas of skin with specific flora are the external auditory meatus, axillae, toe clefts, vulva, perineum and groin.

Chapter contents
Bacterial infections
Viral infections
Fungal infections

1 Furuncles (boils) and carbuncles

Furuncles or common boils are acute, usually necrotic infections of a single hair follicle, caused by S. aureus. Uncommon in early childhood, their incidence increases in puberty, adolescence and early adulthood. In the UK they are more common during the early winter months. The factors responsible for outbreaks and persistence are unknown. It is uncommon to find evidence of impairment of immune response in affected individuals. The organism may be isolated from the nose or perineum.

Carbuncles are deep inflammatory nodules resulting from infection of a group of contagious follicles with S. aureus. The condition includes intense inflammation of the underlying connective tissue and subcutaneous fat.

Management options

1. Systemic treatment with oral antibiotics until resolution of acute inflammation.
2. Bacteriology culture to confirm diagnosis, without prescription of empirical antibiotics.
3. Bacteriology culture to confirm diagnosis, with prescription of empirical antibiotics.
4. Take a good clinical history. Bacteriology culture to confirm diagnosis and assess the carrier status of the patient, with prescription of empirical antibiotics. Blood glucose levels also requested.

Option 1. Systemic treatment with oral antibiotics until resolution of acute inflammation.

Advise the patient to seek help if there is no improvement over the next 48 hours.

✓ Cheap option – no investigations.
✓ Fast – no increase in waiting times.
✓ Most likely pathogen is covered with first-line therapy.
✓ Most patients respond well to oral antibiotic therapy for an isolated episode of infection.
✓ Patient is reassured that the infection is short-lasting and likely to resolve within the next few days.

✗ Assessment of individual risk factors are not considered – e.g. diabetes.
✗ Carriage of S. aureus by patient or other members of the household is not assessed.

Option 2. Bacteriology culture to confirm diagnosis, without prescription of empirical antibiotics.

✓ Avoidance of prescription of antibiotic to which pathogen may be resistant.
✓ Antibiotic therapy is more specifically directed against the organism isolated.
✓ Follow-up ensures review of lesion.

✗ Culture results ready in 48 hours. Considerable deterioration of clinical picture may take place by this stage.
✗ Risk factors (e.g. diabetes, cardiac failure or drug addiction) are not considered.
✗ Follow-up increases waiting times.
✗ Carrier status is not assessed.

Option 3. Bacteriology culture to confirm diagnosis, with prescription of empirical antibiotics.

✓ Most likely pathogen is covered by first-line therapy.
✓ Most patients benefit from oral antibiotic therapy.
✓ Avoids risk of further deterioration of the infection.
✓ Antibiotic therapy is directed against a specific pathogen.

✗ Risk factors are not considered.

✗ Increase in waiting times, as the patient needs follow-up.
✗ Carrier status is not assessed.

Option 4. Take a good clinical history. Bacteriology culture to confirm diagnosis and assess the carrier status of patient, with prescription of empirical antibiotics. Blood glucose levels also requested.

✓ Most likely pathogen is covered by first-line therapy.
✓ Most patients benefit from oral antibiotic therapy.
✓ Risk of deterioration of infection is avoided.
✓ Risk of pathogen being resistant to antibiotic therapy is avoided.
✓ Risk factors are considered (e.g. diabetes and systemic steroid treatment).
✓ Carrier status is assessed.

✗ Expensive – several cultures and other investigations are necessary.
✗ Increase in waiting times due to follow-ups.

Management options for S. aureus carriage
1. Do nothing.
2. Treat carriage taking into consideration that permanent eradication is not possible (for details, see 'Hints for investigators and prescribers', p. 228).

Option 1. Do nothing.

✓ Carriage is not in itself an indication for treatment.
✓ Cheap – no prescription involved.
✓ Waiting times are not increased with follow-ups.

✗ Recurrences are more likely.
✗ Other members of household may eventually become infected.
✗ Prophylaxis in health workers, such as operating theatre and neonatal nursery staff, may not be performed.

Option 2. Treat carriage taking into consideration that permanent eradication is not possible (for details, see 'Hints for investigators and prescribers', p. 228).

✓ Risk of recurrence is decreased.
✓ Patients with recurrent staphylococcal infections are likely to improve.
✓ Infection of other members of the household is avoided.
✓ Prophylaxis is necessary in health workers or staff in high risk units.

✗ More expensive, as it involves prescription of antibiotics and in some instances further assessment of carriage.
✗ Some patients with no need for treatment will receive antibiotics.

History checklist

General
• For how long has the lesion been present? The rate of development varies greatly. Necrosis may occur from 2–14 days. It may occur in crops.

Specific
• Where did the lesion appear? Lesions may appear anywhere on the body except palms and soles. Sites commonly involved are face, neck, arms, wrists, fingers, buttocks and anogenital region.
• Is the patient otherwise well? Occasionally, fever and mild constitutional symptoms may

be present. Malnutrition may favour the presence of pyaemia and septicaemia. In HIV patients furuncles may coalesce with the formation of violaceous plaques. Diabetes, cardiac failure, drug addiction, generalized dermatoses and prolonged steroid therapy are considered predisposing factors.

- Constitutional symptoms are common with carbuncles, and may be severe.
- Consider other conditions. Lesions may correspond to infected epidermoid cysts. If there is a previous history of acne, consider nodular acne. If painful nodule on the vulva consider Bartholin gland infection.
- Any previous episodes? Recurrent attacks are not infrequent and present a management problem.

Examination checklist

- What is the appearance of the lesion? Lesions commonly present as small (single or multiple) follicular, tender nodules (larger lesions may produce throbbing pain).
- Which stage of development has the lesion reached? Nodules eventually become pustular and necrotic with posterior discharge of necrotic material (core). These leave a purplish macule and resolve with a scar.

Hints for investigators and prescribers

- The concomitant use of a topical antibacterial agent reduces contamination of the surrounding skin.
- In recurrent cases of infection, exclusion of diabetes or other possible underlying condition is advisable.
- Carriage of S. aureus in the nasal and perineal area of patients and other members of the household should also be sought.
- The following regimen can be used for temporary eradication of carriage or reduction of a heavy bacterial load:
  (i)   Daily hygiene with soap and water. Patient must use their own separate towel and flannel.
  (ii) Long-term topical application of chlorhexidine to anterior nares, axillae and perineum and/or its use in daily bathing or showering.
  (iii) Bed linen and underwear should be laundered at high temperature and should be changed daily.
  (iv) Oral or topical antibiotics may contribute to the reduction or elimination of carriage but recolonization occurs soon after therapy.
  (v)   Intranasal mupirocin eliminates the organism in 5 days.
  (vi) Refractory cases may be treated with oral rifampicin.

Further reading

Becker, B.A., Frieden, I.J. and Odom, R. et al. (1989) Atypical plaque-like staphylococcal folliculitis in human immunodeficiency virus-infected persons. J. Am. Acad. Dermatol. 21: 1024–1026.
Editorial. (1985) Recurrent staphylococcal furunculosis. Lancet ii: 81–82.
Noble, W.C. (1981) Microbiology of Human Skin, 2nd Edn. Lloyd-Luke Medical Books, London.
Roodyn, L. (1960) Epidemiology of staphylococcal infections. J. Hyg. 58: 1–10.
Savin, J.A. (1974) Bacterial infections in diabetes mellitus. Br. J. Dermatol. 91: 481–487.

2 Impetigo

Impetigo is a contagious superficial bacterial infection of the skin which may manifest clinically in one of two forms:

- Non-bullous impetigo which may be caused by S. aureus, or by streptococci (commonly Lancefield group A β-haemolytic streptococci, e.g. Streptococcus pyogenes).
- Bullous impetigo which is considered a staphylococcal disease although streptococcal bullous impetigo has been reported.

Impetigo is a relatively frequent condition in everyday practice and throughout the world, and outbreaks are common.

Management options

1. Do nothing.
2. Topical treatment only. No investigations.
3. Skin is sampled by swabbing, followed by culture and antibiogram. Topical treatment followed by systemic treatment when results are available.

Option 1. Do nothing.

✓ Some cases clear spontaneously.
✓ Cheap – no cost for either investigations or medication.
✓ Patient reassured about mildness of condition.

✗ Possibility of missing a nephritogenic strain of streptococcus. The latent period for the development of nephritis after streptococcal pyoderma is 18–21 days.

Option 2. Topical treatment only. No investigations.

✓ Topical antiseptic (chlorhexidine, povidone-iodine) and antibiotic (mupirocin) normally suffice in mild and localized infection. Fusidic acid is also effective.
✓ Cheap option – no investigations involved.

✗ Because of its value in systemic infection, fusidic acid should be avoided as a first-line therapy whenever possible to reduce the risk of development of resistance.
✗ Oral antibiotic is indicated in more severe infections. Possibility of missing a nephritogenic streptococcus.

Option 3. Skin is sampled by swabbing, followed by culture and antibiogram. Topical treatment followed by systemic treatment when results are available.

✓ Topical treatment is usually effective.
✓ Organism responsible may be isolated, guiding systemic treatment.
✓ Systemic treatment instituted as and when necessary.

✗ Expensive – mainly due to investigations and switch to systemic treatment.
✗ Increase in waiting time due to follow-up.

History checklist

General
- Age of patient? Increased incidence in pre-school and school-age children.

Specific

- Onset of symptoms? Days or weeks?
- Similar cases in other family members or at school? Outbreaks often occur.
- Time of year? The peak incidence of non-bullous impetigo is in late summer whereas bullous impetigo is more frequent in summer months.
- Duration of symptoms? There is a tendency to spontaneous cure (2–3 weeks) but a prolonged course is not uncommon.
- Overcrowding, poor hygiene and existing skin disease (e.g. eczema, scabies) predispose to infection.

Examination checklist

- Distribution of lesions? The sites more commonly affected are the face, especially around the mouth and nose, and the limbs. Involvement of mucous membranes is rare.
- Lymphadenopathy may be present.
- Non-bullous impetigo usually presents as a short-lived thin-walled vesicle on an erythematous base, followed by the formation of a yellowish crust. The lesions extend peripherally with no central healing; multiple lesions may be present and some may coalesce. This is followed by dryness of crusts which eventually come off leaving an area of mild erythema without scarring.
- In bullous impetigo the vesicles and bullae are larger, take longer to rupture and may persist for 2–3 days. Crusts are thicker.

Pitfalls

- Many cases occur in previously healthy individuals with good standards of living.
- Bullous impetigo is usually sporadic. It may be particularly widespread in the newborn.
- Cases demonstrating positive pemphigus-like antibodies on direct or indirect immunofluorescence have been reported.

Hints for investigators and prescribers

- Antiseptics are less effective than antibiotics but would be a useful adjunct to systemic treatment.
- Complications are uncommon. However, scarlet fever, urticaria and erythema multiforme may follow streptococcal impetigo.
- Streptococcal impetigo is responsible for the majority of cases of post-streptococcal acute glomerulonephritis.
- Rheumatic fever is not known to be a complication of streptococcal impetigo.

Further reading

Dajani, A.S., Ferrieri, P. and Wannamaker, L.W. (1972) Natural history of impetigo II. Etiologic agents and bacterial infections. *J. Clin. Invest.* **51**: 2863–2871.

Dajani, A.S., Ferrieri, P. and Wannamaker, L.W. (1973) Endemic superficial pyoderma in children. *Arch. Dermatol.* **108**: 517–522.

Dillon, H.C. (1979) Post-streptococcal glomerulonephritis following pyoderma. *Rev. Infect. Dis.* **1**: 935–943.

Dillon, H.C. (1980) Topical and systemic therapy for pyodermas. *Int. J. Dermatol.* **19**: 443–451.

El Tayeb, S.H.M., Nasr, E.M.M. and Attallah, A.S. (1978) Streptococcal impetigo and acute glomerulonephritis in children in Cairo. *Br. J. Dermatol.* **98**: 53–61.

Guillet, G. and Fizet, D. (1984) Immune findings in staphylococcal bullae – cross-reactivity between epidermal and staphylococcal antigens. *Clin. Exp. Dermatol.* **9**: 515–517.

Helsing, P. and Gaustad, P. (1992) Bullous impetigo caused by group A streptococci. *Acta. Derm. Venerol. (Stockh.)* **72**: 90–91.

Lissauer, T.J., Sanderson, P.J. and Valman, H.B. (1981) Re-emergence of bullous impetigo. *Br. Med. J.* **283**: 1509–1510.

Mertz, P.M., Marshall, D.A., Eaglstein, W.H. *et al.* (1989) Topical mupirocin treatment of impetigo is equal to oral erythromycin therapy. *Arch. Dermatol.* **125**: 1069–1073.

Noble, W.C. (1981) *Microbiology of Human Skin*, 2nd Edn. Lloyd-Luke Medical Books, London.

3 Ecthyma

Ecthyma is a pyogenic infection of the skin characterized by formation of superficial adherent crusts over an area of necrotic ulceration. The causative organisms are similar to those of impetigo. S. pyogenes and/or S. aureus may be isolated.

Management options
1. Do nothing.
2. Look for predisposing factors. Improve hygiene and nutrition. Start on antibiotic treatment.

Option 1. Do nothing.
✓ Cheap – no investigations or prescription.
✓ Some patients may clear of infection without antibiotics.
✓ Patients who are not keen on using antibiotics will be pleased.

✗ A number of new lesions may develop by inoculation over a long period.
✗ Unlike impetigo, ecthyma heals with scars. A number of them may be left without treatment.
✗ Predisposing factors (e.g. malnutrition, poor hygiene) are not considered.

Option 2. Look for predisposing factors. Improve hygiene and nutrition. Start on antibiotic treatment.
✓ Correction of predisposing factors and treatment of underlying disease are important.
✓ Patient recovers quicker with appropriate antibiotic treatment.
✓ Scarring process may be less prominent.

✗ More expensive – due to laboratory investigations and systemic treatment.
✗ Increase in waiting times due to follow-ups.

History checklist

General
- Onset of symptoms? Hours or days ago?

Specific
- Age of patient? In Europe most cases occur in children. In the tropics, where the disease is more common, it may occur at any age.
- Predisposing factors? Poor hygiene and malnutrition are considered predisposing factors. Site of minor injury, insect bite, other skin condition (e.g. scabies) and drug addiction may determine the site of lesions.

Examination checklist
- Presenting signs? Most lesions consist of small bullae or pustulae on an erythematous base. This soon changes to a dried exudate and hard crust which increases in size. Removal of the crust exposes an area of purulent punched-out ulcer.
- Site and number of lesions? Most commonly affects buttocks, thighs and legs. It usually follows an insect bite on the leg of a child. One or two lesions is the norm. New lesions may develop by autoinoculation.

Hints for investigators and prescribers
The antibiotic of choice should be active against both S. pyogenes and S. aureus.

Further reading
Kelly, C., Taplin, D. and Allen, A.M. (1971) Streptococcal erythema. *Arch. Dermatol.* **103**: 306–310.

4 Staphylococcal scalded skin syndrome

Staphylococcal scalded skin syndrome (SSSS) is an exfoliative dermatosis which affects most of the body surface. The skin becomes erythematous and the necrotic superficial epidermis peels off. Although originally described in children, adults may also be affected.

Clinical signs and symptoms are produced by the exfoliative (or epidermolytic) toxins of the staphylococci. These are most commonly phage group II, but other phage groups have been described. Two of the toxins (A and B) have been shown by immunofluorescence to bind to keratohyalin granules.

Management options
1. Take a good clinical history. Start empirical antibiotics with no investigations.
2. Take a good clinical history, skin swabs and blood cultures. Start empirical antibiotics. Adjust treatment according to culture results.

Option 1. Take a good clinical history. Start empirical antibiotics with no investigations.

✓ In children the prognosis is generally good. Early antibiotic treatment decreases the mortality rate.
✓ Patients without underlying cause recover more rapidly.
✓ No delay in starting treatment which may be critical to the outcome.
✓ Identification of predisposing factors through clinical history.
✗ Culture results are not available to guide therapy.
✗ No identification of potential predisposing factors, such as alcoholism or immunosuppression.

Option 2. Take a good clinical history, skin swabs and blood cultures. Start empirical antibiotics. Adjust treatment according to culture results.

✓ Improvement of prognosis as mortality rate decreases with the use of systemic antibiotics.
✓ Identification of predisposing factors with correction may improve outcome.
✓ Culture results are available to guide antibiotic therapy.
✓ In adults, blood cultures are usually positive.

✗ In children, blood cultures are usually negative.
✗ More expensive – due to investigations and in-patients' systemic treatment.
✗ Swabs and skin culture are usually negative as the blisters are toxin mediated.

History checklist

General
• Age of patient? More common in children.

Specific
• Presenting symptoms? Fever, irritability and skin tenderness are typical.
• When did the symptoms start? Hours or days ago?
• Where did the lesions start? Localized staphylococcal infection on the skin? Original lesion may be at a distant 'occult' site.
• Underlying predisposing factors? In adults consider renal failure, malignancy, immunosuppression and alcohol abuse.

Examination checklist
• Widespread erythematous eruption, rapidly followed by the development of blisters which on rupture leave raw, extremely painful areas.

Hints for investigators and prescribers

- A 'wait and see' approach is not acceptable as deterioration in this condition occurs fairly rapidly.
- The toxin is disseminated haematogenously. Staphylococci are more likely to be isolated from the original site of infection.
- The condition usually heals within 7–14 days.
- SSSS differs from toxic epidermal necrolysis (TEN) in that cell necrosis does not occur in SSSS. To confirm diagnosis, frozen sections of peeled skin will confirm the split in the granular layer seen in SSSS.
- Tzank preparation may also be helpful in differentiating between the two conditions: in SSSS there is presence of a number of epithelial cells with large nuclei and no inflammatory cells, whereas in TEN there are only a few epithelial cells but many inflammatory ones.

Further reading

Bailey, C.J. and Smith, TP. (1990) The reactive serine protease residue of epidermolytic toxin A. *Biochem. J.* **269**: 1989–1991.

Cribier, B., Piemont, Y. and Crosshans, E. (1994) Staphylococcal scalded skin syndrome in adults. *J. Am. Acad. Dermatol.* **30**: 319–324.

Melish, M.E and Glasgow, L.A. (1970) The staphylococcal scalded skin syndrome. *N. Engl. J. Med.* **282**: 1114–1119.

Murono, K., Fujita, K. and Yoshioka, H. (1988) Detection of staphylococcal exfoliative toxin by slide latex agglutination. *J. Clin. Microbiol.* **26**: 271.

5 Cellulitis and erysipelas

Cellulitis is an acute, subacute or chronic inflammation of subcutaneous tissue for which an infective agent (usually bacterial) may be responsible.

Erysipelas is a bacterial infection of the dermis and superficial subcutaneous fat which manifests a well-defined raised plaque. There is, however, considerable overlap and cellulitis may extend superficially and erysipelas deeply. Most authors regard erysipelas as a form of cellulitis and therefore definition of cellulitis would include inflammation of the dermis and subcutaneous tissue.

Lancefield group A β-haemolytic streptococci is the commonest cause of cellulitis, but groups G and C may occasionally be responsible. Group B is more common in neonatal infections especially under the age of 3 months. S. aureus has also been implicated alone or together with a streptococcus in cellulitis.

Management options
1. Observe severity of signs and symptoms. Prescribe oral antibiotics and advise rest. No investigations.
2. Advise in-patient treatment with further investigations.

Penicillin remains the treatment of choice for suspected streptococcal infections. Mild or early cases may be managed as out-patients with oral penicillin V (or amoxycillin, which is more reliably absorbed) and flucloxacillin.

In-patient treatment with i.v. therapy is indicated in infants, adults with severe constitutional symptoms and cases involving limbs in which circulation may be impaired.

Option 1. Observe severity of signs and symptoms. Prescribe oral antibiotics and advise rest. No investigations.

✓ May be appropriate for mild or early cases.
✓ Cheap – no investigations or in-patient treatment.
✓ Patient reassured about mildness of condition.

✗ Rapidly spreading infections may deteriorate within the next 48 hours.
✗ Patient may be deterred from seeking further advice, as they are already on treatment.
✗ Most infants require in-patient treatment.

Option 2. Advise in-patient treatment with further investigations.

✓ Most patients with moderate to severe infection may need i.v. therapy.
✓ May enable bed rest with elevation of the affected limb to 45°.
✓ May help to identify a possible site of entry – e.g. superficial wound, inflammatory lesion including bacterial or fungal infection or an ulcer.
✓ Further investigations may help in the exclusion of septicaemia.
✓ May prevent further impairment of circulation. Venous insufficiency may predispose to recurrent erysipelas of the leg.

✗ Expensive.

History checklist

General
• When did the symptoms start? More or less than 3 days ago? This is mostly an acute infection.

Specific

- Which is the affected area? The leg is the commonest site of infection. Other localizations include the face, ear and periorbital region. Facial cellulitis has been reported in children due to Haemophilus influenzae type b, unilateral and often associated with otitis media. The affected skin presents with a purplish blue discoloration.
- What are the circumstances? Previous history of trauma? Associated skin pathology?
- Is the patient unwell? Constitutional symptoms are often present with fever, rigors and malaise. Headache, nausea and back pain may also be present.

Examination checklist

- The physical signs include erythema, heat, oedema (swelling), and pain or tenderness. Blistering is common, particularly in erysipelas. Severe cellulitis may also show bullae formation and progression to dermal or subcutaneous necrosis.

Pitfalls

- More often than not, the site of entry is not obvious.
- The general belief that in cellulitis the edge of the lesion is diffuse and in erysipelas is raised and well-demarcated is not always true.
- Lymphangitis and lymphadenopathy are common occurrences.
- Cultures from biopsy material, from swabs at biopsy sites, from needle aspiration of saline injected tissue or from fluid from blisters are often unsuccessful due to the small number of bacteria present in affected tissues. Diagnosis is usually made on the characteristic clinical picture.
- Investigations including blood cultures and swabs from possible entry sites only occasionally yield the relevant organisms.
- Recurrent cellulitis is attributed to lymphatic damage which may initially be clinically inapparent. Further infection may produce further lymphatic impairment that may manifest as lymphoedema.

Hints for investigators and prescribers

- Observe severity of signs before advising in-patient treatment.
- Look for a possible site of entry.
- Recurrent cases benefit from long-term antibiotic treatment. Patients allergic to penicillin should be started on erythromycin as soon as recurrence is suspected.
- In all cases it is advisable to start with an antibiotic that covers streptococci. Mixed infections benefit from combination therapy (e.g. flucloxacillin plus amoxycillin or penicillin V).
- Cases of penicillin allergy are managed with oral erythromycin or first generation cephalosporins. Do not use tetracyclines, as the condition does not respond to this form of treatment.
- Mild cases of H. influenzae cellulitis may be treated with oral amoxycillin-clavulanic acid. Severe cases need in-patient treatment.
- Remember that cellulitis is one of the main causes of pain associated with gravitational ulcers.
- Resistance of S. pyogenes to penicillin has yet to be reported. If the patient is not responding to treatment, consider mixed infection or lack of compliance.
- Cellulitis of the tongue in neutropenic patients has been reported to cause upper airway obstruction.
- In facial infection, the responsible organism should be sought from nose, throat, conjunctiva and sinuses.
- Consider anticoagulant therapy if associated thrombophlebitis.
- Some patients may require lifelong prophylactic treatment.

Further reading

Baker, C.J. (1982) Group B streptococcal cellulitis-adenitis in infants. *Am. J. Dis. Child.* **136**: 631–633.

Bernard, P., Bedane, C., Mounier, M. *et al.* (1989) Streptococcal cause of erysipelas and cellulitis in adults. *Arch. Dermatol.* **125**: 779–782.

Chartier, C. and Grosshans, E. (1990) Erysipelas. *Int. J. Dermatol.* **29**: 459–467.

Hauger, S.B. (1981) Facial cellulitis: an early indicator of group B streptococcal bacteraemia. *Paediatrics* **67**: 376–377.

Hook, E.W., Hooton, T.M., Horton, C.A. *et al.* (1986) Microbiologic evaluation of cutaneous cellulitis in adults. *Arch. Intern. Med.* **146**: 295–297.

Musher, D.M. and McKenzie, S.O. (1977) Infections due to Staphylococcus aureus. *Medicine* **56**: 383–409.

Smith, O.P., Prentice, H.G., Madden, G.M. *et al.* (1990) Lingual cellulitis causing upper airways obstruction in neutropenic patients. *Br. Med. J.* **300**: 24.

6 Herpes simplex virus infections

This infection is caused by Herpesvirus hominis also known as herpes simplex virus (HSV). The common antigenic types are HSV type 1 (HSV-1) mostly responsible for facial infections and HSV type 2 (HSV-2) classically associated with genital disease. Both types have the ability to persist in sensory nerve ganglia after primary infection (latency) and may travel along the nerve fibre to the periphery of the skin or mucous membranes where, if it replicates, it causes recurrent disease.

The mode of infection is by direct contact with infected secretions. Primary infections with HSV-1 (often subclinical) are more common in infants and young children. Infections with HSV-2 (commonly symptomatic) are more common after puberty and often sexually transmitted. After primary infection, humoral and cellular immunity develops without full protection against primary or recurrent disease. Immunodeficiency status increases the incidence and severity of disease.

Management options

These refer mainly to recurrent or reactivated HSV infection as most of the other forms of infection are not seen by dermatologists, and this chapter deals solely with skin infections.

1. Do nothing.
2. Take a good clinical history (most patients will refer to previous episodes in recurrent infections). Treat all patients with topical antiviral cream.
3. Request viral culture (culture of virus from vesicle fluid takes 1–5 days) and/or electron microscopy (EM) and/or polymerase chain reaction (PCR). Treat all patients with systemic antiviral drugs.

Option 1. Do nothing.

Tell the patient that the infection resolves spontaneously in 1 or 2 weeks and advise only analgesia.

✓ Mild infection requires no treatment.
✓ Symptomatic medication with common analgesics is the correct management for uncomplicated viral infections.
✓ Cheap – no investigations or prescription involved.
✓ Old fashioned remedies may suffice for mild attacks of recurrent HSV-1 infections, e.g. dabbing with surgical spirit.

✗ If the lesions are infected, the patient's condition may deteriorate and they may become unwell.
✗ In herpetic gingivostomatitis, drinking and eating are very painful. Parents will find it difficult to accept that nothing needs to be done.
✗ No consideration of immunosuppression may be detrimental, as disseminated or systemic infection may occur.

Option 2. Take a good clinical history (most patients will refer to previous episodes in recurrent infections). Treat all patients with topical antiviral cream.

✓ Reduces the need for laboratory investigations.
✓ Useful in more severe and frequent attacks.
✓ It may cut down the length of attacks.
✓ It may increase the interval between attacks.

✗ In primary infections it is important to exclude other pathologies, e.g. thrush, aphthosis, coxsackie infection including herpangina, Behcet's and Stevens–Johnson syndrome.

✗ It is no help in primary gingivostomatitis.

Option 3. Request viral culture (culture of virus from vesicle fluid takes 1–5 days) and/or electron microscopy (EM) and/or polymerase chain reaction (PCR). Treat all patients with systemic antiviral drugs.

✓ Moderate infections require oral aciclovir. For severe infections, aciclovir by i.v. infusion is the drug of choice.

✓ Helpful in preventing possible complications, e.g. eczema herpeticum in atopic patients and herpes encephalitis or meningitis or recurrent dendritic ulcers that may result in corneal scarring.

✓ Isolation of the virus may help in excluding other serious conditions, e.g. Stevens–Johnson syndrome.

✗ Expensive. Most cases require no investigations.
✗ EM and PCR are not widely available.
✗ Mild infections do not need systemic treatment.

History checklist

General
- Age of the patient? Infants and young children are more likely to have a primary infection, whereas adults and adolescents more commonly develop recurrences.

Specific
- When did the symptoms start? Days or hours ago? This is more relevant in recurrent infections.
- What are the presenting symptoms?
  (i) Primary HSV-1 infection: fever, malaise and excessive dribbling followed by painful oedema and erythema of the gums which may bleed easily. Gingivostomatitis is the most common clinical manifestation of primary HSV-1 infection after a 4–5 day incubation period.
  (ii) Genital herpes infection with HSV-2 occurs mainly after the onset of sexual activity. The most frequent clinical presentation is with painful ulceration of the genitalia.
- Are there any triggering factors for recurrent infection? Minor trauma, febrile illnesses, trivial upper respiratory tract infections and ultraviolet radiation. Some women have reported an increase in the number of episodes in the premenstrual period. In many cases, however, it is not possible to identify a responsible factor.

Examination checklist
- Primary HSV-1 infection. Vesicles may be present on tongue, pharynx, palate and oral mucous membranes and may evolve into ulcers. Enlargement of regional lymph nodes is not uncommon. Resolution is usually complete after 2 weeks.
- Primary genital HSV-2 infection. Ulcer is usually present on glans, prepuce or shaft on the penis in men and vulval mucosae, vagina or cervix in women. It usually resolves in 2–3 weeks.
- In recurrent infection with HSV-1, the clinical presentation is a cluster of small vesicles frequently on the face, preceded by an itching or burning sensation, in the absence of constitutional symptoms. These vesicles normally heal in 1 week without scarring.
- Recurrent infections with HSV-2 are fairly common with clusters of small vesicles that evolve into non-indurated ulcers. They are present on glans or shaft of the penis, labia, vagina or cervix. They can cause painful, distressing symptoms.

Hints for investigators and prescribers
- Most primary infections are subclinical. However, if clinical lesions develop, the severity is generally greater than in recurrent infections.

- Primary genital infection is often more symptomatic than oral infection.
- Seroconversion (complement-fixation test) is only valuable in primary infections.
- Rapid diagnosis can be obtained by EM of vesicle fluid or detection of antigen by immunofluorescence in scrapings from lesions.
- PCR is also useful in diagnosis, especially in erythema multiforme (65% of all patients with this condition have a history of herpes labialis).
- Perianal infection can cause chronic ulceration in male homosexuals with AIDS.

Further reading

Brett, E.M. (1986) Herpes simplex virus encephalitis in children. *Br. Med. J.* **293**: 1388–1389.

Bryson, Y.J, Dillon, M., Lovett, T. *et al.* (1983) Treatment of first episodes of genital herpes simplex virus infection with oral aciclovir. *N. Engl. J. Med.* **308**: 916–921.

Corey, L. (1988) First-episode, recurrent and asymptomatic herpes simplex infection. *J. Am. Acad. Dermatol.* **18**: 169–172.

Corey, L. and Spear, P.G. (1986) Infections with herpes simplex viruses. I. *N. Engl. J. Med.* **314**: 868–891.

Corey, L. and Spear, PG. (1986) Infections with herpes simplex viruses. II. *N. Engl. J. Med.* **314**: 749–757.

Corey, L., Adams, S.G., Brown, Z.A. *et al.* (1983) Genital herpes simplex virus infections: clinical manifestations, course and complications. *Ann. Intern. Med.* **98**: 958–972.

Goldberg, L.H, Kaufman, R., Conant, M.A. *et al.* (1986) Oral aciclovir for episodic treatment of recurrent genital herpes. *J. Am. Acad. Dermatol.* **15**: 256–264.

Huff, J.C. and Weston, W.L. (1989) Recurrent erythema multiforme. *Medicine* **68**: 133–140.

Saral, R., Burns, W.H., Laskin, O.L. *et al.* (1981) Aciclovir prophylaxis of herpes simplex virus infections. *N. Engl. J. Med.* **305**: 63–67.

7 Varicella-zoster virus infections

Varicella and zoster are caused by Herpesvirus varicellae also known as varicella-zoster virus (VZV). The clinical expression of the disease is as varicella (chicken pox) after a primary infection following which the virus persists in nerve ganglia in a latent form. Zoster (shingles) is the result of reactivation of the latent virus. It occurs throughout the world.

Management options for varicella and zoster
1. Do nothing.
2. Request viral culture and/or EM and/or PCR. Treat all patients with systemic antiviral drugs.

Option 1. Do nothing.

Tell the patient that all that is required is rest and ordinary painkillers.

✓ In otherwise healthy individuals varicella only requires symptomatic treatment: rest and analgesics plus topical applications of soothing antiseptic preparations.
✓ Cheap – no investigations or prescription involved.
✓ Patient feels reassured about the severity of the condition.

✗ If secondary infection is present, oral antibiotics are required.
✗ Severe varicella, zoster or high-risk patients have indication for systemic aciclovir treatment to be started within the first 1–2 days.
✗ There is some evidence that a course of aciclovir may have some protective effect in the development of post-herpetic neuralgia.

Option 2. Request viral culture and/or EM and/or PCR. Treat all patients with systemic antiviral drugs.

✓ Good outcome in severe cases of varicella or zoster.
✓ Relatively less incidence of post-herpetic neuralgia.
✓ Less damage in complicated infections, e.g. ophthalmic.

✗ Most cases of varicella require no treatment.
✗ Some patients may benefit from topical treatment without the need for systemic drugs.
✗ Expensive – typical infection presents few diagnostic difficulties once the eruption has developed.

History checklist

General
*   Age of patient? Varicella is more common in children. It provides lasting immunity with second mild episodes reported only occasionally in healthy subjects. Zoster is uncommon in children, affecting mostly adults and the incidence increases with age.

Specific
*   Has the patient been in contact with an infected individual recently? Varicella is readily transmissible, principally via infected droplets from the nasopharynx.
*   How long after contact did the symptoms appear? The incubation period of varicella is usually 14–17 days.
*   In varicella, after an incubation period of 2–3 weeks, patients develop fever and malaise, followed by the appearance of a scarlatiniform or morbiliform erythema.
*   Pain is usually the first manifestation of zoster and may be accompanied by fever and malaise.

Examination checklist

Varicella
- Are there any papules or vesicles? The development of papules takes place rapidly becoming tense vesicles which develop in crops. The content of the vesicles becomes turgid after a few hours, drying in 2–4 days with crust formation and generally heals without scarring.
- What is the distribution of the lesions? Centripetal mainly on the trunk, then affecting face, scalp and limbs.
- Is there any mucous membrane involvement? Vesicles may be seen in the mouth and occasionally on other mucous membranes.
- Is the patient very ill? Severity and duration of fever is variable as are constitutional symptoms. Recovery is usually complete in 2 weeks.

Zoster
- Are there any papules or vesicles? After 1–3 days of pain, grouped red papules that rapidly become vesicular appear in the area of one or two dermatomes. The lesions become pustular and may develop in an uninterrupted band accompanied by enlargement and tenderness of local lymph nodes.
- What is the distribution of lesions? Commonly thoracic but it may also be trigeminal including ophthalmic and lumbosacral. The incidence of ophthalmic zoster increases with age.
- Is there any mucous membrane involvement? Mucous membranes within affected dermatome are involved. In ophthalmic nerve zoster, eye involvement occurs in approximately two in three cases. Complications include keratitis, uveitis, conjunctivitis, scleritis and chemosis.

Hints for investigators and prescribers
- In everyday practice most diagnoses of this condition are made on clinical grounds.
- Systemic aciclovir is more effective if given within 48 hours of the onset.
- If there is widespread involvement, look for an underlying cause: Hodgkin's lymphoma, chronic lymphocytic leukaemia (CLL), HIV or AIDS. Patients with lymphoma or otherwise immunocompromised may develop disseminated zoster which may be haemorrhagic.
- Post-herpetic neuralgia, the commonest sequel of zoster, is the persistence of recurrence of pain more than 1 month after the onset of the infection. Elderly patients are more likely to develop post-herpetic neuralgia than the young.
- For post-herpetic neuralgia amitriptyline is useful. Clonazepam and carbamazepine have been of value in the elderly with stabbing pain. Topical capsaicin 0.025% is reported to relieve pain. Beware of burning sensation after application.

Varicella-zoster in pregnancy

Immunological factors as well as nutritional state and quality of care of patients play an important role in the outcome of viral infections in pregnancy.

There is a suggestion that a large gravid uterus may compromise pulmonary ventilation facilitating the development of varicella pneumonia. Varicella is also potentially more severe in adults. Therefore pregnant women should be given varicella-zoster immunoglobulin in an attempt to attenuate the severity of the condition, if given within 72 hours of exposure.

Varicella is potentially more severe in late pregnancy. Admission to hospital may be advisable if breathlessness is present, as this may indicate onset of pneumonia. Aciclovir treatment is indicated once the infection has developed. There is evidence that aciclovir treatment does not increase the incidence of birth defects.

This may be effective if given up to 10 days after exposure. Indications are:

- Non-immune individuals after exposure.
- Immunodeficient children under 15 years of age.
- Neonates born to mothers with chicken pox.
- Non-immune pregnant women.
- Bone marrow transplant recipients.

It is of no use once varicella has developed. In this case, patients should be treated with systemic aciclovir.

Further reading

Gershon, A.A., Steinberg, S.P., Gelb, L. *et al.* (1984) Clinical reinfection with varicella-zoster virus. *J. Infect. Dis.* **149**: 137–142.

Juel-Jensen, B.E. (1970) The natural history of shingles. *J. R. Coll. Gen. Practit.* **20**: 232.

Vonderheid, E. and van Voorst Vader, P.C. (1980) Herpes zoster-varicella in cutaneous T-cell lymphomas. *Arch. Dermatol.* **116**: 408–412.

Weller, T.H. (1983) Varicella and zoster. I. *N. Engl. J. Med.* **309**: 1362–1368.

Weller, T.H. (1983) Varicella and zoster. II. *N. Engl. J. Med.* **309**: 1434–1440.

8 Pityriasis versicolor

This is a common, usually asymptomatic, chronic infection of the stratum corneum caused by the lipophilic yeast Malassezia furfur, characterized by discrete scaly depigmented areas of skin mainly on the trunk.

M. furfur is part of the normal flora of the skin, and mechanisms by which its overgrowth is regulated are not well understood. It has a preference for colonization of some areas of the body which include scalp, upper trunk and flexures.

Management options
1. Do nothing.
2. Use Wood's lamp on skin (fluoresces pale yellow if positive) and treat all patients topically.
3. Request direct microscopy of skin scrapings. Treat all patients with systemic antifungals (azoles).

Option 1. Do nothing.

✓ Some cases resolve spontaneously.
✓ Certainly very cheap.
✓ No increase in waiting time as patient does not need follow-up.
✓ Patient is reassured about the mildness of the condition.

✗ Most patients need at least a topical preparation to clear the condition.
✗ Relapses are more common.

Option 2. Use Wood's lamp on skin (fluoresces pale yellow if positive) and treat all patients topically.

✓ Most cases settle with topical preparations.
✓ Wood's lamp usually reveals that the infection is affecting wider areas of skin.
✓ Cheap – the lamp is not expensive and a useful topical treatment is 2.5% selenium sulphide in a detergent base which is also very cheap.

✗ Some patients may request a quicker option.

Option 3. Request direct microscopy of skin scrapings. Treat all patients with systemic antifungals (azoles).

✓ This is the correct way to confirm the presence of infection.
✓ The possibility of relapses appears to decrease with systemic treatment.
✓ Almost all cases of infection are positive.

✗ Cost.

History checklist
- When did the lesions appear? Weeks or months ago?
- Is it recurrent? Does it have seasonal variation? The condition tends to recur in the summer.
- Has the patient been abroad? It is more common in tropical climates.
- Are there any predisposing factors? It has been claimed that the condition is commoner in various diseases. However, the evidence so far shows this to be the case only in Cushing's syndrome and possibly in malnutrition.
- What are the symptoms? Does it bother the patient? The condition is mostly asymptomatic. Occasionally there is mild inflammation and pruritis. Most patients seek medical opinion because of the 'look' of it.

Examination checklist
- The main clinical sign is the change of skin colour which varies according to the degree of pigmentation of the patient's skin.
- The lesions are non-inflammatory brown patches with fine scaling, localized or widespread, affecting mainly the trunk and upper limbs. In dark skin the lesions produce a whitish discoloration.
- Vitiligo, melasma and pityriasis rosea need to be excluded.

Hints for investigators and prescribers
- Erythrasma and pityriasis versicolor may coexist.
- Warn the patient that residual depigmentation may remain for many months after treatment.
- Selenium sulphate shampoo 2.5%, applied overnight twice weekly, is usually enough to clear the condition, but relapses are common.
- In some cases the use of short courses of itraconazole may be justifiable.

Further reading
Borelli, D. (1985) Pityriasis versicolor por Malassezia ovalis. *Mycopathologia* **89**: 147–153.

Del Palacio Hernanz, A., Delgado Vicente, S., Menendez Ramos, F. *et al.* (1987) Randomized comparative clinical trial of itraconazole and selenium sulphide shampoo for the treatment of pityriasis versicolor. *Rev. Infect. Dis.* **9** (suppl. 1): 121–127.

Gueho, E., Midgley, G. and Guillot, J. (1996) The genus Malassezia with description of four new species. *Antonie van Leeuwenhoek* **69**: 337–355.

Roberts, S.O.B. (1969) Pityriasis versicolor: a clinical and mycological investigation. *Br. J. Dermatol.* **81**: 315–326.

Roberts, S.O.B. (1986) Pityriasis versicolor. In: *Superficial Fungal Infections* (ed. J.L. Verbov). MTP Press Ltd, Lancaster, pp. 47–72.

9 Tinea (ringworm)

These infections are caused by a group of organisms called dermatophytes that have the ability to invade the non-living cornified tissues of skin, hair and nail. Dermatophytes are classified in three genera: Epidermophyton, Microsporum and Trichophyton. Epidemiologically they may be divided into three groups:

- Anthropophilic, with normal habitat on man, e.g. Trichophyton rubrum.
- Zoophilic, acquired from infected animals, e.g. Trichophyton verrucosum.
- Geophilic, saprophytes in the soil from which infection may be contracted, e.g. Microsporum gypseum.

Management options
The treatment of dermatophyte infections varies according to the severity and localization of the infection.
1. Do nothing.
2. Treat all patients topically. Do not request mycological examination of clinical specimens.
3. If scalp ringworm is suspected, use Wood's light on the scalp and treat all patients topically.
4. Request mycological examination of clinical specimens (skin scrapings, nail clippings and hairs). Await results. Prescribe treatment according to type, severity and distribution of lesions.

Option 1. Do nothing.

✓ Some cases may resolve spontaneously.
✓ Certainly very cheap.
✓ No increase in waiting time as patients do not need follow-up.
✓ Patient is reassured about the mildness of the condition.

✗ Most patients need at least a topical preparation to clear the condition.
✗ Some infections will not clear even with topical preparations, e.g. scalp, nail and foot ringworm.

Option 2. Treat all patients topically. Do not request mycological examination of clinical specimens.

✓ Topical treatment mainly with imidazole derivatives is useful in localized forms of tinea corporis, tinea cruris and acute forms of tinea pedis.
✓ Cheap.

✗ Widespread or chronic ringworm, particularly tinea capitis, tinea unguium and tinea pedis (moccasin type), require systemic treatment with oral antifungal drugs, e.g. terbinafine, itraconazole or griseofulvin.
✗ With no culture result, the possible source of infection may be overlooked.

Option 3. If scalp ringworm is suspected, use Wood's light on the scalp and treat all patients topically.

✓ Wood's light is helpful in the diagnosis of Microsporum infections (green) and favus (dull greenish colour).
✓ The lamp is not expensive.

✗ It is of considerable importance to discover the species involved. A small much-loved pet may be the source of infection.
✗ Most cases do not settle with topical preparations.

Option 4. Request mycological examination of clinical specimens (skin scrapings, nail clippings and hairs). Await results. Prescribe treatment according to type, severity and distribution of lesions.

✓ Accurate diagnosis is made. Direct microscopy of skin scrapings and nail clippings reveals the organism. Culture of the same clinical specimens identifies the species.
✓ Possible source of infection may be identified.
✓ Less possibility of recurrence as infection is treated with topical or systemic treatment as necessary to ensure clearance.

✗ Delay in starting treatment may upset the patient as culture results are only available after 3 weeks.
✗ Expensive – particularly if systemic antifungal drugs are necessary.

History checklist
- When did the lesions appear? Weeks or months ago?
- Are there any predisposing factors? Warm climates, sweating and corticosteroid therapy are considered predisposing factors. In general they are more common in tropical climates. Tinea corporis and tinea cruris are commonest in tropical developing countries.

Examination checklist
What are the clinical signs?
- Tinea corporis (tinea circinata or ringworm of the body). Clinically, lesions vary from mild scaling to very inflammatory lesions with papules and vesicles. Classically the lesions are eczema-like, circular and well demarcated with an erythematous border and some degree of scaling and inflammation which tends to subside in the centre of the lesion.
- Tinea cruris (ringworm of the groin). The typical lesion which usually begins below the fold and spreads down to the thigh is well demarcated with a raised, erythematous active border, some degree of scaling and tendency to central clearing.
- Tinea capitis (scalp ringworm). This infection presents mainly in children as chronic non-inflammatory patches of alopecia with very short broken off hairs. It may present with severe inflammation known as kerion.
- Tinea pedis (ringworm of the feet, athlete's foot). The infection is restricted to the feet, especially toe webs and soles. It varies in its clinical presentation from mild chronic scaling lesions, that may be associated with interdigital maceration, to an acute inflammatory disease.
- Tinea unguium (onychomycosis or nail ringworm). Nail involvement may occur alone but commonly accompanies tinea pedis, with the development of thickening, discoloration and friability (nail dystrophy).
- Tinea manuum (ringworm of the hands). Eruption is unilateral in half of cases. Diffuse, fine scaling, often hyperkeratotic, is seen. It is often associated with nail or body involvement.
- Tinea barbae and tinea faciei (ringworm of the beard and face). Tinea barbae is a fungal infection of the bearded area of the face and neck. It presents with papulo-pustules scattered or grouped into kerion-like, reddish-purple lesions that may cause scarring and alopecia. Tinea faciei may affect any part of the face, commonly with vesiculopustular rings and partial central clearing.

Are there any other conditions to be considered?

- Tinea corporis should be differentiated from pityriasis rosea, contact dermatitis, and lichen simplex. Tinea cruris may be confused with candida intertrigo and erythrasma. Tinea pedis should be differentiated from contact dermatitis, pompholyx and plantar psoriasis.

Hints for investigators and prescribers

- All three genera of dermatophytes affect the skin. Epidermophyton affects the nails but not the hairs. Microsporum seldom involves the nails. Trichophyton affects skin, nails and hairs.
- Infections by dermatophytes are highly prevalent in the tropics and subtropics.
- Tinea capitis caused by Microsporum species tends to heal spontaneously at puberty. Trichophyton infection tends to persist indefinitely.
- Any scaling alopecia on a child's scalp should be considered ringworm until proven otherwise.
- Tinea manuum is often a 'one hand, two feet' disease.
- Tinea barbae is more commonly a rural disease contracted from infected animals. It is rare in the tropics, where tinea faciei is more common.
- Use of topical corticosteroid preparations produces atypical clinical lesions – 'tinea incognito' or steroid-modified tinea.
- Griseofulvin is effective against dermatophytes and at present the only drug licensed for oral treatment of scalp ringworm in children. Terbinafine may be available in the near future.

Further reading

Blank, F., Mann, S.J. and Peak, P.A. (1974) Distribution of dermatophytes according to age, ethnic group and sex. *Sabouraudia* 12: 352–361.

Clayton, Y.M. (1984) Scalp ringworm (tinea capitis). In: *Superficial Fungal Infections* (ed. J.L. Verbov). MTP Press Ltd, Manchester, pp. 1–8.

Clayton, Y.M. and Midgley, G. (1977) Tinea capitis in school children in London. *Hautarzt* 28: 32–34.

De Vroey, C. (1985) Epidemiology of ringworm (dermatophytosis). *Semin. Dermatol.* 4: 185–200.

English, M.P. (1976) Nails and fungi. *Br. J. Dermatol.* 74: 697–701.

Hay, R.J. (1982) Chronic dermatophyte infections. I. Clinical and mycological features. *Br. J. Dermatol.* 106: 1–6.

Hay, R.J. (1988) New oral treatments for dermatophytosis. *Ann. N.Y. Acad. Sci.* 544: 580–585.

Ive, F.A. and Marks, R. (1986) Tinea incognito. *Br. Med. J.* iii: 216–221.

Roberts, S.O.B. (1980) Treatment of superficial and subcutaneous mycoses. In: *Antifungal Chemotherapy* (ed. D.C.E. Speller). John Wiley & Sons, Chichester, pp. 255–283.

10 Superficial candidosis (thrush)

Candidosis is an infection caused by the genus Candida in which clinical manifestations vary from acute, subacute and chronic forms involving skin, nails and mucous membranes, to deep infection, localized or disseminated in one or more organs especially in the immuno-suppressed and AIDS patients.

The organisms are part of the microflora of the oral cavity and gut of normal individuals, therefore disease occurs only when there is a localized or generalized abnormality of the host. The species most commonly responsible for infection is Candida albicans.

Management options

1. Prescribe topical treatment to all patients. No investigations.
2. Prescribe topical treatment to all patients. Consider most common predisposing factors and request laboratory investigations.
3. Request relevant investigations. Start with topical treatment. Change to a systemic anti-fungal as necessary when results are available.

Option 1. Prescribe topical treatment to all patients. No investigations.

✓ In many cases topical therapy is enough. In infants, suspensions of nystatin or micona-zole gel applied several times a day are usually adequate for oral thrush.

✓ Cheap – no investigations involved.

✗ No consideration for predisposing factors. Serious underlying condition may be missed, e.g. diabetes or Cushing's syndrome.

✗ No consideration of the role of local trauma or tissue damage. In adults, removal of den-tures with careful hygiene at night is important.

✗ Oral candidosis in chronic mucocutaneous candidosis (CMC) or the immunosuppressed patient frequently fails to respond to topical treatment.

Option 2. Prescribe topical treatment to all patients. Consider most common predisposing factors and request laboratory investigations.

✓ Many patients respond to topical treatment.
✓ This may pick up patients with diabetes.
✓ Not too expensive.

✗ Some clinical syndromes do not respond to topical treatment, e.g. CMC.
✗ Patients with more serious or rare underlying conditions may be missed.

Option 3. Request relevant investigations. Start with topical treatment. Change to a systemic antifungal as necessary when results are available.

✓ Patients are adequately treated.
✓ Cases of immunodeficiency, either congenital or acquired, may be detected.
✓ Consideration of predisposing factors other than immune defects is made.
✓ CMC, candida onychomycosis and candida septicaemia require systemic treatment.
✓ Some patients may need long-term prophylactic treatment, e.g. CMC and HIV.

✗ Expensive.

History checklist

- When did the symptoms start? Days or weeks ago?
- Age of the patient? Oral thrush is common in infants, the elderly and the seriously ill patient.

- Is the patient well otherwise? Predisposing factors vary from wearing of dentures, pregnancy, malnutrition, antibiotics or corticosteroid therapy to underlying disease such as diabetes or HIV infection.
- What is the patient's occupation? Candidal paronychia and onychia are often seen in individuals whose hands are constantly wet as a result of their occupation, e.g. housewives and chefs.

Examination checklist

What are the presenting features?

- Oral thrush is characterized by a creamy-white to grey curd-like membrane, which can easily be removed, exposing a red, oozing base. Angular cheilitis presents with moisturizing, reddish fissures at the corners of the mouth.
- Genital candidosis may present as vulvovaginitis with discharge that may be scant and watery or profuse and cheesy. In male patients it produces balanoposthitis when the glans of the penis becomes red, tender and covered by superficial vesicles and erosions. A mild urethral discharge may be present. Phymosis may develop.

Skin involvement is usually as candida intertrigo affecting the great folds of the body (i.e. groin, inframammary, axilliary and perianal). The interdigital area may also be affected. The lesions are bright 'beefy' red and oozing, with a macerated centre and a festooned, scaly border. At the periphery of the lesions vesiculopustules may be present. Nail involvement is often chronic.

- What is the localization or distribution of the lesions? This should take into consideration all possible clinical syndromes:

> Acute pseudomembranous candidosis (oral thrush)
> Acute atrophic oral candidosis
> Chronic hyperplastic candidosis (candidal leukoplakia)
> Median rhomboid glossitis
> Chronic atrophic candidosis (denture-sore mouth)
> Angular cheilitis (perleche)
> Candidal intertrigo
> Genital and perineal candidosis (vulvovaginal thrush)
> Candidal balanitis
> Perianal and scrotal candidosis
> Napkin candidosis (diaper candidosis)
> Candidal paronychia
> Onychomycosis due to Candida spp.
> Congenital candidosis
> CMC

Hints for investigators and prescribers

- In most instances the diagnosis is made on a clinical basis. Direct microscopy of skin scrapings examined in potassium hydroxide shows a characteristic mixture of yeast-like cells and pseudohyphae. Cultures develop in 24–48 hours. Creamy, yeast-like colonies develop.
- Be aware of susceptibility factors.
- In cases precipitated by medication, this should be discontinued whenever possible.
- In infants, candidiais may complicate nappy rash.
- Antibiotics of the polyenes group including amphotericin B, nystatin and natamycin are all effective against Candida spp. Fluconazole and itraconazole also produce good response.
- In AIDS and HIV patients fluconazole is used in prophylaxis.
- Systemic disease includes involvement of the urinary tract, endocarditis, meningitis and septicaemia, all with serious prognosis.

Further reading

Arendort, T.M., Walker, D.M, Kingdom, R.H. *et al.* (1983) Tobacco smoking and denture wearing in oral candidal leukoplakia. *Br. Dent. J.* **155**: 340–343.

Aronson, I.K. and Soltani, K. (1976) Chronic mucocutaneous candidiasis. A review. *Mycopathologia* **60**: 17–25.

Fergusson, A.G., Fraser, N.G. and Grant, P.W. (1966) Napkin dermatitis with psoriasiformide. A review of 52 cases. *Br. J. Dermatol.* **78**: 289–293.

Hay, R.J., Baran, R., Moore, M. *et al.* (1988) Candida onychomycosis – an evaluation of the role of Candida species in nail disease. *Br. J. Dermatol.* **118**: 47–58.

Chapter 14
SOFT TISSUE, SURGICAL AND TRAUMATIC INFECTIONS

E.S.R. Darley and M.P. Wilson

Soft tisssue, surgical and traumatic wound infections are common presentations both among hospitalized patients and those in the community. This chapter considers the aetiology and management of a wide range of such infections, from the relatively frequent presentation of a 'sticky' post-operative wound to the rather less common exotic animal bites.

A thorough history detailing the circumstances in which the injury was sustained is essential. Specific points of relevance are raised in each section as applicable. Inevitably, the choice of antibiotics will reflect both the nature of the wound as well as the established antibiotic policy in use. Cellulitis and erysipelas are covered in Chapter 13 (p. 234).

Chapter contents

1 Animal bites, domestic and exotic

Mammalian bites are often perceived to be fairly minor injuries. Many who sustain a bite do not seek medical attention at the time of the injury for this reason. Other individuals may simply feel embarrassed to present to casualty with what is clearly a human bite wound. However, infection of such wounds is both common and potentially very serious. Although fortunately rare, fatalities have been reported following dog bites – particularly among patients who fall into an 'at risk' group, e.g. splenectomized patients.

The following section considers the management of infection in animal bites sustained at home or abroad. Insect bites etc. are not discussed here.

Management options

These alternative management plans are based on the presentation of a bite wound which does not initially appear to be infected on clinical examination. It is assumed that clinicians, faced with an obviously infected wound, would commence empirical antibiotic therapy as part of the treatment and therefore the option not to treat these types of injuries is not considered here.

1. Clean the wound superficially and observe. Patient advised to seek help again if it does not begin to heal over the next 48 hours.
2. Debride and irrigate wounds. Collect appropriate culture specimens but do not prescribe antibiotics empirically. Clinic/GP to review with results.
3. Debride and irrigate all wounds. Prescribe empirical antibiotics to 'at risk' patients or those with 'at risk' bites.
4. Debride and irrigate all wounds. Prescribe antibiotics. No culture specimens collected. Review as indicated.
5. Debride and irrigate all wounds. Prescribe antibiotics after culturing from all but trivial wounds. Review with results.
6. Debride and irrigate all wounds. Prescribe empirical antibiotics to 'at risk' patients or those with 'at risk' wounds. Collect culture specimens in all but very superficial wounds. Review with results.

Option 1. Clean the wound superficially and observe. Patient advised to seek help again if it does not begin to heal over the next 48 hours.

✓ Cheap option – no antibiotics or investigations.
✓ Quick – keeps accident and emergency (A&E) waiting times down.
✓ Patient feels reassured that this is not a serious injury, but is encouraged to return if necessary.
✓ Some early (<8 hours ago) trivial bites may require no further management than this.

✗ Thorough examination of the wound is not carried out. Irrigation and debridement are required in all but the most trivial wounds.
✗ Assessment of individual's risk factors is not considered. There is a recognized mortality associated with bite wounds in, for example, post-splenectomy patients.
✗ Site/type/age of wound is not considered.
✗ Without prophylaxis some bite wounds may progress to severe infection before the patient re-presents.

Option 2. Debride and irrigate wounds. Collect appropriate culture specimens but do not prescribe antibiotics empirically. Clinic/GP to review with results.

✓ Unnecessary prescribing is avoided.

✓ Antibiotics may be directed towards the pathogens isolated.

✓ Follow-up of all patients ensures review of the wound.

✗ Minimum 48 hour delay exists while awaiting results from infected bites. Infection may progress considerably in this time.

✗ Individual risk status is not considered.

✗ Site of wound etc. is not considered.

✗ Culture of all bites is expensive. Many results will be negative, while others will identify flora that would have been covered adequately by first-line empirical therapy.

✗ Some pathogens, despite their presence, may not be cultured. False negatives may misguide therapy.

✗ Patient is required to attend for review. Increased pressure on GP/out-patient clinic.

Option 3. Debride and irrigate all wounds. Prescribe empirical antibiotics to 'at risk' patients or those with 'at risk' bites.

✓ Most patients requiring antibiotics are likely to receive them.

✓ Unnecessary prescribing is largely avoided.

✓ Patient is reassured by individual consideration.

✓ Time and expense of microbiological investigation is not incurred.

✓ Most likely pathogens can be covered by first-line therapy.

✗ Some patients not perceived to be at risk may subsequently develop infection. No follow-up arrangements have been made for these cases.

✗ No culture results, therefore no additional information available for those who do not respond to empirical therapy.

Option 4. Debride and irrigate all wounds. Prescribe antibiotics. No culture specimens collected. Review as indicated.

✓ Patient is treated for a potential wound infection.

✓ Time and expense of microbiological investigation is not incurred.

✓ Review arranged on an individual basis.

✗ Many patients will receive antibiotics who do not require them. This increases the incidence of associated side-effects unnecessarily.

✗ Widespread prescribing in blanket fashion encourages antimicrobial resistance.

✗ No culture results are available if treatment fails.

Option 5. Debride and irrigate all wounds. Prescribe antibiotics after culturing from all but trivial wounds. Review with results.

✓ Patient is treated for a potential wound infection.

✓ Culture results are available to adjust therapy if indicated.

✓ Patient feels reassured by thorough management.

✗ Increased pressure on clinic time.

✗ Many patients receive antibiotics who do not require them. Increased incidence of unwanted side-effects.

✗ Culture results may give false negatives. Stopping antibiotics in these patients may result in partially treated infections and late complications.

✗ Expensive option.

✗ Patient required to attend for review. Increased pressure on GP/out-patient clinic.

Option 6. Debride and irrigate all wounds. Prescribe empirical antibiotics to 'at risk' patients or those with 'at risk' wounds. Collect culture specimens in all but very superficial wounds. Review with results.

✓ Patients likely to benefit from antibiotics receive them immediately.
✓ Patient is reassured by thorough management.
✓ Therapy may be adjusted in the light of results.
✓ Option to review wound in more serious bites.
✓ Those dealing with bite wounds, e.g. A&E staff, become aware of the usual pathogens isolated and sensitivity patterns from results.

✗ Time-consuming and relatively expensive approach.
✗ Patient is required to attend for review. Increased pressure on clinic/GP.
✗ False negative results may misguide therapy.
✗ Some untreated superficial wounds may develop infection. No culture results available.

History checklist

General, for any bite

- When did the bite occur? More than 8 hours ago increases the likelihood of infection developing.
- What animal was the patient bitten by? Was it provoked? Note: patients may be reluctant to admit to a human bite, therefore ask this directly.
- Is the patient otherwise well? Previous splenectomy, immunocompromised state, history of alcoholic liver disease, mastectomy or age >50 years (i.e. 'at risk' patients) increase the risk of developing serious infection following bites.
- Any concurrent antibiotic therapy?

Specific for domestic bites

- All bites. Ascertain tetanus immunization status (consider giving tetanus toxoid or immunizing as indicated).
- Human bites. Is the biter known to be hepatitis B (HBV), hepatitis C (HCV) or HIV positive, or likely to fall into the 'high risk' category, e.g. i.v. drug user?

Specific for exotic bites

- In which country did the bite occur?
- When did the bite occur – how many days ago?
- Was the animal:
  - (i) A domestic pet? Was it well at the time? Is it still well?
  - (ii) A wild animal – bats, foxes etc?
- Was the bite a provoked attack?
- Has the wound been licked by any other animals since the bite?

Specific for venomous bites

- When did the bite occur?
- Has the animal been caught/identified?
- Has the individual been bitten before? What were the sequelae on that occasion?

Examination checklist

- Type of wound. Crush, puncture or superficial injury. Crush and puncture wounds are more likely to become infected (i.e. they are 'at risk' bites).
- Depth of wound. Superficial, to tendon sheaths or to bone (see 'Pitfalls', p. 255).
- Clinical signs of infection.
  None.
  Localized cellulitis.

Tracking, lymphangitis, lymphadenitis.

Evidence of a collection of pus/blood.

Systemic involvement, pyrexia, malaise, tachycardia – shock.

- Radiographs. Baseline films if osteomyelitis is a possible complication.
- Site of wound. Extremity bites have poorer blood supply and are therefore more likely to develop infection, particularly bites to the hand.

Referrals

- Exotic animal bites may be sustained abroad (though these are less likely to present for the first time in the UK), or at home, by the owners of unusual pets.
  - (i) All exotic bites should be treated for potential infection, as in 'Management options', p. 252.
  - (ii) The possibility of the animal transmitting rabies should be considered in all cases of mammalian bites. Seek specialist advice from a medical microbiologist or infectious diseases physician regarding the need for post-exposure prophylaxis.
- Venomous bites tend to present early! Often the victim will be the owner or know the owner of the snake and will therefore know the species. Snake venom is usually sterile, but the prey of the snake often defecates during ingestion and faecal type flora may therefore be present in the bite. Consider antibiotics, particularly in puncture or crush wounds.
  - (i) Seek immediate advice from Guy's Poisons Unit while instituting first aid management. (Tel: 0171 635 9191)
  - (ii) Consider empirical antibiotic cover for potentially infected wounds or those considered at risk (see 'Management options', p. 252).
- Deep or complicated wounds may require surgical review, i.e. excision and debridement of necrotic tissue, under anaesthetic if necessary.
- If transmission of hepatitis or HIV is a concern, save the patient's serum and discuss further management with a medical microbiologist or infectious diseases physician regarding HBV immunization. Occasionally, HIV post-exposure prophylaxis may also be appropriate.

Pitfalls

- Almost all bites severe enough to present to A&E require formal debridement and irrigation, regardless of whether or not antibiotics are to be prescribed.
- Bites occurring more than 8 hours before presentation are very likely to become infected, even though the wound may look relatively clean at the time.
- Facial bites have a good blood supply, however the cosmetic effect of a wound infection may be devastating. Consider a lower threshold for prescribing antibiotics in these cases.
- Human bites to a clenched fist are particularly likely to become infected. Often the bite will penetrate the superficial metacarpophalangeal and proximal interphalangeal joint capsules despite appearing to be quite trivial. Antibiotics are recommended for these bites – consider potential complications.
- Legal action may follow some bites – details should be well documented. Photographs will be required in cases of suspected non-accidental injury or assault.
- Review should be arranged for all potentially infected bites by GP or in an out-patient clinic.

Hints for investigators and prescribers

- Where there is clinical evidence of infection, or the bite was sustained more than 8 hours ago, attempts should be made to culture the wound – either a deep swab or debrided tissue culture.
- Blood cultures should be taken from all patients with marked inflammation or systemic illness.
- Co-amoxiclav is likely to cover most common pathogens implicated in human and animal bites. A cephalosporin and metronidazole is an alternative for human bites but

animal bites should not be treated with a cephalosporin because Pasteurella spp. may be resistant. Doxycycline or erythromycin with metronidazole are recommended as second and third line therapies, respectively.

Further reading

Barnham, M. (1991) Once bitten twice shy: the microbiology of bites. *Rev. Med. Microbiol.* **2**: 31–36.

Cumming, P. (1994) Antibiotics to prevent infection in patients with dog bite wounds. *Ann. Emergency Med.* **23**: 535–540.

Feder, H.M. *et al.* (1987) Review of 59 patients hospitalized with animal bites. *Paediatr. Infect. Dis. J.* **6**: 24–28.

Goldstein, E.J.C. (1992) Bite wounds and infection. *Clin. Infect. Dis.* **14**: 633–640.

Mellor, D.J. (1997) Man's best friend: life threatening sepsis after minor dog bite. *Br. Med. J.* **314**: 129–130.

Moore, F. (1997) I've just been bitten by a dog. *Br. Med. J.* **314**: 88–89.

Zubovicz, Z.N. and Cravier, N. (1991) Management of early human bites of the hand. *Plas. Reconstr. Surg.* **81**: 111–114.

2 Burns

A burn describes the tissue damage that follows excessive topical exposure to heat, chemicals, electricity or radiation. It may also be applied to friction trauma and, occasionally, damage caused by severe cold, although these are not considered here.

Human burns are subdivided into three broad categories according to the depth of the tissue damage:

- 1st degree – affecting only the outer layer of skin.
- 2nd degree – involving the epidermis and deeper dermis.
- 3rd degree – a 2nd degree burn with further damage to the underlying tissues, e.g. fascia and/or muscle.

Eschar is necrotic scab-like tissue resulting from a burn injury. It may slough off, but while *in situ* remains an excellent medium for bacterial proliferation.

Local infection and subsequent septicaemia are the major causes of death in patients admitted to hospital with burn injuries.

Excluding those who do not survive beyond the initial resuscitation period, up to 75% of patients who then succumb will do so because of infectious complications. The survival rate has increased in recent years with improved resuscitation and better nutritional support. However, there remains a significant fatality rate, particularly among those sustaining ≥70% burns. Ideally, treatment of serious burns should be managed in a tertiary referral centre in order to optimize outcome.

Management options

1. Clean burn and apply dressings as appropriate. Observe for any signs of infection at dressing changes.
2. Clean and dress burn. Commence prophylactic penicillin immediately for 5 days. Then observe the wound at dressing changes for signs of infection.
3. Clean burn. Dress and swab regularly at dressing changes (e.g. every 48 hours). No antimicrobials unless there are signs of infection.
4. Clean burn. Culture burn regularly with swabs (± full thickness biopsy). Use topical antimicrobials according to swab results and knowledge of the organisms predominant in a particular unit. Further antibiotics if indicated by the patient's clinical condition.

Superficial burns may be managed on an out-patient basis, in which case the principles of the following options may still apply. All other burns will require in-patient therapy, and in these cases the ultimate goal is to close the wound completely as quickly as possible, thus preventing further infectious complications. Management is tailored in each individual by the surgeon's decision regarding the timing and method of closing the wound.

Option 1. Clean burn and apply dressings as appropriate. Observe for any signs of infection at dressing changes.

✓ May be appropriate management for small burns.
✓ Patient does not have to take antibiotics, therefore suffering no side-effects.
✓ No exposure to possible toxic effects of topical antimicrobials.

✗ Burn wounds will become significantly colonized with bacteria within 48 hours of injury if topical therapy is not applied.
✗ Eschar acts as culture medium for rapid, but concealed, proliferation of organisms.
✗ Burn wound sepsis may develop before there are any visible signs of infection. There are no culture results immediately available if this does occur.

Option 2. Clean and dress burn. Commence prophylactic penicillin immediately for 5 days. Then observe the wound at dressing changes for signs of infection.

✓ No exposure to possible toxic effects of topical antimicrobials.

✗ Some Gram-positive organisms will not be covered by penicillin.
✗ There is no evidence to support routine use of penicillin prophylaxis.
✗ Streptococcus pyogenes infection is relatively easy to treat should it occur.
✗ No consideration of local environmental flora in this approach.

Option 3. Clean burn. Dress and swab regularly at dressing changes (e.g. every 48 hours). No antimicrobials unless there are signs of infection.

✓ Regular surveillance of colonizing and potentially pathogenic organisms.
✓ Resistance not encouraged by blind use of antimicrobials. No unnecessary side-effects.

✗ Wound will become rapidly colonized, but there may be no signs of infection developing, for example under the eschar, until invasive infection is present.
✗ Swabs indicate colonization but, as above, they are not necessarily representative of infecting organisms.

Option 4. Clean burn. Culture burn regularly with swabs (±full thickness biopsy). Use topical antimicrobials according to swab results and knowledge of the organisms predominant in a particular unit. Further antibiotics if indicated by the patient's clinical condition.

✓ Colonization by potential pathogens kept to a minimum, thereby decreasing the risk of burn wound sepsis.
✓ Likely colonizing/infecting organisms are known and guide the choice of antimicrobials.
✓ Use of tissue biopsy accurately indicates the presence of deep wound infection/invasive infection before conventional signs are observed.
✓ Topical antimicrobials may penetrate eschar, unlike systemic therapy.
✓ Topical antimicrobial usage has been shown to decrease mortality significantly in up to 40% of burn patients.

✗ Patient is exposed to potentially toxic side-effects of topical preparations (e.g. haematological, pain, skin staining, etc).
✗ Use of a single agent may encourage resistant organisms.
✗ Application of cream with occlusive dressing may prevent free movement of a joint, which is necessary for rehabilitation.
✗ Impaired visualization of wound healing.

History checklist

General
- When were the burns sustained? More or less than 3 days ago?
- What caused the burn, e.g. electricity, chemicals, heat etc?
- What were the circumstances? If fire, consider the complications of smoke inhalation in the initial management.
- Has any first aid treatment been given? (e.g. creams, ice packs, prolonged cold water immersion). The latter treatment may constrict the local vascular supply to a large burn and compromise healing further.

Specific
- How old is the patient? Poorer healing is seen at extremes of age.
- Any underlying medical disorders? Peripheral vascular disease, diabetes mellitus or immunocompromised state?

- Current drug therapy? Antibiotics, cardiovascular drugs, e.g. β-blockers?
- Scald/electrical/cigarette burns? Take a very clear history, particularly in paediatric patients. Photograph all wounds if non-accidental injury is suspected, e.g. a child who 'fell backwards' into a hot bath.

Examination checklist

Immediate assessment followed by full examination is required for all but the most superficial burns.

- Severity of burns. 1st, 2nd or 3rd degree.
- Extent of burns. Percentage of body surface area involved (a diagram illustrating the rule of nines (percentage) is displayed in most A&E departments or in clinical handbooks).
- Cardiovascular status. Profound fluid loss may occur very rapidly following extensive burns – early and aggressive replacement may be needed to prevent shock.
- General health and nutrition of patient (e.g. an alcoholic who has collapsed into a fire). Burn wound healing creates a hypercatabolic state – supplemental nutrition may be needed.
- Site of burns. Impaired healing of extremities in patients with peripheral vascular disease.
- Facial burns/chemical splash. Look for corneal scarring. Consider early ophthalmological review. A scarred cornea is particularly liable to infection, which may result in blindness.
- Clinical signs of infection. Local erythema, frank pus in wounds, fever, tachycardia, hypotension, etc.
- Local signs of infection. Discoloration of the wound (may be fungal).
    Oedema at margins of viable skin.
    Green pigmentation of subcutaneous tissue (associated with Pseudomonas aeruginosa).
    Rapid separation of eschar from base (Gram-positive or fungal infection).
    Central necrosis with surrounding oedema (may be fungal).
    Vesicles in wound (herpes simplex virus (HSV)).
    Partial thickness burn becoming full thickness (any infection).

Referrals

Significant burn injuries will be under the care of the plastic surgeons. Some centres advocate the use of selective digestive tract decontamination for a period of approximately 7 days following major burns. This controversial method of bowel decontamination should be discussed with the local microbiologist and is beyond the scope of this chapter.

Good nutritional support is fundamental for wound healing. It may be helpful to arrange dietetic review in some cases.

Rituals and myths

- Penicillin should be prescribed empirically for 5 days for all significant burns. There is no clinical evidence to support this practice.
- First aid measures should include prolonged immersion in cold water or application of ice packs. In large burns this may promote vasoconstriction and decrease local vascularity.
- The eschar is protective and should not be dislodged until it falls off naturally. Infection or collections of blood may accumulate underneath an eschar – the necrotic tissue provides a culture medium and should be debrided early.
- Burn wounds should be left open to heal. Desiccation only encourages infection in these sites – burns should be kept clean and moist.
- Systemic antibiotics are the best treatment for burn wound infections. These are necessary, although topical antimicrobials may exhibit superior penetration into the eschar. In other cases, wide excision – even down to muscle – is required to treat the infection (see below).
- Wound swabs suffice for the diagnosis of burn wound infections. At best, these indicate colonization and potential pathogens. Tissue biopsy is the gold standard for diagnosing deep infection.

Pitfalls

- There may be no local signs of infection in early burn wound sepsis.
- Fever is commonly observed in the first 48 hours after a burn in adults and children. This is not invariably caused by infection.
- Hypovolaemic shock is not confined to the initial resuscitation period. Always consider this as a cause of hypotension in the burned patient.
- Infection is the major cause of graft failure (autologous, allograft or xenograft). Staphylococuss aureus and haemolytic streptococci are most frequently implicated, but any pathogen can cause this.
- Invasive fungal infection may develop into fungaemia relatively quickly. Therefore, extensive excision may be necessary to treat this type of burn wound infection.

Hints for investigators and prescribers

- Initially, a burn wound is most likely to become colonized with Gram-positive organisms, for example, staphylococci and streptococci. Late colonization (>5 days) on the other hand, is more likely to reflect a Gram-negative flora, although inevitably there is some overlap. Wound swabs may be useful in indicating possible causal organisms where there are features of burn wound infection. However, the significance of such isolates will not always be clear. In all cases of burn wound sepsis, advice should be sought from a medical microbiologist. Fungal infection may prove difficult to manage without wide excision of affected tissue. Occasionally, burns may become infected by viruses, e.g. HSV or cytomegalovirus (CMV).
- Prophylaxis of burns with systemic antibiotics is not recommended routinely, but is advised for any surgical manipulation of burn wounds and following autografting (when wounds are left undisturbed for several days).

Further reading

Childs, C. (1988) Fever in burned children. *Burns* 14: 1–6.

Dasco, C.C., Luterman, A. and Curreri, P.W. (1987) Systemic antibiotic treatment in burned patients. *Surg. Clin. N. Am.* 6: 57–68.

Deitch, E.A. (1990) The management of burns. *N. Engl. J. Med.* 323: 1249–1252.

Lowbury, E.J. (1996) Burn infection studies. *J. Hosp. Infect.* 32: 167–173.

Luterman, A., Clifford, G.D. and Curreri, P.W. (1986) Infections in burn patients. *Am. J. Med.* 8 (suppl. A): 45–50.

3 Infected sinuses

A sinus is an infected tract that connects a focus of infection to the surface of the skin or to a hollow organ.

In practice, these are most commonly seen in orthopaedic patients – complicating osteomyelitis or deep infection around a prosthetic joint. (Joint and bone infections are covered in Chapter 8.) Less frequently, sinus formation complicates infection with Mycobacterium tuberculosis, Actinomyces spp., Nocardia spp., and Chlamydia trachomatis (in the context of lymphogranuloma venereum (LGV)).

Hidradenitis suppurativa is an inflammatory condition causing obstruction of the apocrine sweat glands. In particular, it affects skin in the axillae, buttocks and groin, and may present acutely or as a chronic abscess with sinus formation.

LGV is a 'tropical' sexually transmitted condition, caused by C. trachomatis, which is occasionally encountered in this country. Painless ulceration of genitalia, tender lymphadenopathy and, later, matting of lymph nodes (buboes) with discharge of contents are the principle features (see 'Genital infections', p. 119).

Management options

These are determined on an individual basis in each case, according to the underlying cause and the patient's general state of health.

1. Take a full history and examine thoroughly. Collect pus or a sinus tract swab for culture and sensitivity. Start empirical therapy based on the most likely diagnosis for the individual patient. Review antibiotics in the light of culture results.
2. Take a full history and examine thoroughly. Collect pus from the sinus tract for culture and sensitivity. Discuss with a radiologist the appropriate imaging needed to outline the extent of the infection. Consider early surgical exploration. If microscopy and culture of pus are negative or equivocal, proceed to diagnostic biopsy which may be performed during formal exploration and drainage. Treat with antibiotics as indicated by results.

Option 1. Take a full history and examine thoroughly. Collect pus or a sinus tract swab for culture and sensitivity. Start empirical therapy based on the most likely diagnosis for the individual patient. Review antibiotics in the light of culture results.

✓ The history and examination may point to the correct diagnosis, and appropriate therapy may be commenced, even when culture results are incomplete.

✓ Antibiotic therapy, when appropriate, is not delayed while awaiting culture results.

✓ Gram or Ziehl-Nielsen (ZN) stain may be negative even when the clinical diagnosis is correct. This does not affect antibiotic administration here.

✗ Microscopy and culture results may be negative whether or not the clinical diagnosis is correct. With this approach there is no indication to change antibiotics at this stage. (Note: LGV is not diagnosed routinely by microscopy and culture.)

✗ Attempts to repeat equivocal or negative pus/swab cultures may be confounded when antibiotics have already been commenced. Results may remain negative or be of little significance.

✗ In chronic infections there may be no visible signs to indicate whether the antibiotics are effective or not. A prolonged course of inappropriate antibiotics may be administered before it is evident that the infection is not resolving, or even progressing.

Option 2. Take a full history and examine thoroughly. Collect pus from the sinus tract for culture and sensitivity. Discuss with a radiologist the appropriate imaging needed to outline the extent of the infection. Consider early surgical exploration. If microscopy and culture of

pus are negative or equivocal, proceed to diagnostic biopsy which may be performed during formal exploration and drainage. Treat with antibiotics as indicated by results.

✓ Pus collected from the sinus may identify causal organism(s) (not in LGV).
✓ Radiology may support the clinical diagnosis while awaiting culture results and enable guided aspiration and biopsy. Extent of tissue involvement can be visualized.
✓ Surgical assessment is made early in the management course. Exploration may yield diagnosis when initial culture results are equivocal or negative.
✓ Formal drainage is a necessary part of effective treatment in many cases and should not be delayed.
✗ A time-consuming and labour intensive approach.
✗ Antimicrobial therapy may be delayed for several days.
✗ Not all patients are fit enough for surgery.
✗ ZN stains may be negative in up to 50% of cases of spinal tuberculosis (TB). Culture of mycobacteria takes weeks rather than days, during which time the patient may deteriorate considerably without antituberculous chemotherapy.

History checklist

• Immunocompromised state? This predisposes to TB reactivation and nocardial infection. Diabetes mellitus, lymphoma, leukaemia, alcoholic liver disease, cardiac transplantation and underlying lung disease all predispose to M. tuberculosis and nocardiosis.
• Previous surgery? Gastrointestinal surgery or dental extraction are associated with actinomycosis, which may have been several months or even years ago. Spinal surgery, complicated by post-operative wound infection? Metalwork *in-situ* following orthopaedic surgery?
• Previous TB?
• Respiratory symptoms? Consider M. tuberculosis and nocardiosis.
• Genital ulceration? May have passed unnoticed as the primary ulcer is painless in cases of LGV and resolves spontaneously before lymphadenopathy develops. Pelvic inflammatory disease (PID)?
• Use of an intra-uterine contraceptive device? Associated with pelvic actinomycosis.
• Known history of hidradenitis suppurativa?
• Travel history? LGV is endemic in South East Asia, Africa, India, South America and the Caribbean.
• Drug history? Immunosuppressive therapy, e.g. steroids or cytotoxic chemotherapy?

Examination checklist

Table 1 highlights the diagnoses that should be considered depending on the site of the infected sinus and other clinical features.

Table 1. Conditions to be considered depending on the site of the infected sinus and other features

Site of infected sinus	Considerations
Foot (or hand)	Nocardia infection? e.g. 'Madura foot', with swelling and destruction of soft tissues and bone in the foot. Multiple tracts discharging pus are present.
Axilla	Hidradenitis suppurativa, nocardia
Neck, chest wall	TB, actinomycosis, nocardiosis
Abdominal wall	Actinomycosis (exclude fistula secondary to inflammatory bowel disease)
Perianal/natal cleft	Pilonidal sinus, hidradenitis suppurativa
Inguinal or femoral region	LGV, TB, hidradenitis suppurativa
Over-lying joint/bone	Osteomyelitis (see Chapter 8)
Other features:	
Local lymphadenopathy	Non-specific sign – associated with TB, nocardiosis
	LGV (tender lymphadenopathy ± buboes)
Disseminated lymphadenopathy	In immunocompromised patients with TB
	In advanced LGV
Palpable abdominal mass	May be a finding in gastrointestinal actinomycosis or TB.

Referrals

- Early review by a surgical team is recommended in all cases of discharging sinuses.
- Patients with TB should be managed by a physician experienced in the use of antituberculous drugs. In practice, this will usually be an infectious diseases or chest physician.
- Patients with pulmonary nocardial infection should receive medical review or out-patient follow-up where there is underlying pulmonary pathology.
- Patients presenting with LGV should be referred for further investigation to a GUM clinic.

Rituals and myths

- Tonsil swabs are useful to identify the source of infection in a patient with actinomycosis. Actinomycetes are, in fact, present in the oral flora of 50% of healthy individuals, and their presence does not affect management or prognosis.
- Presence of actinomycete-like organisms on a cervical smear implies PID and warrants treatment. While actinomycosis can cause PID, it may be a commensal organism in the female genital tract and does not need to be eradicated in the absence of relevant symptoms.
- A negative Heaf test effectively excludes TB from the differential diagnosis. This is not true for immunocompromised patients (e.g. AIDS patients with TB) or the very old. Also, a BCG scar does not imply absolute immunity to mycobacterial infection.
- A superficial swab of the sinus tract opening is helpful when no pus is expressed. This is likely to reveal skin flora or colonizing organisms only. In the latter case this can be misleading when potential pathogens (e.g. coliforms) are isolated, as significance is then questionable.

Pitfalls

- Negative stain results (i.e. ZN and Gram stain) do not exclude tuberculous infection. Culture results should reveal the causal organism if repeat specimens are collected on two or three occasions.
- A past history of TB does not immediately point to a diagnosis of reactivation (though it must be considered in context).
- Painful genital ulceration is a feature of HSV infection and chancroid. It is not a feature of LGV, but should prompt a search for other sexually transmitted diseases (STD).
- Consider underlying immunosuppression (e.g. HIV) in patients presenting with TB.
- The chlamydia causing LGV cannot be demonstrated by microscopy of expressed pus or cultured in most microbiology laboratories. Diagnosis is largely clinical with supporting serology.

Hints for investigators and prescribers

- The infections described in this section are not encountered in everyday practice. Therefore, it is recommended that cases should be discussed on an individual basis with an infection specialist (microbiologist or infectious diseases physician). Ideally, this should be done before collecting specimens so that appropriate investigations are requested (including serology for LGV) and, if necessary, transport medium can be provided. Laboratory staff need to be made aware of the differential diagnosis so that the relevant staining and culture procedures are employed.

Further reading

Arya, O.P. (1996) Tropical STDs. *Medicine* 24: 1019–1020.
Burden, P. (1989) Actinomycosis. *J. Infect.* 19: 95–99.
Lerner, P.I. (1996) Nocardiosis. *Clin. Infect. Dis.* 22: 891–905.

4 Necrotizing fasciitis and gas gangrene

This section covers two distinct clinical entities, necrotizing fasciitis and gas gangrene, that are fortunately rare in everyday practice. As most doctors will be relatively unfamiliar with these presentations, they are considered together here, highlighting the particular discriminating features.

If undiagnosed, clostridial gas gangrene can be rapidly fatal – there is almost 100% mortality within 48 hours in untreated cases. It is therefore essential to make the correct diagnosis promptly and proceed to urgent excision and debridement when indicated. In difficult cases, where doubt remains, a surgical exploration may be needed to give the pathological and microbiological diagnosis.

Necrotizing fasciitis is a deep soft tissue infection that results in the progressive necrosis of fascia and fat. There are various forms of fasciitis, but it may broadly be described as:

- Type I. Non-streptococcal necrotizing fasciitis, caused by mixed anaerobes, Gram-negative aerobes, enterococci, etc., that is, gut type flora. It is associated with recent surgery, diabetes mellitus and peripheral vascular disease. Type I includes Fournier's gangrene which classically affects male genitalia.
- Type II. Streptococcal necrotizing fasciitis is caused by S. pyogenes (dubbed by the media, the 'flesh-eating killer bug' in recent years), sometimes present with other organisms, e.g. Staphylococcus aureus. It causes rapid and extensive necrosis, may cause myonecrosis and may be associated with streptococcal toxic shock-like syndrome. It tends to follow recent trauma, even very minor trauma.

Gas gangrene is a rapidly progressive myonecrosis and systemic toxicity is associated with gas production, usually by anaerobic pathogens. Skin and subcutaneous tissue tend to be spared early in the course, unlike necrotizing fasciitis.

While gas gangrene is classically associated with clostridial infection, several forms of non-clostridial gas gangrene are also recognized, including:

- Anaerobic streptococccal myonecrosis. This is usually a post-traumatic infection. Swelling and erythema over the muscle occurs early, prior to the onset of pain.
- Synergistic necrotizing cellulitis. Myonecrosis and cutaneous involvement are secondary to underlying subcutaneous infection. It is most often seen in diabetic and elderly patients or those with peripheral vascular disease, and is caused by a mixture of aerobes and anaerobes.
- Infected vascular gangrene. By definition, this occurs in areas of poor tissue perfusion, e.g. in patients with peripheral vascular disease or diabetic vasculopathy.
- Aeromonas hydrophila myonecrosis. Classically follows freshwater exposure.

By definition there is destruction of muscle in gas gangrene (in contrast to clostridial cellulitis, a superficial infection with which it should not be confused). Gas gangrene may complicate traumatic wounds and surgery (particularly pelvic and large bowel) but occasionally there are no predisposing factors at all (spontaneous gas gangrene).

Management options

1. Collect cultures, swabs and treat as for uncomplicated cellulitis with i.v. antibiotics. Adjust therapy according to culture results, if necessary. If there is deterioration, seek further advice and/or surgical review.
2. Collect blood cultures and swab lesions (vesicular/discharge fluid for Gram stain and culture if possible). Start empirical antibiotics to cover likely pathogens. Request X-rays of affected areas if the patient is systemically unwell, or there is crepitus or other signs suggestive of gas gangrene or fasciitis. Request urgent surgical review if there is evidence of gas in soft tissue on X-rays or rapid spread of the cellulitis.

3. Collect blood cultures and swab lesions. Start empirical antibiotics to cover possible pathogens. Request X-rays of affected parts and request urgent surgical review while awaiting films if examination or history suggest the possibility of necrotizing fasciitis or gas gangrene. Diagnostic biopsy/laparotomy may be needed to establish the diagnosis, as decided by the surgical team. Hyperbaric oxygen (HBO) therapy may be considered at this point for clostridial gas gangrene, according to local policy and availability of HBO chambers.

Option 1. Collect cultures, swabs and treat as for uncomplicated cellulitis with i.v. antibiotics. Adjust therapy according to culture results, if necessary. If there is deterioration, seek further advice and/or surgical review.

✓ Systemic antibiotics may be adequate for severe cellulitis that may clinically mimic fasciitis or early gangrene. They are a necessary adjunct for deep infection.

✓ Culture results may identify a pathogen to guide ongoing therapy.

✗ No consideration is given to the site of infection, predisposing factors or local signs that may indicate a diagnosis of fasciitis (e.g. recent childbirth) or gangrene (e.g. gas in soft tissues).

✗ Antibiotics commonly prescribed for cellulitis may not cover the wide range of pathogens implicated in fasciitis and gangrene.

✗ A 'wait and see' approach is not acceptable for the management of rapidly advancing deep tissue infections – a delay of even 6 hours may prove fatal.

✗ Immediate Gram stain results are not available to guide therapy.

Option 2. Collect blood cultures and swab lesions (vesicular/discharge fluid for Gram stain and culture if possible). Start empirical antibiotics to cover likely pathogens. Request X-rays of affected areas if patient is systemically unwell, or there is crepitus or other signs suggestive of gas gangrene or fasciitis. Request urgent surgical review if there is evidence of gas in soft tissue on X-rays or rapid spread of the cellulitis.

✓ Immediate antibiotics to cover all likely pathogens are a useful adjunct if surgery is needed, and may provide adequate treatment if not.

✓ Relevant points from history and examination findings are considered, enabling a more accurate provisional diagnosis.

✓ X-rays may reveal gas in tissue planes when crepitus has not been elicited in some cases of gangrene.

✓ The more serious cases are reviewed early in management by the surgical team.

✗ Not all cases of gas gangrene will show gas on X-rays or produce demonstrable crepitance. The rate of spread of early necrotizing fasciitis may not be evident on initial presentation and may be missed during the period of initial assessment.

✗ A delay of a few hours may exist between requesting X-rays and receiving the films to review. This period may be critical.

Option 3. Collect blood cultures and swab lesions. Start empirical antibiotics to cover possible pathogens. Request X-rays of affected parts and request urgent surgical review while awaiting films if examination or history suggest the possibility of necrotizing fasciitis or gas gangrene. Diagnostic biopsy/laparotomy may be needed to establish the diagnosis, as decided by the surgical team. Hyperbaric oxygen (HBO) therapy may be considered at this point for clostridial gas gangrene, according to local policy and availability of HBO chambers.

✓ Broad-spectrum antibiotics are commenced immediately.

✓ Possibility of a severe, potentially life-threatening infection is considered from the outset and managed accordingly.

✓ Diagnosis is established as early as possible by surgical means in equivocal cases (with Gram staining of tissue).

✓ Surgical excision and debridement is possible within hours of presentation when indicated.

✗ In some cases a patient may be subjected to surgical exploration/laparotomy when it is not required for treatment. In practice this is unlikely, as both gangrene and necrotizing fasciitis warrant early and extensive debridement, and, after considering all the factors, are unlikely to be confused with uncomplicated cellulitis.

✗ If HBO therapy is to be used in the management, transfer to a unit may delay surgical intervention. As a general rule, surgery should never be delayed more than an hour because of transfer to a unit with HBO.

History checklist

General
- Onset of symptoms? Days or hours ago?
- First presenting symptom? Pain, swelling, redness or other symptoms?
- Recent surgery? Especially abdominal, pelvic or amputation.
- Recent trauma? Accidental (e.g. road accident) or non-accidental (e.g. gunshot wound).
- Recent injections? Medical or social drugs? What was injected? (Adrenaline is associated with gas gangrene arising from local ischaemia at the injection site.)
- Where is the injection site? Any local signs?
- Underlying medical conditions? Peripheral vascular disease, large bowel malignancy, leukaemia, diabetes mellitus, chronic renal failure or chronic ischaemic ulcers/bed sores.
- Age of patient? Increased mortality is statistically associated with those over 60 years old.

Specific
- Female of reproductive years. Exclude recent childbirth or gynaecological instrumentation.
- Children. Recent varicella infection may predispose to secondary bacterial infection, including streptococcal necrotizing fasciitis.
- Drug history. Use of non-steroidal anti-inflammatory drugs may reduce initial features of streptococcal infection and mask the severity.
- Freshwater sports/exposure? Aeromonas spp. infection.

Examination checklist

Local signs of infection
- Absent or minimal signs with marked tenderness is characteristic of early clostridial gangrene.
- Localized erythema, tenderness, warmth with systemic toxicity, and tachycardia are characteristic of necrotizing fasciitis.
- Tense oedema, pallor of skin, progressing to a bronzed appearance with vesicles and bullae is associated with advanced gas gangrene. Crepitus may be present but is not always elicited and is not pathognomic of gas gangrene.
- Purple discolouration of skin, clear vesicles becoming haemorrhagic and an area of local anaesthesia is associated with necrotizing fasciitis. Skin mottling is often patchy, unlike gas gangrene.
- Look for a trauma site if it is not obvious, e.g. broken skin, insect bite, etc.
- Delineate edges of advancing cellulitis with a marker pen at presentation (for later comparison).

Systemic signs of infection
- Cardiovascular/general state of patient. Otherwise well (indicating another diagnosis), unwell or septic shock?
- Fever, malaise, tachycardia, hypotension or jaundice? Marked tachycardia and jaundice (massive haemolysis) are associated with clostridial gangrene.
- High fever early in presentation is more consistent with necrotizing fasciitis.
- Mental status? Patients with gas gangrene remain anxious and alert throughout until coma ensues in fatal cases. (Any mental clouding is therefore a very poor prognostic feature.)
- Evidence of streptococcal toxic shock syndrome (malaise, vomiting, diarrhoea, tachycardia, tachypnoea and shock).

Rituals and myths
- Names given to different types of fasciitis do not necessarily infer a different pathology or treatment, e.g. Fournier's gangrene and Meleney's synergistic gangrene.
- HBO use in anaerobic infection is neither a ritual nor a myth! However, it is not as yet considered part of the standard management universally. Opinions appear to vary from centre to centre: consider on an individual basis.

Pitfalls
- The presence of gas in tissues on X-ray, or crepitus on examination is not only found in gas gangrene, but occasionally occurs in severe necrotizing fasciitis or with non-infective aetiologies. Similarly, myonecrosis, though always a feature of gas gangrene, is sometimes seen with necrotizing fasciitis. Inevitably there is some overlap between the two conditions, though this should not affect the ultimate management.
- Excision and drainage may need to be repeated several times before the infection is finally eradicated. Daily review of the margins is indicated.
- For treatment purposes, necrotizing fasciitis may usefully be defined as streptococcal or non-streptococcal – descriptive terms may be less helpful. Similarly, gas gangrene should be defined as clostridial or non-clostridial to indicate severity and prognosis.
- Early presentations of gas gangrene may mimic necrotizing fasciitis (bullae, discoloured skin and fever) and early necrotizing fasciitis may resemble cellulitis (erythema, warmth and tenderness). However, full examination and assessment of the rate of spread should point to the correct diagnosis. Further specific features are outlined above. An index of suspicion is sometimes needed, but uncertainty should not delay exploratory surgery.
- Absence of physical signs may encourage a 'wait and see' approach. Do not miss early clostridial gas gangrene when pain is elicited that is out of proportion with the visible findings.

Hints for investigators and prescribers
- Early diagnosis and urgent extensive debridement are both vital components in the successful treatment of necrotizing fascitis and gas gangrene. Antibiotic therapy should be commenced prior to surgery or the receipt of positive culture results, and be sufficiently broad-spectrum to cover streptococci, Gram-negative aerobes and anaerobes and clostridial species. Traditionally, a combination such as ampicillin, gentamicin and metronidazole has been used, or, more recently, meropenem monotherapy.
- Where S. pyogenes has been identified as the cause of a necrotizing fasciitis, the spectrum may be narrowed to benzyl penicillin with clindamycin, for example.
- Despite these measures the mortality rate remains high, particularly in cases where there are predisposing risk factors or a delayed presentation.

Further reading
Burge, T.S. and Watson, J.D. (1994) Necrotising fasciitis. *Br. Med. J.* **308**: 1453–1454.
Efem, S.E.E. (1994) The features and aetiology of Fournier's gangrene. *Postgrad. Med. J.* **70**: 568–571.

Elliott, D.C., Kufera, J.A. and Myers, R.A. (1996) Necrotising soft tissue infections. Risk factors for mortality and strategy for management. *Ann. Surg.* **224**: 672–683.

Rudge, F.W. (1993) The role of hyperbaric oxygen in the treatment of clostridial myonecrosis. *Mil. Med.* **158**: 80–83.

Shibuy, G.H. *et al.* (1994) Gas gangrene following sacral pressure sores. *J. Dermatol.* **21**: 518–523.

Swartz, M.N. (1995) Subcutaneous tissue infections and abscesses. In: *Principles and Practice of Infectious Diseases* (eds G.L. Mandell, J.E. Bennett and R. Dolin). Churchill Livingstone, New York, NY, pp. 922–927.

5 Post-operative wound infections

There are many different causes of post-operative infections including chest infection, urinary tract infection, wound infection, drip site infection and intra-abdominal collection. Post-operative pyrexia can also be caused by various non-infective complaints, such as a pulmonary embolus, deep vein thrombosis and drug or transfusion reactions. This section will focus on post-operative wound infections.

Management options
1. Do nothing.
2. Treat with local cleansing only.
3. Treat all patients with suspected wound infection with flucloxacillin.
4. Surgically explore and debride any infected wound.
5. Collect a swab and prescribe antibiotics. If no improvement, intervene surgically.

Option 1. Do nothing.

Tell the patient the wound is infected but will improve without treatment.

✓ If it is a minor wound and the patient is not systemically unwell it may get better without treatment.

✗ The infection may get worse, with the patient becoming systemically unwell and a life-threatening condition developing.

Option 2. Treat with local cleansing only.

Tell the patient that it is a minor wound infection which will improve with local cleansing and that there is no need for antibiotics which may in themselves have side-effects.

✓ If the wound is minor it may improve with saline washes.
✓ No antibiotic side-effects will occur (such as diarrhoea, rash etc.).

✗ The wound and the patient may deteriorate.

Option 3. Treat all patients with suspected wound infection with flucloxacillin.

Tell the patient that there is a wound infection which requires antibiotics.

✓ The commonest cause of post-operative wound infections is S. aureus which will hopefully be sensitive to flucloxacillin. Therefore, the patient should improve clinically with this.

✗ There could be another organism infecting the wound, or the S. aureus may be resistant to flucloxacillin.
✗ If there is a stitch abscess or a collection of pus associated with the wound infection, antibiotics will not penetrate this and will not work effectively.
✗ If specimens are not taken, there will be no local knowledge of what organisms are causing infections (or their sensitivity patterns), nor any indicators of cross-infections.
✗ If the patient clinically deteriorates, and specimens have not been taken, you will have no idea as to which antibiotic is appropriate.

Option 4. Surgically explore and debride any infected wound.

Tell the patient that the wound is infected and that the best option is to take him to theatre to look at the wound and remove any dead tissue.

✓ This means that the wound can be explored to see how deep it is and whether there is an abscess, a haematoma or a fistula associated with it.

✓ This is particularly useful if the wound is extensive or the patient is systemically unwell.

✓ The wound can be drained if there is a collection, or debrided if there is necrosis present.

✓ If the wound is surgically cleaned and any collection drained, the patient may get better without antibiotics, and thus without any drug side-effects.

✓ Useful specimens can be taken in theatre. If deeper tissue or pus is taken it is more likely to be representative of a true infection rather than superficial colonization.

✗ If the wound is very minor, surgery may not be necessary and has complications associated with it.

Option 5. Collect a swab and prescribe antibiotics. If no improvement, intervene surgically.

Tell the patient that clinically the wound looks infected but because you do not know what is causing the infection you need to take a swab. However, because he seems unwell, you will start antibiotics before the results come back, by making an educated guess.

✓ Intelligent, rational approach. You will know what organism is causing the infection and so can change the treatment if necessary when the results come back.

✓ In the meantime, the patient is getting some treatment.

✓ If the patient is not responding to antibiotics, the wound is extensive or a collection is suspected, then surgical treatment is indicated.

History checklist

General

- A general history should be taken, including questions about a predisposition to infection such as diabetes or immunosuppression.

Specific

- What type of operation was it? Whether the operation was clean, clean contaminated or contaminated helps determine increased likelihood of infection.
- Was appropriate antimicrobial prophylaxis given peri-operatively? There is an increased chance of infection if the correct antibiotics were not given at the right time.
- Where is the site of the wound?
- What does the wound look like, and is the patient complaining of pain?

Examination checklist

- Examine for general signs of infection, taking the patient's temperature, pulse and blood pressure.
- Look for potential sources of infection other than the wound (e.g. chest, catheter) and for non-infective causes of fever (e.g. pulmonary embolism).
- Examine the wound looking for evidence of infection such as warmth, erythema, swelling, tenderness, crepitus and purulent discharge.
- Is there suspicion of a wound haematoma or a spreading cellulitis?

Referrals

- Refer to a general surgeon for wound exploration and debridement.

Rituals and myths

- There is a myth that a wound is best kept covered, and medical staff can be reluctant to remove the dressings to inspect it. This means that an infected wound can go unnoticed.

Pitfalls

- It is often thought that any organism cultured from a wound swab must be causing a wound infection. This is not true because organisms can colonize a wound without causing an infection. If the wound does not appear infected, there is no need for treatment.

Hint for investigators and prescribers

- A superficial swab may not correlate with the infective organism. Pus or deeper specimens taken while in theatre can be more useful.

Further reading

Anon. (1992) *The Wound Programme*, 1st Edn. University of Dundee Centre of Medical Education, Dundee.

Dellinger, P.E. (1994) Peri-operative infection. In: *Surgical Infections: Diagnosis and Treatment* (ed. J.L. Meakins). Scientific American, Inc., New York, NY, pp. 217–220.

Kernodle, D.S. and Kaiser, A.B. (1995) Post-operative infections and antimicrobial prophylaxis. In: *Principles and Practice of Infectious Diseases*, 4th Edn (eds G.L. Mandell, J.E. Bennett and R. Dolin). Churchill Livingstone, New York, NY, pp. 2742–2756.

6 Pressure sores

Pressure sores, or 'bed sores', occur where there is prolonged pressure, usually from the patient's own body weight, over a localized area of skin (e.g. sacrum, buttocks or heels in a bed-bound patient). The ischaemia and ulceration that develop are often a consequence of prolonged immobility and may be compounded by morbid obesity, cachexia or incontinence in many cases. Treatment can be difficult and must take into account the underlying medical problems. Conscientious nursing care is a mainstay in the treatment and prevention of bed sores.

The following section considers the place of antibiotics in treatment. Other important measures, such as appropriate bedding, patient aids (e.g. hoists), application of various dressings and skin grafting, are not included here. Similarly, advice regarding prevention and risk assessment of pressure sores should be sought elsewhere.

Management options

1. Clean ulcer, apply dressing and leave to heal by primary intention. District nurse to review progress at dressing changes.
2. Clean ulcer and collect swabs from deep in the ulcer base if there are clinical signs of infection (local or systemic). Treat according to the results of swabs and refer for specialist advice if ulceration fails to respond or advances further.
3. Clean wound and assess the size and depth of the pressure sore. Consider the factors required for healing with respect to the individual's nutritional status and medical history. Collect culture swabs if there are clinical signs of infection and discuss the significance of the results with a medical microbiologist. Chronic ulcers, or those proving difficult to treat with conservative management may be discussed with a relevant specialist regarding in-patient management and possible grafting.

Option 1. Clean ulcer, apply dressing and leave to heal by primary intention. District nurse to review progress at dressing changes.

✓ No hospital admission required. A prolonged in-patient stay can be very debilitating and demoralizing, particularly for elderly patients.
✓ No requirement to take antibiotics, therefore no related side-effects.
✓ District nurse can review the wound regularly and liaise with the GP regarding progress.

✗ No consideration is made of individual factors that may impair healing.
✗ No assessment or treatment of potential infection.
✗ No culture results available if the patient subsequently develops systemic signs of infection.
✗ Chronic and deep ulcers may never heal with a conservative approach.
✗ Advancing ulceration or infection may be missed.
✗ At home, the patient may be unable to avoid exerting further pressure on the ulcer.

Option 2. Clean ulcer and collect swabs from deep in the ulcer base if there are clinical signs of infection (local or systemic). Treat according to the results of swabs and refer for specialist advice if ulceration fails to respond or advances further.

✓ Patient may remain at home.
✓ Cultures may indicate infecting organisms, which can be targeted with appropriate antibiotics, if clinically indicated.
✓ Regular review by a district nurse optimizes dressing care and enables assessment of progress.
✓ Specialist advice is sought when necessary.

✗ No consideration has been made of individual factors that may impair healing.

✗ Size of ulcer is not considered here. Deep and chronic ulcers may not heal with this approach.
✗ Pressure sores are invariably colonized with local flora. These may be isolated from culture swabs but do not necessarily indicate infection. Such results may prompt inappropriate use of antibiotics and encourage resistant organisms to colonize the ulcer.
✗ Many patients will require regular turning by trained nursing staff to prevent further pressure on the ulcer. This can only be achieved in hospital.

Option 3. Clean wound and assess the size and depth of the pressure sore. Consider the factors required for healing with respect to the individual's nutritional status and medical history. Collect culture swabs if there are clinical signs of infection and discuss the significance of the results with a medical microbiologist. Chronic ulcers, or those proving difficult to treat with conservative management may be discussed with a relevant specialist regarding in-patient management and possible grafting.

✓ All relevant factors are considered with respect to each individual case.
✓ The possibility of infection is considered and may be treated with appropriate antibiotics when indicated.
✓ Specialist advice is sought early rather than waiting until the ulcer has become wider, deeper and therefore more difficult to treat.
✓ A multidisciplinary approach optimizes the management of the ulcer.
✓ In-patient therapy facilitates nursing care of the patient with regular turning, attention to nutrition, management of incontinence, etc.

✗ Admission to hospital may entail a long in-patient stay. This can be very detrimental in some cases, for example, an elderly patient who wishes to maintain independence in their own home.
✗ Chronic pressure sores are relatively common in the community. Busy surgeons and geriatricians do not have time to discuss all 'problem patients' with bedsores!
✗ In some cases, surgery or aggressive therapy may be necessary to heal the ulcer, but may be inappropriate in view of the individual's general condition and expectations.
✗ It is not always possible to ascertain the significance of isolates from a colonized ulcer even when signs of infection are present.

History checklist

General
• How long has the ulceration been present? Longer duration corresponds with difficulty in achieving healing.
• What are the predisposing factors?
   Immobility – chronic or recent?
   Bedridden patient?
   Urinary incontinence?
   Obesity?
   Relative local ischaemia?
• What is the nutritional status of the patient?
   Diabetic?
   Malabsorbing/hypoproteinaemic?
   Anaemic?
• Where does the patient live? At home, in a nursing home, residential home, or a hospital in-patient?
• What care is provided regarding handling and turning the patient?
• Does the hospitalized patient have a special mattress or bed?
• What is the normal activity level of the patient? A young, previously active person

rehabilitating from acute trauma or a bed-bound patient with marked residual impairment after a stroke?

Specific
- Any symptoms of infection? Localized pain, discharge, swelling, systemic malaise, fevers, etc.
- Any previous episodes of related infection?
- Any self-medication or topical applications being used?

Examination checklist
- Site of pressure sore? Over bony prominence/ischaemic area?
- Size of pressure sore (measure and record)? Note: ulceration tends to become far more extensive under the skin than is visible superficially.
- Depth of ulceration? To muscle or bone?
- Any discharge or pus present?
- Malodorous or not?
- Surrounding erythema or cellulitis?
- Local vascularity?
- Any visible healing or granulation of base?
- It is important to record the mobility of the patient on presentation and make an assessment of the nutritional status clinically.

Referrals
- As above. Discussion with geriatrician and/or plastic surgeon will be helpful in certain cases.
- A multidisciplinary approach will optimize management, e.g. for diabetic patients to tighten diabetic control and dietetic review for those with poor nutritional status.
- Some hospitals will have a wound nurse who should be able to offer advice on the appropriate dressings and applications to use.

Rituals and myths
- Slough or creamy discharge in the base of an ulcer indicates infection. This slough may be necrotic debris and exudate only.
- Chronic ulcers should be swabbed regularly to avoid missing undiagnosed infection. Without clinical signs of infection, culture of the wound is unhelpful, as colonization with local flora is inevitable.

Pitfalls
- Vascular compromise, a predisposing factor for the development of pressure sores may lessen the visible inflammation expected in an infected ulcer (as in diabetic foot ulcers).
- Always consider osteomyelitis when bone or tendon is visible at the base of a heavily colonized or infected ulcer.
- Methicillin-resistant S. aureus isolated from an ulcer may indicate infection or merely colonization – a clinical judgement has to be made. Advice should be sought from infection control experts regarding the prevention of cross-infection, particularly with regard to in-patients.
- Alcohol-based products should not be used to clean open wounds. Preparations such as chlorhexidine or povidone iodine are more appropriate here. Cotton wool, which produces lint and fluff on contact, should also be avoided.

Hints for investigators and prescribers
- As outlined above, culture results from an ulcer swab are of questionable benefit, except when there is clear evidence of clinical infection, locally or systemically. Choosing appropriate therapy for recognized pathogens may be straightforward, e.g. S. aureus infection.

When the significance of isolates is less certain, treatment is best discussed with a medical microbiologist.

- Unfortunately, despite prompt treatment of infection, scrupulous nursing care and attention to nutrition, bed sores can be difficult to manage. As always, prevention is better than cure.

Further reading

Anon. (1992) *The Wound Programme,* 1st Edn. University of Dundee Centre of Medical Education, Dundee.

Ward, A.B. (1990) Pressure sores. *Prescrib. J.* **30**: 253–264.

7 Traumatic wounds

Traumatic injuries can be very varied depending on (among other things) the mechanism of the injury, and this needs to be taken into consideration when assessing the patient.

Management options
1. Prescribe tetanus prophylaxis only.
2. Irrigation of the wound.
3. Treat with antibiotics.
4. Surgical exploration and debridement, antibiotics and tetanus prophylaxis.

Option 1. Prescribe tetanus prophylaxis only.

Tell the patient that the wound will heal but you want to protect against tetanus.

✓ The patient will not get tetanus.
✓ If the wound is minor and clean, this is all that is required.

✗ There is a chance that the wound may become infected and complications will arise.

Option 2. Irrigation of the wound.

Tell the patient that the wound is mucky and that cleaning is all that is necessary.

✓ Removes debris so that the wound may then be able to heal by itself.

✗ Even though the wound is cleaned there might still be necrotic tissue present which will stop the wound improving.
✗ Antibiotics may be necessary and tetanus is a risk.

Option 3. Treat with antibiotics.

Tell the patient the wound is infected and requires antibiotic treatment.

✓ Appropriate antibiotic therapy can help: this might be all that is required for a minor wound.

✗ If dead tissue is present, antibiotics will not be able to penetrate into this and so will not work effectively.
✗ There is a risk of tetanus if the patient is not up to date with immunizations.

Option 4. Surgical exploration and debridement, antibiotics and tetanus prophylaxis.

Tell the patient that this is the best treatment.

✓ The surgery removes necrotic tissue and foreign bodies and allows the wound to heal.
✓ The extent of the wound can be discovered and assessed.
✓ Useful microbiological specimens can be taken in theatre.
✓ Antibiotics are indicated, especially if the patient has signs of sepsis.
✓ The patient will be protected from tetanus.

History checklist

General
A general history needs to be taken, noting any underlying conditions which may predispose to infection.

Specific
- What were the circumstances, and what was the mechanism, of the injury? This will give clues as to the suspected injuries.
- When did it happen? Has it only just occurred or is the injury days or even weeks old?
- Where did it happen? This will help assess what organisms may infect the wound. Did the injury occur in water, for instance, or perhaps it was contaminated with soil?
- Was it a blunt or sharp mode of injury?
- Is there debris or a foreign body present in the wound?
- What other injuries are there? Ask about the extent of injuries and haemorrhage.

Examination checklist
- Do a thorough general examination, noting the conscious state, temperature, pulse, blood pressure and checking the extent of the injuries.
- The site, size and depth of any injury and the presence of fractures must be ascertained.

Referrals
- Refer to the general surgeons or orthopaedic surgeons as appropriate, depending on the type of injury involved.

Pitfalls
- It is often thought that if a wound appears minor, the patient will not be at risk of tetanus. However, even small, seemingly innocent wounds or scratches have caused tetanus. Therefore, tetanus prophylaxis is always recommended, especially if the wound has had soil contact.

Hints for investigators and prescribers
- When advising on tetanus prophylaxis, a history of the immunization status and the type of wound needs to be taken into account. For 'clean' wounds, if the patient has not had a three dose course of tetanus vaccine, these are commenced. If the patient has had the course, but no booster in the last 10 years, a booster is then required. If the patient has had both of these, no vaccination is necessary.
- If the wound is 'tetanus prone', the same advice applies, but human tetanus immunoglobin is advised in addition to the vaccine.

Further reading
Bleck, T.P. (1995) Clostridium tetani. In: *Principles and Practice of Infectious Diseases*, 4th Edn (eds G.L. Mandell, J.E. Bennett and R. Dolin). Churchill Livingstone, New York, NY, pp. 2173–2178.

Department of Health (1996) *Immunisation Against Infectious Diseases*. HMSO.

Fiore, A.E. Joshi, M. and Caplan, E.S. (1995) Approach to infection in the multiply traumatized patient. In: *Principles and Practice of Infectious Diseases*, 4th Edn (eds G.L. Mandell, J.E. Bennett and R. Dolin). Churchill Livingstone, New York, NY, pp. 2756–2760.

8 Ulcers

An ulcer is a loss of continuity of an epithelial surface. There are three main categories of ulcer:

- An ischaemic ulcer is caused by an inadequate blood supply; because this is due to arterial insufficiency they are usually manifest at the end of limbs.
- A venous ulcer is caused by a distorted pattern of venous bloodflow and venous hypertension, and usually occurs on the medial side of the lower third of the leg.
- A neuropathic ulcer develops as a result of a patient's insensitivity to repeated trauma. It is commonly associated with neurological disease that causes loss of pain and light touch sensation in weight-bearing areas.

Ulcers in the above categories are not primarily caused by infection, but such ulcers can later become infected, which will make it more difficult for them to heal.

There are a number of rarer causes of ulcers, including certain infections which may directly cause ulcerating skin infection (e.g. cutaneous leishmaniasis and Mycobacterium ulcerans infection).

Management options
1. Do nothing.
2. Treat all ulcers with antibiotics.
3. Treat all ulcers surgically.
4. Assess the patient, then treat with antibiotics and/or surgery, as appropriate.

Option 1. Do nothing.

Tell the patient that nothing more is required than regular dressing of the ulcer and watching it to ensure that it does not get worse.

✓ If the infection is a minor one, or the ulcer is only colonized, then further treatment is unnecessary.
✓ Regular dressing, elevation, rest and weight loss is the correct management for an uninfected venous ulcer.

✗ If the ulcer is infected, it may rapidly deteriorate with spreading cellulitis, and the patient may become very unwell.

Option 2. Treat all ulcers with antibiotics.

Tell the patient that they have an ulcer which is infected, and will be prescribed antibiotics.

✓ If the ulcer is infected, it may improve with appropriate antibiotics.

✗ If the ulcer is colonized rather than infected, antibiotics are not required. In fact, they may be detrimental to the patient in that they will select-out resistant organisms which will colonize, or eventually infect, the ulcer.
✗ If there is an infection, it is advisable to take specimens first, rather than treating blindly.
✗ If the infection is deep, extending into the subcutaneous tissues, or if there is deep tissue necrosis, surgical debridement will be a necessary part of the management.

Option 3. Treat all ulcers surgically.

Tell the patient that the ulcer is infected and that to find the extent of the damage, and thus to treat it, they need to be taken to theatre.

✓ Surgical exploration is helpful. There should be initial unroofing of the crusted areas and the wound should be probed to assess its depth.

✓ If it is a deep ulcer, extending to the subcutaneous tissues, or if there is deep tissue necrosis with suppuration, the debridement of the dead tissue is necessary to promote healing.

✓ Useful microbiology specimens can be taken in theatre, such as deep tissue and pus. Any organisms cultured from these are likely to be more representative of the infective agent than those grown from superficial swabs.

✗ If the ulcer is very minor, then taking the patient to theatre is inappropriate.

✗ Even with surgical intervention, the ulcer and patient may rapidly deteriorate without antibiotic therapy.

Option 4. Assess the patient, then treat with antibiotics and/or surgery, as appropriate.

Tell the patient they need to be assessed and treated as necessary.

✓ This is a rational approach. The patient needs to be clinically assessed and investigated. The investigations should include X-ray to rule out underlying osteomyelitis.

✓ If the ulcer is thought to be infected, especially if it is large or the patient is systemically unwell, the patient can be prescribed antibiotics and further assessed in theatre where the ulcer can be debrided.

History checklist

General
- A general history should be taken including age, nutritional status, smoking and other causes of ischaemia.
- Previous ulcers?
- Known diabetes mellitus or symptoms suggesting this diagnosis?
- Any known connective tissue disease or vasculitis?
- Any haematological problems which could be relevant, such as myeloma or sickle cell disease?
- Any history to suggest neuropathy, or a history of another condition which could lead to this?

Specific
- Description of the ulcer? Should include site, size and colour. Is there a history of trauma.
- Are there any other ulcers?
- How long has it been there?
- Is it getting better, worse, or is it the same?
- Ask if it is painful, hot and/or has red spreading margins? This might indicate infection, as would an offensive discharge.

Examination checklist
- A general examination is needed, looking for evidence of systemic infection such as fever and tachycardia.
- A specific examination of the ulcer includes documentation of site, size and whether the base has healthy granulation tissue present, or necrotic material. Is the edge sloping, flat, undermined or punched out? How deep is it?
- Is there a discharge? Whether it is serous, serosanguinous, purulent and offensive-looking or smelling should be noted. Also, see whether it is copious or only slight with scabbing.
- Local lymph nodes should be examined for signs of enlargement, and the local tissue should be looked at for spreading cellulitis.
- Any evidence of venous or arterial compromise?
- Any evidence of neuropathy?

Referrals

- Refer to a general surgeon or occasionally a vascular surgeon.
- If, at a later stage, skin grafting is considered, then refer to a plastic surgeon.

Rituals and myths

- That any organism found in an ulcer must be causing infection is a common myth. Most uninfected ulcers are colonized with bacteria, but this is not harmful to the patient.

Pitfalls

- Occasionally, infected ulcers can be associated with an underlying osteomyelitis. It is important not to miss this as it alters the management of the patient.

Hints for inv estigators and prescribers

- Deep swabs of the ulcer or tissue, or pus taken in theatre, are preferable to superficial swabs. If the patient is systemically unwell, blood cultures can be useful.
- The initial therapy should cover S. aureus and β-haemolytic streptococci. Antibiotics can then be altered depending on whether the patient responded to initial therapy and laboratory results of ulcer and blood cultures.

Further reading

Anon. (1992) *The Wound Programme*, 1st Edn. University of Dundee Centre of Medical Education, Dundee.

Swartz, M.N. (1995) Cellulitis and subcutaneous tissue infections. In: *Principles and Practice of Infectious Diseases*, 4th Edn, (eds G.L. Mandell, J.E. Bennett and R. Dolin). Churchill Livingstone, New York, NY, pp. 919–920.

Chapter 15
URINARY INFECTIONS

C.L.C. Williams

Urinary tract infection (UTI) is often discussed in terms of the presence or absence of bacteria in the urine (bacteriuria). This is not helpful in a clinical context as the management of the patient will often depend more upon the type of patient and the patient's symptoms than the laboratory findings. The common presentations with urinary tract symptoms are:

- Cystitis. The usual symptoms are of frequency and dysuria. In addition, the patient may have noticed a change in the character of the urine. Infections occur more commonly in women, but only around half of symptomatic women will have infection, and a microbiological examination of urine is the only way to prove a UTI.
- Pyelonephritis. Loin pain and fever in addition to frequency and dysuria are characteristic of pyelonephritis, but in some patient groups, pyelonephritis may be subclinical. Subclinical pyelonephritis, by definition, will remain undiagnosed until serious renal damage has ensued or a urine sample is taken.
- Asymptomatic bacteriuria. In this case the patient has no symptoms. A urine sent for culture, either as a screening test to attempt to intervene in the natural history of asymptomatic bacteriuria, or as an incidental finding, reveals $>10^5$ colony forming units (c.f.u.) ml^{-1}.

Clinical problem-solving must address:

- Whether the patient is symptomatic, and if so, the diagnosis that the symptoms suggest bearing in mind that symptoms of a UTI may vary between women, children and men.
- If the patient is asymptomatic, are they in a risk group which requires intervention for asymptomatic bacteriuria?
- Does the patient require investigation for the underlying causes of the UTI, or is treatment directed at this episode alone, sufficient?

Microbiological examination of urine
Microbiological examination of urine remains the gold standard for the diagnosis of UTI. This consists of two parts:

- Microscopy. Microscopic examination of the urine is performed mainly to identify the presence of white blood cells (WBC) (pus cells) in the urine. The presence of more than 10 WBC mm^{-3} is taken to indicate pyuria, and while the finding of pyuria is not entirely specific for UTI, the vast majority of patients with symptomatic or asymptomatic bacteriuria will have pyuria.
- Culture. The growth of bacteria in urine is usually expressed semi-quantitatively. The main reason for this is that whereas urine in the bladder is normally sterile, the urethra and peri-urethral areas are often colonized with bacteria which may be difficult to remove by cleaning. The aim of the semi-quantitative culture is to separate contamination from infection. Patients with infection usually have at least 10^5 bacteria ml^{-1}, whereas if the patient has sterile urine, a properly collected sample will usually contain less than 10^4 bacteria ml^{-1}. The exception to this is in young women, of whom up to one third, with a symptomatic lower UTI, will have bacterial counts of less than 10^5 bacteria ml^{-1}. These criteria apply only to midstream urine (MSU) containing Enterobacteria, i.e.

Escherichia coli, Proteus spp. etc. Gram-positive organisms such as group B streptococci may be significant at counts of between 10^4 and 10^5 bacteria ml^{-1}.

Chapter contents

1 Acute cystitis in women

In young non-pregnant women, with clear symptoms of UTI, the standard criteria of $>10^5$ c.f.u. ml^{-1} of bacteria present in the urine requires modification. In this group, counts as low as 100 c.f.u. ml^{-1} of uropathogenic bacteria often indicate infection. These low counts are not thought to be due to dilution by the patient's urine or failure of the bacteria to grow in the urine. It is possible that in these cases the infection is not established in the bladder, but represents an early phase in the development of bladder infection.

The microbiological findings must be weighed against clinical symptoms. A low count of bacteria may be of significance in the presence of symptoms of urethritis, but may be of no significance in women with vague symptoms. Thus, while a low count cannot be ignored, treating all patients with low bacterial counts may lead to overtreatment of what is essentially a self-limiting illness.

What remains more controversial is the so-called 'urethral syndrome' where it is proposed that bacteria not normally considered to be uropathogens, such as Gardnerella vaginalis and Lactobacillus spp., cause infection in the urethra and para-urethral glands, leading to symptoms of dysuria and frequency. These bacteria require special cultural conditions and will not be found in urine unless specifically sought.

Management options

1. Do nothing.
2. Treat every symptomatic patient with antibiotics without investigating further.
3. Make a presumptive diagnosis of UTI using leucocyte esterase/nitrite dipsticks and treat with antibiotics, i.e. prescribe selectively. Do not follow up unless symptoms persist or recur.
4. Make a firm diagnosis of UTI by collecting an MSU on each occasion, and treat with antibiotics prior to the culture result becoming available.
5. Make a firm diagnosis of UTI by collecting an MSU on each occasion, and delay treatment with antibiotics until the culture result becomes available.

Option 1. Do nothing.

Tell the patient that cystitis is a common and trivial complaint which will get better on its own.

✗ Up to a quarter of women will be denied effective relief of symptoms and may well be deterred from seeking medical attention in the future.
✗ A small number of patients may have serious underlying problems which will be missed.
✗ You will become unpopular with your colleagues as their clinics grow.

Option 2. Treat every symptomatic patient with antibiotics without investigating further.

Tell the patient that she has an infection and will get better on antibiotics.

✓ About a quarter of patients who have UTI will benefit from rapid relief of symptoms.
✓ The patient may feel that the doctor is taking an appropriate interest and may be reassured. Most patients hope to receive a prescription anyway!
✓ There is no inconvenience or cost of investigations.

✗ At least half of patients will have no infection and therefore cannot benefit from antibiotics. Patients are therefore exposed to unnecessary side-effects and the community as a whole is exposed to large amounts of antibiotics promoting the development of resistant organisms.
✗ This practice will reinforce the patient's belief that antibiotics are 'cure-alls' and may increase the pressure on you to prescribe antibiotics in the future.
✗ You will never learn what is wrong with your patients.

Option 3. Make a presumptive diagnosis of UTI using leucocyte esterase/nitrite dipsticks and treat with antibiotics, i.e. prescribe selectively. Do not follow up unless symptoms persist or recur.

Tell the patient that if the symptoms have not resolved in 3 days to come back for further investigations, i.e. an MSU.

✓ This approach has been shown to be safe and cost-effective when used appropriately.
✓ On each occasion the patient will be fully assessed and offered appropriate treatment. The unnecessary use of antibiotics will be limited.
✓ The patient may feel that the doctor is taking an appropriate interest and may be reassured.
✓ The cost of investigations will be minimized.

✗ Empirical therapy relies on good epidemiological data from the local microbiology laboratory. If all practices adopt the 'dipstick test and treat' approach then no isolates from first cases of cystitis will be tested. This means that the sensitivity data coming from the laboratory will be based upon recurrent infections or treatment failures. This group of organisms may be more resistant, thus encouraging the inappropriate use of more expensive antibiotics as first-line agents.
✗ If empirical therapy fails there will be no sensitivity results upon which to base a modification of therapy.
✗ If empirical therapy fails, the patient will have to return for an MSU, thus possibly increasing the delay in appropriate therapy to 5 days in total.
✗ Around 10% of women who may have pyuria without infection will receive antibiotics unnecessarily.

Because cystitis in young women is caused by a relatively narrow range of organisms whose sensitivities are predictable, dipstick testing of urine, followed by empirical therapy with antibiotics may be proposed. Leucocyte esterase/nitrite dipsticks have a reported sensitivity of 75–96% in detecting pyuria and infection. A positive test, used in conjunction with typical symptoms, is good evidence of a UTI.

Option 4. Make a firm diagnosis of UTI by collecting an MSU on each occasion, and treat with antibiotics prior to the culture result becoming available.

Tell the patient to contact the surgery in 3 days if symptoms persist, and a change in therapy can be made.

✓ The patient will be fully assessed and offered appropriate treatment. The unnecessary use of antibiotics will be limited.
✓ The patient may feel that the doctor is taking an appropriate interest and may be reassured.
✓ Microbiological results are not only of value in treating the individual patient. Over time, they will provide you with information about the likelihood of your patients having an infection, the predominant infecting organisms, and the antibiotics which are effective against these bacteria.
✓ The patient is unlikely to be asked to return for anything other than a prescription for alternative therapy.
✓ In the case of symptom recurrence, a bacterial aetiology is documented.

✗ In a lot of cases the MSU will be negative or the empirical therapy will be appropriate, so unnecessary investigations and expense will be incurred.
✗ By the time lab results are available, the patient is likely to have finished most of a short course therapy so there is still the problem of causing side-effects in patients with no infection, as well as increased drug costs.

The result of sensitivity testing will not be available for at least 24 hours. It is appropriate therefore to start empirical therapy immediately and modify this if necessary on the basis of laboratory results.

Option 5. Make a firm diagnosis of UTI by collecting an MSU on each occasion, and delay treatment with antibiotics until the culture result becomes available.

✓ The use of antibiotics will be restricted. This will reduce the selection pressure for resistant organisms. As there is only around a 50% chance that a woman with symptoms of cystitis will have a bacterial infection you will prescribe antibiotics only on the basis of a positive laboratory result.

✓ There is no risk of unnecessary side-effects.

✗ The patient's requirements are not assessed. The patient came to the surgery for relief of symptoms and nothing is likely to done about this for 2 days.

✗ Seeing each patient twice is time-consuming for both doctor and patient.

History checklist

- A diagnosis of cystitis should be considered in a patient presenting with dysuria, frequency or urgency. However, urethritis and vaginitis may also cause similar symptoms and should be elucidated by specific questioning.
- Is the patient pregnant? This may affect the choice of antibiotics. In addition, due to the increased likelihood of ascending infection in pregnant patients, it is necessary to send an MSU to confirm the presence or absence of bacteriuria.
- Is there any vaginal discharge or are other genito-urinary symptoms present? Does the patient have any vaginal discharge, bleeding or abnormal odour? Is lower abdominal pain present? Has there been any recent change in sexual partner? Unprotected intercourse with a new partner or recent change in sexual partner should prompt the consideration of a sexually transmitted disease and referral to a genito-urinary medicine clinic may be appropriate.
- Have antibiotics been prescribed for any reason in the previous 2 weeks? Antibiotic therapy may cause vaginal candidosis which may be a cause of symptoms.
- Has the patient noticed any vulval soreness, redness or rash? Herpes simplex virus (HSV) infection may cause urethritis. Frequency and dysuria due to urethritis may be of a more gradual onset and less severe than those due to cystitis.
- Have there been any previous urinary tract problems? Urinary tract problems in childhood suggest the possibility of structural abnormalities which may require further investigation.
- Has the patient had antibiotics for cystitis within the past 4 weeks, or a history of repeated episodes of cystitis? If the answer is yes, and the previous episode was not investigated, it is now essential to send an MSU to confirm or refute the presence of bacteria.
- Do the symptoms make sense? Is the effect on the woman's life disproportionate to her symptoms? The patient may be using her symptoms to draw attention to an entirely different problem. Her real concern may lie in other areas.
- Are any unrelated symptoms present? Rarer causes of cystitis should be considered. For example travel abroad may raise the possibility of schistosomiasis.

Examination checklist

- Examination is usually not necessary in the presence of typical symptoms.

Further reading

Carlson, K.J. and Mulley, A.G. (1985) Management of acute dysuria: a decision analysis model of alternative strategies. *Ann. Intern. Med.* **102**: 244–249.

Maskell, R. (1995) Broadening the concept of urinary tract infection. *Br. J. Urol.* **76**: 2–8.

Stamm, W.E. and Hooton, T.M. (1993) Management of urinary tract infection in adults. *N. Engl. J. Med.* **329**: 1328–1333.

2 Recurrent acute cystitis in women

About a fifth of women with an episode of cystitis will have a recurrent infection. Recurrent cystitis is defined as 2–4 episodes more than 4 weeks apart within 1 year. These, in more than 90% of cases, will be separate episodes of re-infection which typically occur between 2–4 weeks following the completion of therapy. In this group of patients anatomical or functional abnormalities are rare and imaging of the genito-urinary tract yields little.

It is possible that predisposition to repeated infections may have some genetic component as women who are blood group antigen non-secretors are more likely to have problems. The presence of uropathogenic strains of bacteria in the bowels of some women may also be relevant.

Management options
1. Make a presumptive diagnosis of UTI using leucocyte esterase/nitrite dipsticks on each occasion and treat with antibiotics, i.e. prescribe selectively. For the pros and cons, refer to Management option 3, p. 284.
2. Make a firm diagnosis of UTI by collecting an MSU on each occasion and treat with antibiotics.
3. Make a firm diagnosis of recurrent UTI by collecting an MSU on at least one occasion and consider prophylactic antibiotics.

Option 1. Make a presumptive diagnosis of UTI using leucocyte esterase/nitrite dipsticks on each occasion and treat with antibiotics, i.e. prescribe selectively. For the pros and cons, refer to Management option 3, p. 284.

Option 2. Make a firm diagnosis of UTI by collecting an MSU on each occasion and treat with antibiotics.

✓ On each occasion the patient will be fully assessed and offered appropriate treatment.
✓ The patient may feel that the doctor is taking an appropriate interest and may be reassured.
✓ Appropriate antibiotic therapy will be assured as evidence from culture will be available on each occasion.

✗ There may be a delay in the patient being able to visit the doctor, during which time unpleasant symptoms may develop. This delay will be compounded if treatment is delayed until the results of culture are available.
✗ Multiple consultations will be time-consuming for both the doctor and patient.

Option 3. Make a firm diagnosis of recurrent UTI by collecting an MSU on at least one occasion and consider prophylactic antibiotics.

✓ Recurrent infection will be prevented and therapy to reduce distressing symptoms can start immediately.
✓ Disruption to the patient's life will be minimized.
✓ The number of consultations will be reduced.
✓ If the strategies are used in appropriate patients, the risk of development of bacterial resistance will be low.

✗ There is a possibility that the patient may develop more serious pathology which could be masked by self-administered antibiotics.
✗ There is a possibility that recurrence may be mistaken for re-infection and that a more serious problem would be masked by prophylactic antibiotics.

In women with recurrent infections who have had at least one bacteriologically proven episode of infection, a strategy for prophylactic antibiotics is often effective. There are several possible strategies and these are summarized in *Figure 1*.

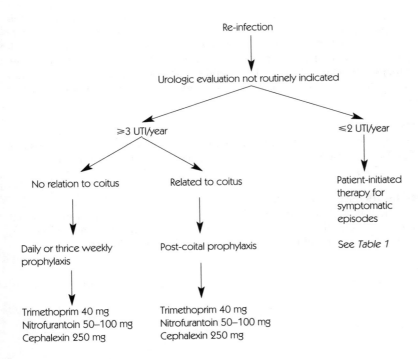

Re-infection

Urologic evaluation not routinely indicated

≥3 UTI/year   ≤2 UTI/year

No relation to coitus   Related to coitus   Patient-initiated therapy for symptomatic episodes

See *Table 1*

Daily or thrice weekly prophylaxis   Post-coital prophylaxis

Trimethoprim 40 mg
Nitrofurantoin 50–100 mg
Cephalexin 250 mg

Trimethoprim 40 mg
Nitrofurantoin 50–100 mg
Cephalexin 250 mg

Figure 1. Strategy for prophylactic antibiotics for recurrent acute cystitis in women. Adapted with the permission of the author from Stamm, W.E. and Hooton, T.M. (1993) Management of urinary tract infections in adults. *N. Engl. J. Med.* **329**: 1328–1333.

Table 1. Treatment regimens for acute uncomplicated cystitis

Condition	Pathogens	Complicating circumstances	Treatment
Acute uncomplicated cystitis	E.. coli S. saprophyticus Coliforms	1. None	3-day regimen of trimethoprim or a quinolone
		2. Diabetes, symptoms for >7 days, age >65, use of diaphragm	7-day regimen of trimethoprim or a quinolone
		3. Pregnancy	7-day regimen of amoxicillin, co-amoxiclav or nitrofurantoin

Adapted with the permission of the author from Stamm, W.E. and Hooton, T.M. (1993) Management of urinary tract infections in adults. *N. Engl. J. Med.* **329**: 1328–1333.

History

Specific

See 'Acute cystitis in women', p. 283. In addition, the following should also be elucidated.

- Does the woman use a diaphragm and spermicide as a contraceptive? Spermicide may increase the likelihood of vaginal colonization with E. coli and has been associated with recurrent infection in some patients.

- Does the development of symptoms relate to intercourse? If symptoms occur after intercourse with a regular partner it is possible that lack of vaginal lubrication could increase friction on the urethra and predispose to the 'milking' of urethral bacteria into the bladder. If the patient feels that vaginal lubrication is inadequate, then the use of a lubricating jelly prior to intercourse may reduce the likelihood of subsequent problems. If this is not seen to be a problem, or the problem persists, then post-coital antibiotic prophylaxis may be appropriate.

Examination checklist
- Examination may not be necessary in the presence of typical symptoms and a positive urine test. If performed, examination should exclude HSV vulvovaginitis and the presence of any vaginal discharge.

Hints for investigators and prescribers
- In addition to the use of antibiotics, consideration should be given in post-menopausal women to the use of topical oestradiol creams. These patients may have altered vaginal microflora with loss of lactobacilli and subsequent colonization with E. coli.

Further reading
Bacheller, C.D. and Bernstein, J.M. (1997) Urinary tract infections. *Med. Clin. N. Am.* **81**: 719–730.

3 Asymptomatic bacteriuria

Asymptomatic bacteriuria is defined as the presence of a bacterial growth of $>10^5$ c.f.u. ml^{-1} from two separate midstream or clean catch urine specimens in the absence of symptoms or pyuria. Its significance varies with the patient group in which it is discovered.

Of high clinical significance
- During pregnancy. Seven per cent of pregnant women have asymptomatic bacteriuria, and of these up to 30% develop pyelonephritis if not treated. As such it is recommended that screening tests are done at the initial booking visit and again at 28 weeks.
- During childhood. Because of the risk of vesicoureteric reflux in children, bacteria in the bladder, regardless of symptoms, may lead to the development of pyelonephritis and as such should be regarded as significant.
- Diabetic patients.
- Prior to urological surgery.

Of debatable clinical significance
- Patients with endo-prostheses. Because of the potential risk of patients with prosthetic heart valves, prosthetic joints or vascular grafts developing infection via blood-borne spread from the urine, it has been suggested that these patients should be treated for any infection. There is no good evidence for this, and as bacteraemias in this group appear to be rare, this approach remains controversial.

Of no clinical significance
- Other adult patients including elderly patients. There have been contradictory studies suggesting an increase in mortality in the elderly with asymptomatic bacteriuria, but the balance of evidence suggests that there is no increased risk and that asymptomatic bacteriuria in the elderly should not be treated.

Management options
1. If the patient is in a high risk group, collect samples for laboratory analysis and treat bacteriuria if it is present.
2. Screen all your patients for bacteriuria and treat everyone who is positive. Decide that all bacteria are harmful to patients and eradicate them whenever possible.

Option 1. If the patient is in a high risk group, collect samples for laboratory analysis and treat bacteriuria if it is present.

✓ You will never have a diagnostic dilemma, as you will not know that your patients in the low risk groups have a bacteriuria.
✓ Treatment will be reserved for those patients who are likely to suffer serious sequelae to asymptomatic bacteriuria. As such, the risk of unnecessary side-effects in the individual, and possible population effects of generating resistant bacteria will be minimized.

Option 2. Screen all your patients for bacteriuria and treat everyone who is positive. Decide that all bacteria are harmful to patients and eradicate them whenever possible.

✓ You will never miss a diagnosis of UTI.
✓ You will single-handedly support your local microbiology department.

✗ Large numbers of patients will be treated with antibiotics for no benefit.
✗ You will see many antibiotic side-effects.

History checklist

- As there are by definition no symptoms, a history is not helpful.

Rituals and myths

Ask yourself why you are performing a urinalysis in an asymptomatic patient who will not benefit from treatment. Two good examples of this are:

- Patients with indwelling catheters. Nearly all patients with indwelling catheters for longer than 1 week will have bacteriuria. There is no good evidence to show that treating these patients with antibiotics will reduce the incidence of febrile illnesses or the amount of bacteriuria. Paradoxically, the opposite is likely to occur in that a more resistant bacterial population will be selected. If the patient does develop a febrile episode related to the urinary tract, then treatment may be more difficult.
- Elderly patients. Bacteriuria is common in the elderly population. The prevalence of bacteriuria in women is around 20% between the ages of 65 and 75, and between 20 and 50% over the age of 80. The evidence suggests that asymptomatic bacteriuria is a benign condition which is not associated with increased morbidity or mortality and therefore does not require treatment.

It would be reasonable, therefore, not to take urine specimens from low risk groups unless the patient has symptoms of UTI.

Further reading

Childs, S.J. and Egan, R.J. (1996) Bacteriuria and urinary infections in the elderly. *Urol. Clin. N. Am.* **23**: 43–54.

4 Urinary catheter-related infections

Urethral catheterization is widely used in both males and females. There is a significant risk of UTI and septicaemia associated with the presence of a catheter, and, for this reason, it is important that their use is minimized. If they do need to be used they should be inserted using aseptic technique. The use of such techniques will minimize the risk of infection following single or short-term catheterization. However, infection is almost inevitable after a catheter has been *in situ* for 7–10 days. No aseptic technique, meatal care or antibiotic prophylaxis can prevent the urine becoming infected. The management of catheter-related infection depends upon the duration of catheterization and the underlying reason for the insertion of the catheter.

Management options
1. Do nothing.
2. Treat with antibiotics.
3. Make a diagnosis of systemic infection. Remove the catheter and where appropriate treat with antibiotics.

Option 1. Do nothing.

Tell your patient with a long-term catheter that cloudy urine containing bacteria is a common complication of catheterization and that unless other symptoms appear it is nothing to worry about.

✓ This is a reasonable approach to take in the majority of patients, and the best approach in long-term catheters. It will prevent the development of resistant bacteria both in the patient and hopefully the community, and reduce patient side-effects from unnecessary courses of antibiotics.

✗ If the patient has infected urine prior to catheterization, and catheterization is due to urological surgery, then not treating the bacteriuria may increase the risk of bacteraemia, which could have been prevented by peri-operative antibiotics.

If the patient is only going to be catheterized for a short time then good catheter insertion technique will probably delay the onset of bladder bacteriuria until the catheter is due to be removed.

Option 2. Treat with antibiotics.

✓ The few patients with systemic symptoms and those who would have benefitted from peri-operative treatment will have been appropriately treated.
✓ You may be the first in your hospital/surgery to generate a totally resistant strain of bacteria.

✗ The majority of patients will have received inappropriate treatment. In addition the antibiotics will have selected out the most resistant bacteria present in the urine which will make subsequent treatment of any invasive infection more difficult.

Option 3. Make a diagnosis of systemic infection. Remove the catheter and where appropriate treat with antibiotics.

✓ This approach will minimize inappropriate therapy but allow treatment for all patients who require it.

Any patient with an indwelling catheter who has symptoms of systemic infection should be treated. Therapy in these cases should be guided by the results of blood and urine culture.

History checklist

- How long has the patient been catheterized? Bladders which have had catheters *in situ* for more than 1 week are almost certain to contain a mixed bacterial flora. Treatment of the infected urine in the absence of any other problems will only result in the development of resistant bacteria which will make subsequent invasive infections more difficult to treat.

- Does the patient have systemic symptoms? If the patient has evidence of systemic infection such as temperature or loin pain, then antibiotics should be prescribed. The treatment is unlikely to eradicate the organisms from the urine.

- Why was the patient catheterized? Certain conditions, such as retention due to bladder outflow obstruction, are unlikely to be managed successfully without catheterization. This makes the option of removing the catheter for the duration of the treatment unrealistic.

- How long is the catheter likely to be in place? If the total duration of the catheterization is likely to be 3–4 days, as in urological or gynaecological surgery, then prophylactic antibiotics could be considered.

Rituals and myths

- Collecting urine samples from catheterized patients who are not systemically unwell. Subsequent treatment of a bacteriuria, which will not be cleared by antibiotics, does nothing but generate resistance in the colonizing organisms.

Further reading

Stickler, D.J. and Zimakoff, J. (1994) Complications of urinary tract infections associated with devices used for long term bladder management. *J. Hosp. Infect.* **28**: 177–194.

Warren, J.W. (1991) The catheter and urinary tract infection. *Med. Clin. N. Am.* **75**: 481–493.

5 Pyelonephritis

Acute pyelonephritis is the clinical syndrome of loin pain and/or tenderness, dysuria and fever. It is a straightforward diagnosis to make except in the very young and the elderly, where it may present atypically.

Chronic pyelonephritis is less clearly defined but is generally accepted as a chronic interstitial nephritis resulting from long-standing or recurrent bacterial infection.

Management options

1. Make a presumptive diagnosis of acute pyelonephritis, assess severity and start oral treatment.
2. Make a presumptive diagnosis of acute pyelonephritis, assess severity, collect an MSU for laboratory analysis and start oral treatment.
3. Make a presumptive diagnosis of acute pyelonephritis and admit to hospital for parenteral therapy. Collect a urine sample on admission.
4. Make a presumptive diagnosis of acute pyelonephritis, collect an MSU and start therapy as appropriate. Following recovery from the initial episode, request further investigations into the underlying cause of the pyelonephritis.

Option 1. Make a presumptive diagnosis of acute pyelonephritis, assess severity and start oral treatment.

✓ The patient will be appropriately assessed, and followed up.
✓ If symptoms and signs resolve or improve within 48–72 hours there are unlikely to be any underlying urinary tract abnormalities.
✓ Treatment is started promptly with a hopefully rapid symptomatic response.
✓ The patient does not require hospital admission.

✗ If symptoms do not resolve in 72 hours, no microbiological results are available to guide a change of therapy.
✗ If nausea or vomiting occur following the initial consultation, oral therapy may be ineffective.

If a patient has symptoms suggestive of pyelonephritis in the absence of nausea and vomiting, empirical treatment with oral antibiotics can be started. The patient should be reviewed at 48 hours to ensure a satisfactory clinical response. Treatment should continue for 2 weeks. Shorter regimens are often effective, but these have not been fully evaluated. The choice of antibiotic will depend upon local sensitivity patterns.

Option 2. Make a presumptive diagnosis of acute pyelonephritis, assess severity, collect an MSU for laboratory analysis and start oral treatment.

✓ As for Option 1, but if symptoms do not resolve within 48 hours, microbiological results are available to guide any change in therapy. In addition, non-response to an apparently sensitive isolate may increase suspicion of an underlying anatomical problem.

A suspected diagnosis, on clinical and dipstick testing grounds, is confirmed by performing urine microscopy, culture and sensitivity testing. The finding of a bacterial count of $>10^5$ c.f.u. in a midstream urine is diagnostic. The usual pathogens are coliform organisms and enterococci. Counts of 10^4 c.f.u. ml^{-1} or less, of a single pathogen, may be significant.

Option 3. Make a presumptive diagnosis of acute pyelonephritis and admit to hospital for parenteral therapy. Collect a urine sample on admission.

✓ The patient will be appropriately assessed, and followed up.
✓ If symptoms and signs resolve or improve within 48–72 hours there are unlikely to be any underlying urinary tract abnormalities.

✓ Treatment is started promptly, hopefully with a rapid symptomatic response.

✗ The patient requires hospital admission.

✗ This is costly.

If a patient has symptoms suggestive of pyelonephritis with nausea and vomiting, empirical treatment with parenteral antibiotics should be started.

Option 4. Make a presumptive diagnosis of acute pyelonephritis, collect an MSU and start therapy as appropriate. Following recovery from the initial episode, request further investigations into the underlying cause of the pyelonephritis.

✓ Treatment is started promptly, hopefully with a rapid symptomatic response.

✓ The patient will be appropriately assessed and followed up.

✗ If symptoms and signs resolve or improve within 48–72 hours there are unlikely to be any underlying urinary tract abnormalities, and investigation of the patient is likely to yield little.

History checklist
- Have there been any previous urinary tract problems? Acute pyelonephritis may be recurrent. This suggests the possibility of structural abnormalities or a renal stone which should be investigated.
- Are any atypical features present? Persistent haematuria or colicky pain may suggest the presence of an underlying urological abnormality.
- Is the patient pregnant? Acute pyelonephritis is more common in pregnancy. In addition, some antibiotics which may be considered for the treatment of pyelonephritis should be avoided in pregnant women, e.g. quinolones.
- Are any unrelated symptoms present? Rarer causes of loin pain should be considered. Staphylococcus aureus infection elsewhere may cause renal abscess via blood-borne spread. Extensive cardiovascular disease may suggest the possibility of renal infarction. Alternatively, epigastric or bone pain could suggest hypercalcaemia and renal stone formation.

Examination checklist
- Take the patient's temperature. Palpation of the abdomen may reveal renal angle tenderness. Visual examination of freshly passed urine may reveal a cloudy sample. This is not always present, and a visually clear urine does not rule out UTI.

Hints for investigators and prescribers
- Women whose symptoms and signs resolve in 48–72 hours are unlikely to have any underlying abnormality requiring investigation. If fever or loin pain persist for more than 72 hours, urine cultures should be repeated and ultrasonography/CT scanning considered to look for perinephric or intranephric abscess formation, or any evidence of urological abnormalities or obstruction.
- Women who have more than one episode of pyelonephritis, or any of the atypical symptoms listed above should also be considered for further investigation.

Further reading
Bereron, M.G. (1995) Treatment of pyelonephritis in adults. *Med. Clin. N. Am.* **79**: 619–649.

6 Acute cystitis in children

A diagnosis of cystitis should be considered in a child with symptoms of lower UTI (i.e. dysuria, urgency, frequency, hesitancy, lower abdominal pain or new onset urinary incontinence) who has little or no fever. If fever is present, a diagnosis of pyelonephritis should be considered, and the management will be different (see p. 293).

Management options

Because of the potentially serious sequelae of childhood UTI and the fact that these may be exacerbated by delays in therapy, the realistic management options are limited.

1. Refer all patients to a paediatrician for specialist assessment and treatment on the basis that all children with UTI will require follow-up.
2. Make a presumptive diagnosis of cystitis using leucocyte esterase/nitrite dipsticks, start treatment, and refer for specialist follow-up.
3. Make a firm diagnosis of cystitis by collecting an MSU, start treatment immediately, and refer for specialist follow-up.

Option 1. Refer all patients to a paediatrician for specialist assessment and treatment on the basis that all children with UTI will require follow-up.

✓ The patient will be appropriately assessed, investigated and followed up.

✗ The patient will be inconvenienced by the need to attend hospital urgently. Non-urgent referral may cause a delay in instituting antibiotic therapy, potentially resulting in renal scarring.

✗ A large number of patients with no confirmed cystitis will be referred.

✗ You will become unpopular with your paediatric colleagues.

Option 2. Make a presumptive diagnosis of cystitis using leucocyte esterase/nitrite dipsticks, start treatment, and refer for specialist follow-up.

✓ Treatment is started immediately so risks associated with delayed therapy are reduced.

✓ A positive dipstick test has a high predictive value and it is therefore unlikely that treatment will be given inappropriately.

✓ Specimen collection is easier, as a sterile specimen is not needed for stick testing.

✗ A negative dipstick test does not absolutely rule out a diagnosis of cystitis. Patients with negative tests and suspicious symptoms will still need to be referred.

✗ If the patient does not respond to initial 'best guess' therapy no bacteriological results will be available.

Option 3. Make a firm diagnosis of cystitis by collecting an MSU, start treatment immediately, and refer for specialist follow-up.

✓ Treatment is started immediately so risks associated with delayed therapy are reduced.

✓ The diagnosis is confirmed, minimizing any uncertainty in future management.

✓ Sensitivity test results are available to guide any changes in therapy which may be necessary if clinical response to empirical therapy does not occur in 48 hours.

✓ Referral to a specialist is accompanied by enough information to allow decisions on further investigation to be taken immediately.

✗ Specimen collection may be difficult.

✗ Interpretation of results may be difficult, especially with bag specimens of urine.

✗ Delays in receiving the report may result in 48 hour follow-up without access to appropriate information.

History checklist

General
Questioning should elucidate any recent change in either urinary habit or change in the nature of the urine.

Specific
- Have there been any previous urinary tract problems? Have any previous UTIs been suspected or diagnosed? Has the child had any problems passing urine or are there abnormalities of urine flow, which may lead to a suspicion of urinary tract obstruction?
- Has the patient any vaginal discharge? Vulvovaginitis in the prepubertal female may present with symptoms of dysuria or hesitancy.
- Are there any symptoms of perianal irritation? Pin worm infections, which may involve the vagina, may cause itchiness and excoriation from scratching which can lead to symptoms of dysuria. Local irritation may also be due to reactions to detergents or irritating fabrics and may lead to local irritation and dysuria.
- Are any unrelated symptoms present? Rarer causes of frequency may be considered, e.g. excessive thirst in diabetes.

Examination checklist
- Take the child's temperature. Cystitis may occur in the absence of an increased temperature but pyelonephritis is unlikely if it is <38° C. Routine examination is not necessary. If the history suggests perineal/perianal irritation, examine the area for signs of excoriation.

Referrals
- Referral to a paediatrician for follow-up, for all children with proven UTI, is recommended.

Hints for investigators and prescribers
- The collection of urine specimens from young children is difficult. Urine collection bags have a high contamination rate. A negative result is reliable, but positive culture results may not indicate infection, especially if a mixed growth of bacteria is found, and repeat samples are often needed. The number of WBCs present in the specimen may aid interpretation.
- Treatment consists of a 5–7 day course of an oral antibiotic such as trimethoprim, nitrofurantoin or nalidixic acid. The patient should be reviewed after 48 hours of therapy to ensure an adequate clinical response. Lack of clinical improvement at this stage is usually due to inappropriate antibiotic therapy or underlying obstruction. Following successful therapy the patient can be routinely referred for follow-up.

Further reading
Hellerstein, S. (1995) Urinary tract infections: old and new concepts. *Paediatr. Clin. N. Am.* **42**: 1433–1455.

Royal College of Physicians (1991) Guidelines on the management of acute UTI in childhood. Report of a Working Group of the Research Unit, Royal College of Physicians. *J. R. Coll. Physicians* **25**: 36–42.

7 Cystitis in pregnancy

Cystitis should be suspected in any woman who has any symptoms of lower UTI, i.e. dysuria, urgency, frequency, hesitancy, lower abdominal pain and little or no fever. If fever is present, a diagnosis of pyelonephritis should be considered (see p. 293).

Management options

Because of the increased risk of pyelonephritis in the pregnant woman, cystitis must always be effectively treated. However, frequency of micturition is a normal feature of pregnancy, and if the MSU shows an absence of infection then the patient can be re-assured.

1. Treat all patients with symptoms.
2. Confirm diagnosis by collecting an MSU, treat immediately and follow up.
3. Refer for specialist assessment and treatment.

Option 1. Treat all patients with symptoms.

Treat all pregnant patients with any symptoms of lower UTI. The patient can be treated with a 3-day course of an appropriate antibiotic such as amoxycillin. All β-lactam antibiotics (penicillins and cephalosporins) are safe to use in pregnancy. Trimethoprim must not be used in the first trimester or nitrofurantoin in the third trimester.

✓ No patient should develop pyelonephritis and symptoms will usually resolve rapidly.
✓ Time is saved by not performing any dipstick or laboratory testing.

✗ Frequency of micturition is common in pregnancy. If this is the only symptom then you will be treating large numbers of people who do not have an infection.
✗ Forty per cent of women with acute pyelonephritis present initially with lower urinary tract symptoms. If other symptoms of pyelonephritis develop, no bacteriology will be available to guide treatment.
✗ If the patient does not respond to initial 'best guess' therapy, no bacteriological results will be available.

Option 2. Confirm diagnosis by collecting an MSU, treat immediately and follow up.

✓ The diagnosis is confirmed, minimizing any uncertainty in future management.
✓ Sensitivity test results are available to guide any changes in therapy which may be necessary if clinical response to empirical therapy does not occur in 48 hours.

✗ Specimen collection and follow-up may be time-consuming.
✗ Delays in receiving the report may result in 48 hour follow-up without access to appropriate information.

Option 3. Refer for specialist assessment and treatment.

✓ The patient will be appropriately assessed, investigated and followed up.

✗ The patient will be inconvenienced by the need to attend hospital.
✗ You will become unpopular with your obstetric colleagues.

History checklist
● Direct questioning should exclude any recent change in urinary habit or change in the nature of the urine. A history of childhood or any prior UTI indicates a higher risk of developing pyelonephritis, as does a history of diabetes mellitus and spinal cord injury with neurogenic bladder.

Examination checklist

- Take the patient's temperature. Pyelonephritis is unlikely if it is <38°C. There are unlikely to be any physical signs present in bacterial cystitis.

Further reading

Cunningham, F.G. and Lucas, M.J. (1994) Urinary tract infections complicating pregnancy. *Baillieres Clin. Obstet. Gynaecol.* **8**: 353–373.

Editorial. (1985) Urinary tract infection during pregnancy. *Lancet* **ii**: 190–192.

8 Acute cystitis in men

Urinary tract infection (UTI) in men is less common than in women and is usually regarded as complicated i.e. likely to be due to a functional or anatomical disorder of the urinary tract, and as such will require investigation. In older men, UTI is usually related to enlargement of the prostate with partial outflow obstruction and residual bladder urine. It can also be secondary to persistent prostatitis. However, in men below the age of 50, infection can still occur, and in this group urological investigation seldom reveals abnormalities.

Management options

1. Make a presumptive diagnosis of UTI and treat empirically with antibiotics.
2. Make a firm diagnosis of UTI by collecting an MSU and treating with antibiotics. Treat empirically as in Option 1 but confirm the diagnosis with an MSU.
3. Collect an MSU and start treatment. Arrange for urological follow-up.

Option 1. Make a presumptive diagnosis of UTI and treat empirically with antibiotics.

Tell the patient that if the symptoms have not resolved in 3 days to come back for review.

✓ This approach may be successful in younger men, but in older men you run the risk of masking or ignoring more serious underlying conditions.
✓ The patient may feel that the doctor is taking an appropriate interest and may be reassured.
✓ The cost of investigations will be minimized.
✓ If you are correct in your choice of empirical therapy and the patient has no underlying abnormalities, the patient will be cured.

✗ A number of patients, particularly in the older age group, will have serious underlying problems which will be missed.
✗ If empirical therapy fails, or underlying abnormalities become apparent, there will be no sensitivity results upon which to base a modification of therapy.
✗ You may delay diagnosis in some young men with underlying structural abnormalities.
✗ The diagnosis has never been documented by a bacterial culture.

Cystitis in young men may be caused by uropathogenic E. coli as is the case in women. The presenting features are usually of cystitis but symptoms of urethritis may also be present. It is recommended that pretreatment urine culture is obtained. Urologic investigation is not required if symptoms resolve.

Option 2. Make a firm diagnosis of UTI by collecting an MSU and treating with antibiotics. Treat empirically as in Option 1 but confirm the diagnosis with an MSU.

✓ This approach may be successful in younger men. Even if the patient does not respond to the initial empirical therapy you will have sensitivity tests upon which to base a modification of therapy.
✓ The patient may feel that the doctor is taking an appropriate interest and may be reassured.

✗ A number of patients, particularly in the older age group, will have serious underlying problems which will be missed.

Option 3. Collect an MSU and start treatment. Arrange for urological follow-up.

✓ The patient may feel that the doctor is taking an appropriate interest and may be reassured.

✓ The patient will be started on treatment immediately which allows early resolution of symptoms. Referring the patient to a urologist will ensure that any underlying problems will be managed effectively.

✗ A few younger patients who may not benefit from referral to a urologist will be referred.
✗ If the infection is related to prostatitis, early antibiotic therapy may make further microbiological sampling more difficult.

History checklist

- A diagnosis of cystitis should be considered in a patient presenting with dysuria, frequency or urgency. However, urethritis or prostatitis may cause similar symptoms and should be elucidated by specific questioning.
- Is there any urethral discharge present? Has the patient noticed any urethral discharge. Has there been any recent change in sexual partner?
- Are any symptoms of prostatism present? Symptoms such as hesitancy, urgency and dribbling are associated with prostatic enlargement and subsequent UTI.
- Have there been any previous urinary tract problems? Such problems in childhood suggest the possibility of structural abnormalities which may require further investigation.
- Previous catheterization should be noted.

Examination checklist

- Examination should include assessment of any urethral discharge and, if indicated by the history, a rectal examination looking particularly for signs of prostatic enlargement or tenderness.

Hints for investigators and prescribers

In cases where there are no obvious complicating symptoms, such as problems with urinary flow or childhood infections, studies suggest that a 7-day course of antibiotics is effective and that urologic follow-up is not required.

Further reading

Krieger, J.N., Ross, S.O. and Simonsen, J.M. (1993) Urinary tract infections in healthy university men. *J. Urol.* **149**: 1046–1048.

INDEX